Principles and Interpretation of

Laboratory Techniques in Pathology

Hematology, Cytology, Histopathology, Museum, and Autopsy Techniques

Principles and Interpretation of Laboratory Techniques in Pathology

Hematology, Cytology, Histopathology, Museum, and Autopsy Techniques

Shameem Shariff MD PhD
Former, Professor and Head
Department of Pathology
St John's Medical College and Hospital
and
MVJ Medical College and Research Hospital
Bengaluru, Karnataka, India

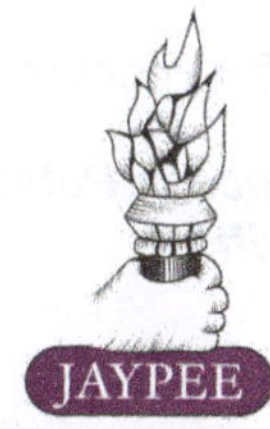

JAYPEE BROTHERS MEDICAL PUBLISHERS
The Health Sciences Publisher
New Delhi | London

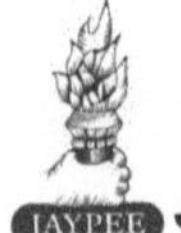

Jaypee Brothers Medical Publishers (P) Ltd

Headquarters
EMCA House
23/23-B, Ansari Road, Daryaganj
New Delhi 110 002, India
Landline: +91-11-23272143, +91-11-23272703
+91-11-23282021, +91-11-23245672
E-mail: jaypee@jaypeebrothers.com

Corporate Office
4838/24, Ansari Road, Daryaganj
New Delhi 110 002, India
Phone: +91-11-43574357
Fax: +91-11-43574314
E-mail: jaypee@jaypeebrothers.com

Overseas Office
J.P. Medical Ltd
83 Victoria Street, London
SW1H 0HW (UK)
Phone: +44 20 3170 8910
E-mail: info@jpmedpub.com

EU GPSR Authorised Representative
Logos Europe, 9 rue Nicolas Poussin
17000, La Rochelle, France
Phone: +33 (0) 6 67 93 73 78
E-mail: contact@logoseurope.eu

Website: www.jaypeebrothers.com
Website: www.jaypeedigital.com

Inquiries for bulk sales may be solicited at: jaypee@jaypeebrothers.com

Principles and Interpretation of Laboratory Techniques in Pathology: Hematology, Cytology, Histopathology, Museum, and Autopsy Techniques / Shameem Shariff

First Edition: **2024**

Reprint: 2026

ISBN: 978-93-5696-520-1

Printed in India

DEDICATED TO

My Husband

Professor MH Shariff

Consultant Radiation Oncologist
Formerly, Professor and Head
Department of Radiation Oncology
St John's Medical College and Hospital, Bengaluru
and Kidwai Memorial Institute of Oncology
Bengaluru, Karnataka, India

For his constant encouragement in all my academic ventures, patience, and endurance for the time spent by me on this book

PREFACE

This book is aimed at providing a comprehensive knowledge on a single platform of all principles and procedures of laboratory medicine in pathology. It is a hands-on detail of all procedures carried out in a laboratory. It comprises two parts. Part 1 deals with hematology and Part 2 is dedicated to cytology, histology, and other sections in the laboratory such as museum techniques, autopsy, photography, and quality control.

Part 1: *Chapters 1 to 9* deal with all techniques used in the hematology laboratory. Simple techniques such as hemoglobin estimation, cell counts, hematocrit, and peripheral smear examination have been outlined in detail. The approach to investigations of all types of anemias, including hemolytic anemias, has been dealt with. Anticoagulants, blood banking, and blood groups have been covered.

Part 2: *Chapters 1 to 14* deal with cytopathology. The methods of specimen collection, processing of material of the various anatomical sites, and fixation and staining are dealt with. Standard and current systems of reporting fine-needle aspiration and fluid cytology on varied anatomic sites have been covered.

Reporting criteria on urine analysis, synovial fluid, and semen analysis as well as The Bethesda System of reporting cervical cytology with recent advances and recommendations have been detailed.

Chapters 15 to 25 outline techniques in histology with the journey of specimens from receipt in the laboratory to the finished report. Fixation, processing of tissue, section cutting, routine staining, and special stains with principles, indications, and time-tested procedures have been provided. Photomicrographs detailing the clarity and results of special stains and other techniques are included. Molecular and advanced laboratory techniques have been outlined. Systematized Nomenclature of Pathology (SNOP) is separately dealt with as a chapter with its modification for Cytology Indexing System. Quality control and quality assurance, accreditation, and methods of laboratory management for both cytology and histopathology are detailed.

Chapters 26 to 31 deal with laboratory procedures intrinsic to any standard institutional department as well as private laboratories. Chapters on microscopy, museum techniques, autopsy techniques, and photography and photomicrography are unique to this book and have been added with the intention of making this a comprehensive reference hands-on book for a surgical pathologist and cytologist. The chapter on autopsy techniques has been introduced for quick reference for the postgraduates.

This book is a hands-on practical manual with detail and precision, based on current concepts amalgamated with years of experience by the author on laboratory procedures. It is extremely useful for all technicians, postgraduates, cytologists, and surgical pathologists.

Shameem Shariff

ACKNOWLEDGMENTS

I acknowledge with gratitude the management of the institutions that I have worked in, for their trust and confidence in me. I have benefitted with the years of experience gained at these institutions—St John's Medical College and Hospital, Bengaluru, and MVJ Medical College and Research Hospital, Bengaluru; these places have helped me mature as a consultant and helped in sharpening and honing my skills and expertise as a cytopathologist and histopathologist.

I extend my sincere thanks to my family for their patience in bearing with the hours of work toward the realization of this book.

I also thank my trainees whose stimulation and curiosity have kept the pursuit of my knowledge alive.

I acknowledge Leica Microsystems for their generosity in the contribution of the various illustrations on their instruments.

My thanks are to my daughter Mariam Shariff (of Pink Lime Web Design) for her help and contribution toward formatting of this manuscript.

I am very grateful to the whole team of M/s Jaypee Brothers Medical Publishers (P) Ltd, New Delhi, India, especially Shri Jitendar P Vij (Group Chairman), Mr Ankit Vij (Managing Director), Mr MS Mani (Group President), Ms Chetna Malhotra (Senior Director – Professional Publishing, Marketing and Business Development), Ms Pooja Bhandari [Director–Production (Books and Journals)], Mr Ajay Kumar Sharma [Deputy General Manager (Books and Journals)], Ms Seema Dogra (Cover Visualizer), Ms Himani Pandey (Senior Development Editor) and the entire Editorial and Production team members, for all their constant support to work in this project and make it a great success.

Shameem Shariff

CONTENTS

PART 1

Hematology

CHAPTER 1

Hemoglobin and Cell Counts

HEMOGLOBIN

Estimation of hemoglobin (Hb) is performed on venous or free-flowing capillary blood that has been anticoagulated with ethylenediaminetetraacetic acid (EDTA). Capillary finger prick blood usually gives higher hemoglobin concentrations compared to venous blood.

The methods to be described are all color or light-intensity matching techniques, which also measure, to a varying extent, any methemoglobin (Hi) or sulfhemoglobin (SHb) that may be present.

The hemiglobincyanide (HiCN; cyanmethemoglobin) method is now in common use, is the principle in manual and most autoanalyzer techniques, and is considered accurate.

Photoelectric Calorimeter Method

Using the cyanmethemoglobin method is the method of choice for the estimation of hemoglobin and is recommended by the International Committee for Standardization in Hematology. This is because all forms of hemoglobin are converted to cyanmethemoglobin (except sulfhemoglobin) and a stable and reliable standard is available.

Principle

The basis of the method is the dilution of blood in a solution containing potassium cyanide and potassium ferricyanide. Blood is mixed with a solution of potassium ferricyanide, potassium cyanide, and nonionic detergent (Drabkin's solution) **(Table 1)**. The erythrocytes are lysed. Potassium ferricyanide converts hemoglobin to methemoglobin and methemoglobin combines with potassium cyanide to form cyanmethemoglobin. The absorbance of the solution is then measured in a spectrometer at a wavelength of 540 nm or in a photoelectric colorimeter with a yellow-green filter, such as Ilford 625 and Wratten 74.

TABLE 1: Drabkin-type reagent.

Reagent	Amount
Potassium ferricyanide (0.607 mmol/L)	200 mg
Potassium cyanide (0.768 mmol/L)	50 mg
Potassium dihydrogen phosphate (1.029 mmol/L)	140 mg
Nonionic detergent	1 mL
Distilled or deionised water	1 L

DRABKIN REAGENT

Other Methods

Other methods of haemoglobin estimation:

- *Sahli's acid hematin method*: It is easy to perform but the acid hematin fades as soon as it is formed.
- *Alkali hematin method*: The alkaline-hematin method gives a true estimate of total hemoglobin concentration even if carboxyhemoglobin (HbCO), Hi or SHb is present; it is less accurate than the cyanmethemoglobin method.
- *Oxyhemoglobin method*: The principle is that the oxygen-combining capacity of blood is 1.34 mL of O_2/g of hemoglobin. The value is always 2% lower than normal. This method is rarely used.
- By estimating the iron content—this is not practical in routine practice
- *Tallquist's hemoglobin chart*: Color comparative method **(Fig. 1)**

This technique of estimating hemoglobin is based on comparing the color of a drop of blood absorbed on chromatography paper (Tallquist's paper) against a printed scale of colors corresponding to different levels

Actual anemia				Suggestive anemia		Normal	
Men and women below 70%				Men: 70–80% Women: 70–80%		Men: Above 85% Women: Above 80%	
30%	40%	50%	60%	70%	80%	90%	100%
4.7 g	6.3 g	7.8 g	9.4 g	10.9 g	12.5 g	14.1 g	15.6 g

FIG. 1: Colors for comparison for Tallquist's method.

of hemoglobin ranging from about 4.7-15.6 g/dL **(Fig. 1)**. After putting a drop of blood on it the test paper is held behind the holes shown in **(Figure 1)**.

SAHLI'S HEMOGLOBINOMETER

Sahli's Acid Hematin Method (Fig. 2)

It is a manual and commonly used method in laboratories that cannot afford auto analyzers.

Sahli's hemoglobinometer consists of the following:

- Comparator which consists of a rack with a standard fixed in front of ground glass.
- A graduated tube with markings in gram (2-22 g) and in percentage (10-160%)
- Hemoglobinometer pipette—glass pipette with 20 mm^3 capacity. Used to pipette blood for hemoglobin estimation.

Procedure

About 20 mL (0.02 mL) of blood is placed in a specially calibrated tube containing N/10 HCl, to the 2 marks. Let the mixture stand at room temperature for 10 minutes, during which time hemoglobin is converted to acid hematin. The solution is diluted with distilled water until the color matches exactly with the standard of the comparator block. The percentage of hemoglobin is read directly from the calibration on the tube to which the solution is diluted.

Advantages

- Simple method
- Small quantity of blood is needed
- No sophisticated equipment is needed
- Can be repeated often

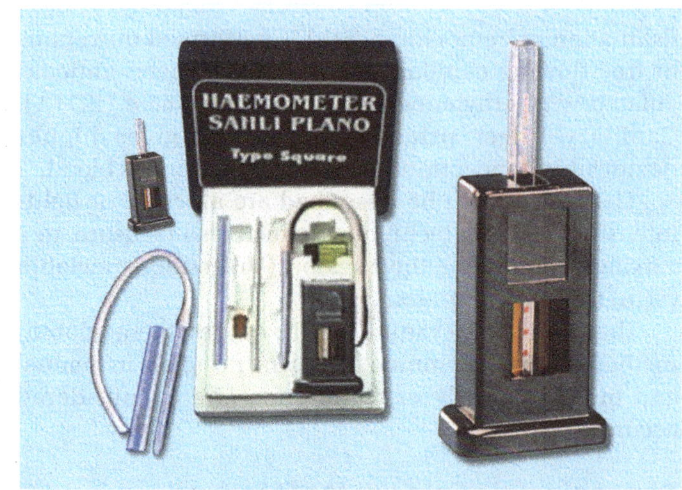

FIG. 2: Various components of Sahli's acid hematin method.

Disadvantages

- Visual error
- Other forms of hemoglobin cannot be estimated (such as sulfhemoglobin and methemoglobin)
- Fading of the standard—false reading
- Time taken for 100% conversion takes 30 minutes; however, the color of acid hematin starts fading after 10 minutes.
- Affected by hyperbilirubinemia

Levels of Hemoglobin

Normal range of hemoglobin:
- Males 14–16 g%
- Females 12–14 g%

Hemoglobin is raised in:
- Polycythemia
- Renal neoplasms (excess production of erythropoietin)
- Dehydration

Hemoglobin is reduced in:
- Anemias
- Hemorrhage
- Blood loss

COMPLETE BLOOD COUNTS

Pipettes for Red Blood Cells, White Blood Cells, and Platelet Counts

Red blood cells (RBCs) pipette is used for:
- Red cell counts
- For white blood cell (WBC) counts in cases of leukemia where a higher dilution is required

Red Cell Counts

- *Using RBC pipette* ***(Fig. 3A)***: Equipment:
- Red cell pipette with a red bead in the bulb (for identification) with markings on it, of '0.5,' '1,' and '101'
- Improved Neubauer chamber **(Figs. 3B and C)**

RBC Fluid

- *Hayem's fluid*:
  - Mercuric chloride: 0.5 g
  - Sodium chloride: 1.0 g
  - Sodium sulfate: 5.0 g
  - Distilled water: 200 mL
- *Dacie's fluid (formal-citrate solution)*: It can also be used. It has an anticoagulant and is an iso-osmotic solution that prevents the shrinkage of RBCs. It also contains formalin to conserve the fluid.
  - Sodium citrate dehydrate: 5.0 g
  - Formalin: 1 mL
  - Distilled water: 100 mL
  - Stock solution is diluted 1 in 10 before use

Method

- Draw EDTA blood to exactly 0.5 mark of RBC pipette. Wipe the tip of the pipette to remove excess blood on the sides of the tip.
- Dip the tip of the pipette in the diluting fluid and draw it up to the mark 101, past the bulb.
- Rotate the pipette in its long axis to ensure the thorough mixing of blood and diluents; facilitated by the *red bead* present in the bulb.
- Place the cover slip on the ruled area of the Neubauer chamber.
- Discard the first drop from the pipette since the blood and diluents are not mixed in the long nozzle of the pipette. Charge the chamber till it is completely charged by the capillary action.
- Wait for 2–4 minutes for cells to settle.
- Locate the central ruled area under the microscope using a low-power objective.
- Count RBCs using *high power objective* in the 5 red squares and add them together (*N*).

Calculation of RBC count:

$$\text{RBC count} = \frac{N}{1/5 \times 1/10 \times 1/200}$$
$$= \text{counted cells} \times 10{,}000$$

Depth of the chamber = 1/10 (0.1 mm)
Dilution = 1 in 200
N = Number of RBCs in 5 small squares
1/5 mm^2 area counted (5 × 1/5 × 1/5 mm^2)

WBC Pipette and Counts

Principle

Whole blood is diluted with WBC diluting fluid that hemolysis the red cells. Nucleated cells—WBCs stained by Gentian Violet are counted in the Neubauer chamber.

Equipment

The hemocytometer set consists of the following:
- *WBC pipette (Thoma pipette)*: It has a white bead in the bulb and markings of 0.5, 1, and 11 **(Fig. 3A)**
- *Improved Neubauer chamber* ***(Fig. 3C)***: It has a shiny surface which makes the lines very clearly visible even after charging it. It has a total area of 3 mm × 3 mm with a central ruled area of 1 mm × 1 mm. The central area consists of 25 groups of 16 small squares separated by bold lines. Corner 1 mm × 1 mm squares have 16 smaller squares each, which are used for total leukocyte count (TLC). The depth of the chamber is 0.1 mm.

WBC Fluid (Turk's Fluid)

Composition
- *Glacial acetic acid*: 2 mL to lyse RBCs
- *1% gentian violet*: Five drops to stain the WBC nuclei
- *Add water*: 100 mL

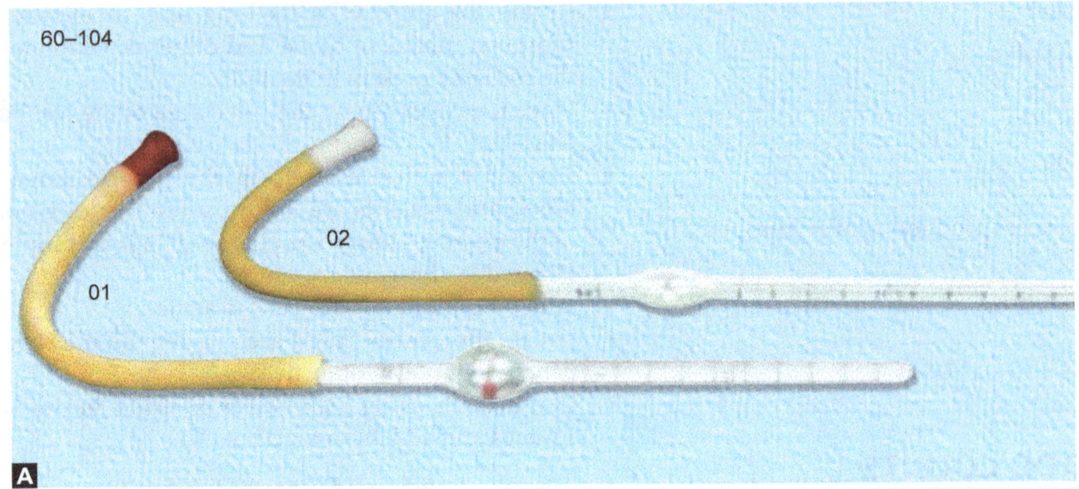

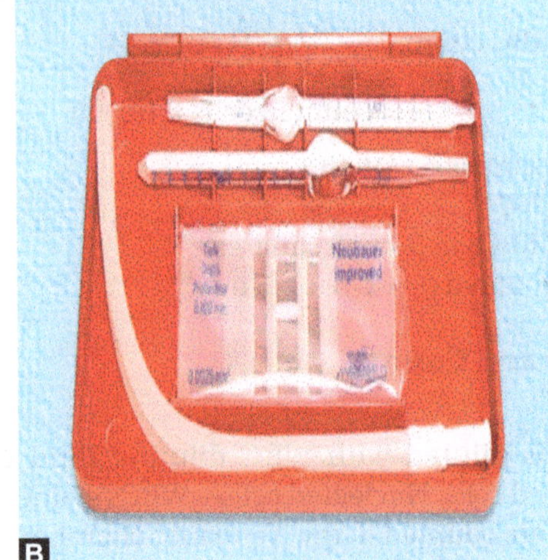

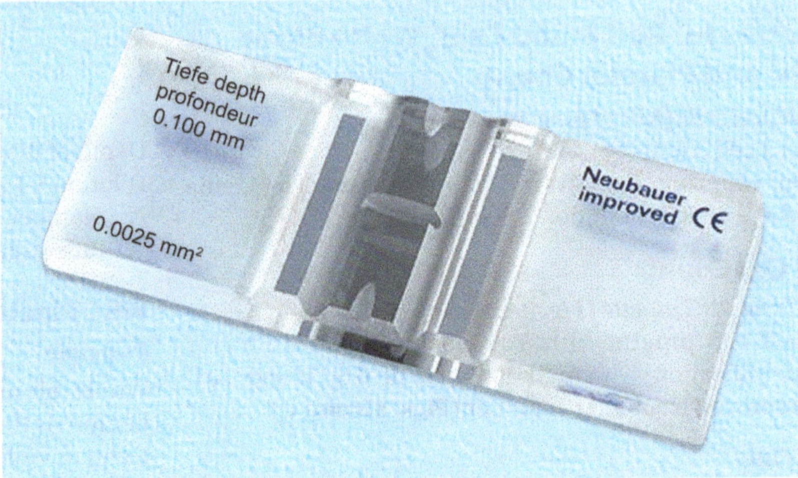

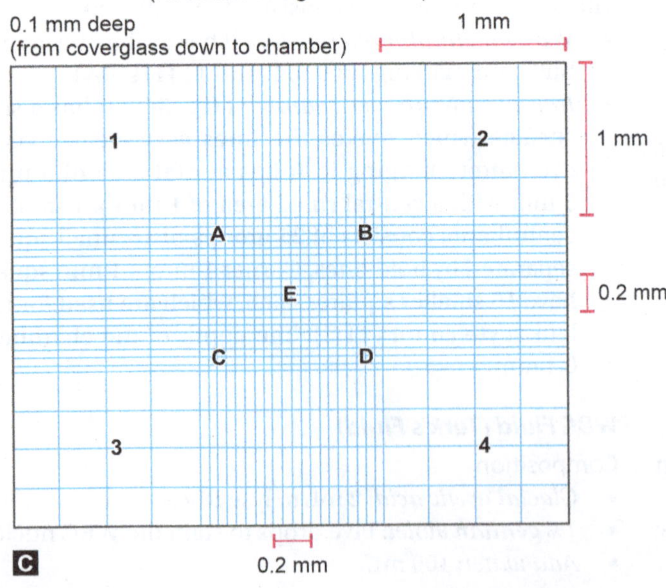

FIGS. 3A TO C: (A) RBC pipette with a red bead (01) within and WBC pipette (02) with a white bead within; (B) Neubauer counting chamber as available in packing (left) and opened out (right) for use; and (C) Neubauer chamber ruling, microscopic view.

Method

- Mix the EDTA anticoagulated blood gently by shaking the vial.
- *Dilution of blood*: Fill the blood in the WBC pipette up to mark 0.5 and wipe off excess blood on the sides of the pipette nozzle. Fill the pipette with Turk's fluid up to mark 11 by taking the fluid from the bottle. Diluting factor is 1:20. (When blood is sucked up to 0.5 mark and the diluting fluid up to 11 marks, gives the 1:20 dilution of blood:diluting fluid and when the blood is sucked up to 1 mark and the diluting fluid up to 11, gives the 1:10 dilution of blood:diluting fluid which less commonly used.)
- Rotate the pipette slowly so that blood and fluid mix thoroughly in the bulb of the pipette; mixing is facilitated by the *white bead* present in the bulb.
- Discard 1 drop of WBC fluid since fluid up to mark 1 has not mixed with the blood.
- Clean the chamber and place the thick cover slip on the ruled area.
- Charge the chamber by placing the tip of the pipette just under the coverslip and fluid flows under it by capillary action till the counting chamber is just filled.
- Wait for 2–3 minutes for cells to settle.
- Examine the ruled area under the microscope using a low-power objective. White cells are easily recognized since their nuclei are stained by gentian violet.
- Count white cells in 4 corner large squares (1 × 1 mm each) (shown as 1, 2, 3, 4 in **Fig. 3C**)

Calculation of TLC:

$$\text{TLC} = \frac{N \times 20}{4 \times 0.1}$$

Depth of the chamber = 0.1 mm
Dilution = 1 in 20
4 corner squares are counted
N = Number of WBCs in 4 large squares
Normal range of TLC

Adults: 4,000–11,000 cells/mm^3

Platelet Count

The platelet count can be done in an automated cell counter or manually.

Principle

Anticoagulated blood is diluted with a diluent that hemolyze the red cells, leaving platelets, e.g., in 1% ammonium oxalate.

Diluting Fluids

- *Brecher-Cronkite fluid*: 1% of ammonium oxalate solution is filtered and stored at 4°C.
- *Rees-Ecker fluid*: It is an aqueous solution of sodium citrate, sucrose, and brilliant cresyl blue, used in platelet counts. Brilliant cresyl blue stains platelets pale blue.
    - Composition:
        - Sodium citrate 3.8 g
        - Formalin 0.2 mL
        - Brilliant cresyl blue 50 mg
        - Distilled water 100 mL

Equipment

- *Improved Neubauer chamber*: The most commonly improved Neubauer's Chamber is used but, in some laboratories, other types of chambers are also employed, such as the Burker's chamber, Levy's chamber, and Fuchs-Rosenthal chamber.
- WBC pipette
- RBC pipette

Method Using White Blood Cell Pipette and Improved Neubauer Chamber

- *Dilution of blood*: Fill the blood up to the mark 0.5 on the WBC pipette. 1% of ammonium oxalate diluents is filled up to mark 11 of the WBC pipette thus making a dilution of 1 in 20.
- Charge the chamber as given for TLC count.
- Place the charged chamber in a moist petri dish (wet filter paper at the bottom) for 5 minutes so that the platelets settle down.
- Platelets are counted in the central 1 × 1 mm square. Platelets are recognized more readily if the focus of the light microscope is altered carefully with the fine adjustment and if the illumination is reduced by closing the iris diaphragm.
- The condenser should be lowered. Platelets appear as highly *refractile* particles.

Calculation of Platelet Count

$$\text{Platelet count} = \frac{\text{No. of platelets counted (N)} \times \text{dilution}}{1 \times 1\ \text{mm}^2 \times 1/10\ \text{mm (depth)}}$$

$$= \frac{N \times 20}{1/10\ \text{mm (depth)}}$$

$$= N \times 200\ \text{platelets/mm}^3$$

Normal Range

- 150,000–400,000 platelets/mm^3 (1.5–4.0 lakhs/mm^3)
- *Platelet counts are reduced in*: Thrombocytopenia, autoimmune diseases, pregnancy, heavy alcohol consumption, or certain medications like anticancer drugs.
- *Platelet counts are increased in*: Reactive thrombocytosis and idiopathic thrombocythemia.

CHAPTER 2

Packed Cell Volume, Red Cell Indices, and Erythrocyte Sedimentation Rate

HEMATOCRIT/PACKED CELL VOLUME

Packed cell volume (PCV) is the volume occupied by the red cells when a sample of anticoagulated blood is centrifuged. It is the ratio of the volume of red blood cells (RBCs) to the total volume of blood. It indicates a relative proportion of red cells to plasma and is expressed as a percentage of the volume of the blood sample. Plasma is approximately 92% water, and the rest includes suspended particles, such as proteins, minerals, electrolytes, and hormones.

The cellular portion of the blood includes erythrocytes, leukocytes [white blood cells (WBCs)], and thrombocytes (platelets).

The normal value of PCV in men is about 42–50% and in women, it is about 36–45%; in infants 45–60%.

Hematocrit is reduced in anemias.

The hematocrit is increased in dehydration; burns and in polycythemia.

Uses of Packed Cell Volume

- Presence or absence of anemia or polycythemia.
- PCV is used to estimate the severity of anemia and to calculate the absolute value of mean corpuscular volume (MCV) and classify anemia as microcytic, macrocytic, and normocytic.
- Estimation of red cell indices.
- Three zones are distinguished in the Wintrobe's tube after centrifugation from above downward—plasma, buffy coat layer (a small grayish layer of white cells and platelets), and packed red cells.

METHODS OF ESTIMATION

There are two methods for the estimation of PCV, i.e., (1) macro method and (2) microhematocrit method.

Macro Method

The macro method includes Wintrobe and microhematocrit method.

Wintrobe Tube or Hematocrit Tube

It is a thick-walled tube with a narrow lumen, one end of the tube closed **(Fig. 1)**. Total length is 11 cm, diameter 2.5 cm. The tube is graduated from 0 to 100 mm. Wintrobe's tube has two measurements along its stem; one for erythrocyte sedimentation rate (ESR) and one for PCV. Markings on one side are above downward and on the other side below upward. The below upward markings are used for hematocrit and the above downward for ESR.

The anticoagulant used is a double oxalate, dry ammonium oxalate mixture (2 mg/mL).

A special pipette, Wintrobe's pipette, or Pasteur's pipette is used to fill the tube.

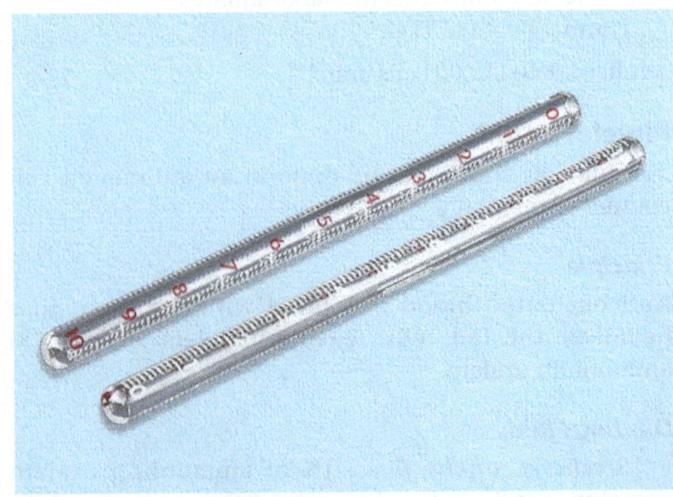

FIG. 1: Wintrobe tube with double markings.

Uses

- For PCV
- ESR

Wintrobe Method of PCV

Figure 1 shows a Wintrobe tube with double markings and **Figure 2** shows the tube with layers after centrifugation.

Principle: Anticoagulated whole blood is centrifuged in a Wintrobe tube to completely pack the red cells. The volume of packed red cells is read directly from the tube.

The advantage of this method is that before performing PCV, a test for erythrocyte sedimentation can also be done.

Equipment

- *Wintrobe tube*: This is about 110 mm in length and has 100 markings each at the interval of 1 mm. The internal diameter of 3 mm. The tube is graduated from 0 to 100 mm. Markings on one side are above downward and on the other side below upward. The below upward markings are used for hematocrit and the above downward for ESR.
- Pasteur pipette with a rubber bulb and a sufficient length of the capillary to reach the bottom of the Wintrobe tube.
- Centrifuge

Procedure

- Mix the anticoagulated blood sample thoroughly. Double oxalate/ethylenediaminetetraacetic acid (EDTA) is the preferred anticoagulant.
- Draw the blood sample in a Pasteur pipette and with the tip to the bottom of the Wintrobe tube, fill the tube from below exactly up to the mark 100.
- Centrifuge the sample at 3,000 rpm for 30 minutes.

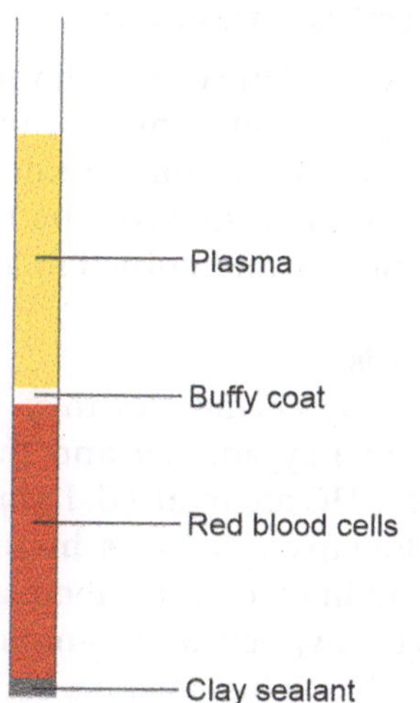

FIG. 2: Various layers after centrifugation in packed cell volume (PCV).

- Take the reading of the length of the column of the red cells.
- Hematocrit is expressed as a percentage or as a fraction of the total volume of blood. Reading is taken from below upward.

Significance of Different Layers Observed in Hematocrit Tube (Fig. 2)

- *Uppermost clear fluid, i.e., plasma layer*: Normal plasma is straw-colored, color is yellow in jaundice, and intravascular hemolysis (pink to brown)
- Increased blood lipids (milky)
- Just below it is a thin layer of platelets.
- Next to the platelet layer in the buffy coat is WBC. Increased thickness of buffy coat layer occurs if white cells or platelets are increased in number, e.g., leukocytosis, thrombocytosis, or leukemia.
- Lower most is the packed cell layer of red cells—hematocrit

(Normally buffy coat is <1% of the total blood volume.)

The thickness of the buffy coat gives an idea of WBC count (1 mm = 10,000/mm^3)

Buffy coat preparation: This preparation of the buffy coat layer is sometimes needed to view the morphology of WBCs especially when the abnormal cell counts are scanty.

- Centrifuge an EDTA-anticoagulated blood sample in a plastic tube for 5–10 minutes at 1,200–1,500g.
- Remove the supernatant plasma carefully with a fine plastic pipette
- With the same pipette, deposit the platelet and underlying leukocyte layers onto one or two slides.
- Mix the buffy coat in a drop of the patient's plasma and then make a smear.
- Allow them to dry in the air and then fix and stain the usual way.

A buffy coat smear is made and has diagnostic value in:

- Aleukemic leukemia
- Kala-azar and trypanosomiasis
- Lupus erythematosus (LE) cells
- Myeloma
- Nucleated RBC
- Malarial parasite

Microhematocrit Method for Packed Cell Volume

Principle

Anticoagulated whole blood is centrifuged in a capillary tube of a uniform bore to pack the red cells. Centrifugation is done in a special microhematocrit centrifuge till the packing is complete and the reading taken.

Equipment

- Microhematocrit centrifuge
- Capillary tube—plain

Procedure

- Fill three-fourths of the plain capillary tube by dipping one end of the tube in the EDTA blood.
- Plug the end of the tube with sealing wax. Care should be taken that there is no air gap between sealing and blood.
- Place the tube in the microhematocrit centrifuge, close and cover the centrifuge.
- Set the speed to 10,000 rpm for 5 minutes.
- Remove the capillary tube, record the hematocrit by placing the tube in the microhematocrit reader scale, or compare it against the standard graph.

Advantage

Only a small quantity of blood is needed (as in case of finger prick/heel prick in infants).

Other Methods

Hematocrit is usually measured in most labs by the above methods; alternatively, hematocrit can be calculated from

- The complete blood cell count (CBC) is done in an automated blood analyzer, (the volume of cells can be calculated by the volume of one cell multiplied by the number of RBCs, which is "MCV" multiplied by the total count of RBCs), *or*
- *By using mean corpuscular hemoglobin concentration (MCHC) and the formula*:

$$\text{Hct}\,(\%) = \frac{\text{ctHb}}{\text{MCHC}} \times 100$$

- It can also be calculated by using calculations from the Hb values. In normal conditions, there is a linear relationship between hematocrit and the concentration of hemoglobin (ctHb). The relationship can be expressed as follows:

$$\text{Hct}\,(\%) = 0.0485 \times \text{ctHb (mmol/L)} + 0.0083 \times 100$$

HEMATOLOGICAL INDICES

Red cell indices are MCV, mean corpuscular hemoglobin (MCH), and MCHC. They are also called *absolute values.* They are derived from values of hemoglobin, PCV/hematocrit, and red cell count. Recently a new parameter called red cell distribution width (RDW) has been introduced.

Red cell indices are accurately measured by an automated hematology analyzer.

Uses of red cell indices:

- In the morphological classes of anemias, e.g., normocytic normochromic, microcytic hypochromic, and macrocytic anemias.
- Differentiation of iron deficiency anemia from thalassemias.

Mean Corpuscular Volume

Mean corpuscular volume is a measure of the average size of the red cells.

$$\text{MCV} = \frac{\text{PCV in \%}}{\text{RBC count in millions/mm}^3\text{ of blood}} \times 100$$

Normal value: 80–94 femtoliters (fL)

MCV: Increased in all macrocytic anemias and decreased in microcytic hypochromic anemias.

Mean Corpuscular Hemoglobin

It is the average amount of hemoglobin in a single red cell.

Mean corpuscular hemoglobin (MCH)

$$= \frac{\text{Hb in g/dL}}{\text{RBC count in millions/mm}^3\text{ of blood}} \times 10$$

Normal value: 27–32 picograms (pg)

Mean Corpuscular Hemoglobin Concentration

The MCHC is a measure of the concentration of hemoglobin in a given volume of packed RBC (it refers to the concentration of hemoglobin in 1 dL or 1 L of packed red cells).

$$\text{MCHC} = \frac{\text{Hb in g/dL}}{\text{PCV in \%}} \times 100$$

Normal value: 33–36 g/dL

MCHC: It is either normal or decreased but not increased.

Red Cell Distribution Width

- It is the measure of the degree of variation in red cell size (anisocytosis). It is helpful in the differential diagnosis of anemias. Among microcytic anemias, RDW is low in the β-thalassemia trait, high in iron deficiency anemia, and normal in anemia of chronic disease.
- Normal RDW is 9–14.5.
- Automated analyzers measure this.
- In iron deficiency anemia and thalassemia MCV, MCH, and MCHC are reduced. In macrocytic anemia and reticulocytosis, MCV is increased. Increased MCH is found in macrocytic anemias, and decreased in microcytic hypochromic anemia. In hemolytic anemias and blood loss anemia, MCH is reduced and MCV and MCC are within normal limits.

ERYTHROCYTE SEDIMENTATION RATE

Erythrocyte sedimentation rate (ESR) is a test done to reveal inflammatory activity in the body. Depending on the value the test helps diagnose or monitor the progress of an inflammatory disease that can be caused by one or more conditions, such as infections, tumors, and autoimmune diseases. A high rate indicates inflammation.

The ESR, or sedimentation (sedimentation rate), denotes the velocity of sedimentation of RBC/unit of time and is expressed in mm at the end of 1 hour. This is an indication of inflammation and increases in many diseases.

Estimation of Erythrocyte Sedimentation Rate

Wintrobe's Method

The anticoagulant is double oxalate. Deliver 5 mL of venous blood into a tube containing 10 mg of dry potassium and ammonium oxalate. Mix the samples well and fill a Wintrobe's hematocrit tube to the 100 mm mark by means of a capillary pipette. Place the tube in exactly a vertical position and observe the point on the scale to which the red cells fall during 1 hour = ESR. For PCV, centrifuge the tube for 30 minutes at 3,000 rpm and read the volume of packed cells.

Normal range:

- *Men*: 0–6.5 mm in 1 hour
- *Women*: 0–15 mm 1 hour

Westergren's Method

It is the preferred method of ESR estimation performed in most of the laboratories **(Table 1)**.

WESTERGREN'S PIPETTE

It is used for ESR alone:

- *Length of the pipette*: 300 mm (30 cm) open at both ends. The lower 20 cm are marked from 0 to 200 mm. Diameter: 2.5 mm **(Fig. 3)**

TABLE 1: The normal range for the sedimentation rate (Westergren method) chart.

Gender and age	Sedimentation rate (mm/h)
Males younger than 50	0 to 15
Males older than 50	0 to 20
Females younger than 50	0 to 20
Females older than 50	0 to 30

Source: emedicine health.com

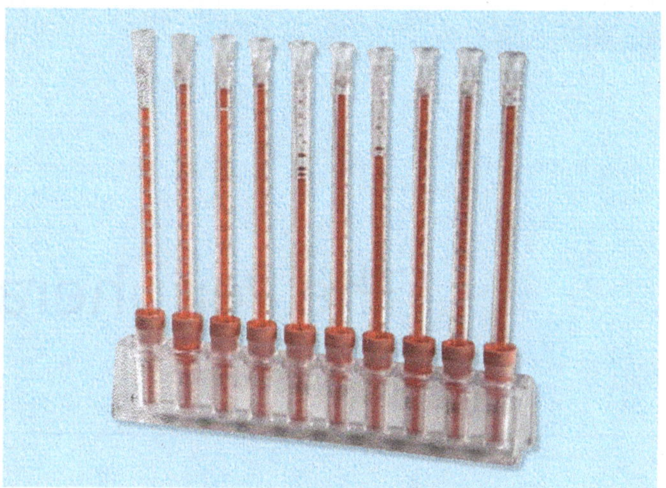

FIG. 3: Loaded Westergren's tube with samples.

- *Uses*: Estimation of ESR
  - Indication for the presence of active diseases: Tuberculosis, subacute bacterial endocarditis.
  - Serial controls on the activity of chronic diseases—arthritis and ankylosing spondylitis.
- *Anticoagulants used*:
  - Trisodium citrate 3.8% 0.4 mL with 1.6 mL of venous blood
  - If EDTA is used, the blood must be diluted with trisodium citrate before testing (4 volumes of blood to 1 volume of citrate)
- *Procedure*: The anticoagulated blood is sucked up to the mark 0 and placed *vertically* in Westergren's stand. The reading is taken at the end of 1 hour, i.e., the distance from the surface meniscus to the top of the column of sedimented red cells.
- *Advantages:* Most sensitive method for serial monitoring of chronic diseases, e.g., tuberculosis.
- *Disadvantages:*
  - A large amount of blood is needed.
  - Involves dilution when collected in EDTA.
- *Precautions*:
  - The tube should be grease-free.
  - Vertically placed in the rack
  - It should be placed on a nonvibrant surface.
  - It should not be exposed to sunlight and heat.
- *Diseases in which ESR is raised*:
  - Tuberculosis
  - Multiple myeloma
  - Rheumatoid arthritis
  - Collagen vascular disease
  - Anemias
  - Renal insufficiency
- *Diseases in which ESR is decreased*: Polycythemia

CHAPTER 3

The Peripheral Blood Smear

INTRODUCTION

A peripheral blood smear study gives important information with regard to the morphology of cells. Also detected on a smear are infections, malignancies, etc.

MAKING OF BLOOD FILMS

For proper assessment a proper procedure of making the blood film is essential.

Thin Film

Thin film is usually made for routine diagnosis in the laboratory (to show newspaper print through it). Clean the patient's fingertip. After allowing the skin to dry, puncture it with a sterile blood lancet or needle with a firm quick jab. Wipe away the first drop that appears. After this take a small drop of blood on a clean slide about 1/2" from the end, taking care that the slide does not touch the skin. Place the edge of a second slide against the first slide at an angle of about 35° and draw it up against the blood drop which will immediately run across the slide edge filling the angle between the slides **(Fig. 1)**. Push the upper slide forward along the other slowly to get a thin film. Dry the blood film in the air.

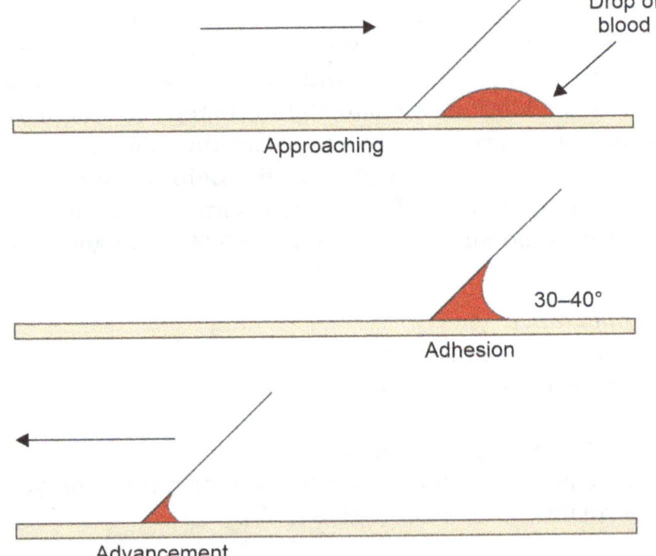

FIG. 1: Making of a peripheral smear.

Requisites of an ideal smear ***(Fig. 2)***:

- Should be tongue-shaped with head, body, and tail.
- Should not cover the entire slide.
- Should be thin enough between the body and tail to show red blood cells (RBCs) one cell thick.
- Gradual transition from thick to thin.
- Should have no windows (or holes).

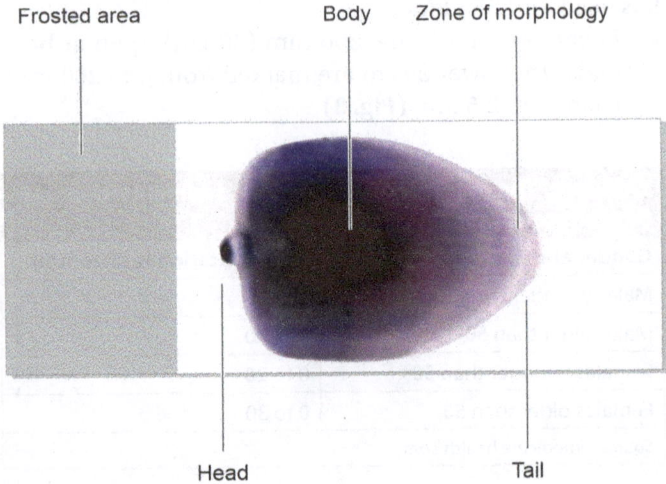

FIG. 2: Parts of an ideal smear.

Thick Film

Thick films are generally made to look for malarial parasites. Take 2–3 drops of blood close together on the slide and with the spreader spread them out enough to show a "hands-on watch" through the film. Dry in the air for 0.5–1 hour.

Fixation

Blood films are dried rapidly in air and fixed by immersing in methyl alcohol for 3 minutes or in ethyl alcohol for 5 minutes. A Leishman's stain has inbuilt methyl alcohol as a fixative.

Staining Blood Films

Romanowsky Stains

Principle

The principle consists of a combination of acidic and basic dyes and after staining various intermediate shades between the two polar stains (red and blue) appear. They depend for their action on the compounds formed by the interaction of methylene blue and eosin. A cationic or basic dye (methylene blue or Azure B) binds to anionic sites in the nucleus and gives a blue-gray color to the nucleic acids [deoxyribonucleic acid (DNA) or ribonucleic acid (RNA)] and nucleoproteins, also granules of basophils. An anionic or acidic dye such as Eosin B or Y binds to cationic sites such as proteins and gives an orange-red color to the hemoglobin and eosinophil granules. There are several combinations of stains available, examples of these are May-Grunwald, Jenner, Wright's, Giemsa, Leishman's, and Field's stains. The stain gives a reddish-purple color to the nuclear material and also the chromatin of malarial and other parasites. This color is due to the substance that forms when methylene blue is ripened either by age as in polychrome methylene blue or by heating with sodium carbonate. Of all the modifications of the original Romanowsky stains, the well-known and most popular ones are the Leishman's and Giemsa stains.

Leishman's Stain

Leishman stain is a neutral stain first used by the British surgeon WB Leishman.

The Leishman stain is one of the best stains to stain the peripheral blood smear routinely. The stain is usually diluted and buffered during the staining procedure. The buffering acts as a mordant and enhances the staining.

Constituents

It is a methyl alcohol mixture of "polychromed" methylene blue and eosin. It consists of a mixture of eosin (an acidic stain), and methylene blue (a basic stain) in methyl alcohol.

Fixative

The methyl alcohol acts as an inbuilt fixative.

Method

- Pour undiluted stain on a dry, unfixed blood film. Allow 3 minutes. Methyl alcohol in the Leishman's stain fixes the film.
- By means of a pipette with rubber, add buffer solution, equal in quantity to the stain added. Mix by gentle blowing. Allow 7 minutes.
- Wash the film in distilled water allowing the preparation to differentiate until the film appears bright pink in color in about half a minute.
- Dry the film in the air.
- Study under oil immersion.

Examination of Blood Smear

It should be done under oil immersion at the junction of the body and tail where the red cells are not seen overlapping.

A normal peripheral smear shows RBCs which measure approximately 7.2 µ and normally show one-third pallor in the center. They do not overlap at the optimal site of examination (i.e., the junction between the two-thirds to the last one-third of the smear. White blood cells (WBCs) are seen; normally neutrophils (40–70% of leukocytes), eosinophils (0–6%), lymphocytes 20–40%, monocytes 2–8%, and basophils (0–2%). Platelets are seen as single forms and in clusters and measure 2–4 µm in size. The following features should be noted:

- Red cells—morphology, immature forms, inclusion bodies, and arrangement of cells (rouleau formation or otherwise).
- White cells—differential count and abnormal or immature forms.
- Platelet count—number and distribution (aggregates/single)
- Parasites
- Anisocytosis is a variation in the size of RBCs. Poikilocytosis is a variation in the shape of erythrocytes. Anisopoikilocytosis is seen in various anemias. Normocytic normochromic RBCs indicate blood loss anemias and microcytic hypochromic cells are seen in iron deficiency anemias and thalassemia; target cells are seen in iron deficiency, thalassemia, and sickle cell anemias.
- *Target cell*: The central dark dot-like coloration in a target cell is because the cell membrane is very thin and gets folded up; wherever folds appear the staining is dark.
- Abnormal shapes of red cells like *elliptocytosis* [hereditary elliptocytosis (HE), also known as *ovalocytosis*, is a disorder of the red cell membrane inherited usually in an autosomal dominant pattern]; stomatocytosis (a hereditary condition with the cell showing a mouth like a shape as a result of abnormal ionic exchange).

- *Macrocytes* are seen in megaloblastic anemias as well as Cabot rings and Howell–Jolly bodies. *Stomatocytes* are seen in stomatocytosis and schistocytes in microangiopathic hemolytic anemia (MAHA).
- *Polychromatic cells (young red cells)* which show a bluish tint on the Leishman's stain are larger in size than normal RBCs and are seen if the patient is on treatment.
- *Burr cells*: Burr cells, also known as echinocytes, are RBCs with about 10–30 small, uniform, and evenly-spaced spicules distributed over their cell surface. The presence of burr cells indicates only an artifact and is of no diagnostic significance.
- *Schistocytes*: They are fragmented red cells that are seen in MAHA; the two major causes of MAHA are (1) thrombotic thrombocytopenic purpura (TTP) and (2) hemolytic uremic syndrome (HUS).
- *Acanthocytes*: Acanthocytes are red cells with a small number of spicules of inconstant length, thickness, and shape, irregularly disposed over the surface of the cell. Seen in hyposplenism, splenectomy, and in liver disease.
- *Howell–Jolly bodies*: Nuclear remnants or inclusions or aggregates of chromatin seen in red cells in megaloblastic anemias, and postsplenectomy cases.
- *Cabot rings*: They are oval, circular, or figure of eight thin thread-like structures in red cells seen in megaloblastic anemias and other dyserythropoiesis. They are remnants of the mitotic spindle.
- *Pappenheimer bodies*: They are small debris of iron that can be found in RBCs. This debris is normally eliminated by the spleen. Pappenheimer bodies are found in patients having had splenectomy. They are also found in anemia with a defect in the synthesis of the "heme" part of hemoglobin (e.g., congenital sideroblastic anemia), or due to lead poisoning, or in advanced alcoholic cirrhosis. Also seen where there is a congenital defect in the synthesis of one of the two protein chains of hemoglobin, e.g., thalassemia.
- *Heinz bodies*: Heinz bodies ("Heinz–Ehrlich bodies") are inclusions within RBCs composed of denatured hemoglobin as seen in exposure to oxidizing drugs and in glucose-6-phosphate dehydrogenase (G6PD) deficiency. They are demonstrated by supravital staining.
- *Basophilic stippling*: is seen as blue-black granules in red cells precipitated due to ribosomal RNA. Seen in megaloblastic anemia, and other forms of severe anemias where erythropoiesis is disturbed. Also seen in lead poisoning, and thalassemia, infections, liver disease. It does not stain positive for iron.

Figure 3 shows the morphology of normal and abnormal cells as detected in a peripheral smear.

- *Ring sideroblasts*: They are erythrocyte precursors with a ring of hemosiderin granules around the nucleus; they are found in sideroblastic anemias.
- *Downey cells*: They are reactive lymphocytes with typical appearances seen in infectious mononucleosis.
- In most nutritional anemias the treatment is started after the blood film examination.
- *Toxic granules*: They are seen in infections.
- Chédiak–Higashi syndrome there are giant but scanty azurophilic granules, in the neutrophils as well as other leukocyte types. The color of the granules is abnormal. A mutation of a lysosomal trafficking regulator protein leads to a decrease in phagocytosis. Patients manifest with albinism and increased infections.

DIFFERENTIAL COUNT

Differential leukocyte counts are usually performed in most laboratories, by automated instruments. However, they can also be performed by visual examination and counting of cells in blood films that are prepared on slides by the spread or a "wedge" technique. Even in well-made films, the distribution of the various cell types is not totally random. Neutrophils are more concentrated toward the junction of the body and the tail of the smear and lymphocytes along the upper and lower margins.

For a reliable differential count on an ideal film spread on slides, the film should not be too thin and the tail of the film should be smooth. To achieve this, the film should be made with rapid movement using a smooth glass spreader with a smooth edge. Most often a second glass slide is used as a spreader. A smooth movement results in a film in which there is some overlap of the red cells, separation of these near the tail, and in which the white cells in the body of the film are not shrunken.

The cells are counted using a ×40 objective in a zig-zag fashion as shown in **Figure 4**. A horizontal strip running the whole length of the film from the head to the tail may also be chosen so that a minimum of 100 WBCs are counted; if less than this a second horizontal strip is counted by coming down and going in the opposite direction.

Automated Differential Counters

Automated differential counters are now available and use flow cytometry incorporated into a full blood counter. These blood cell counters have a differential counting capacity, providing either a three-part or a five or more-part differential count. Counts are performed on diluted

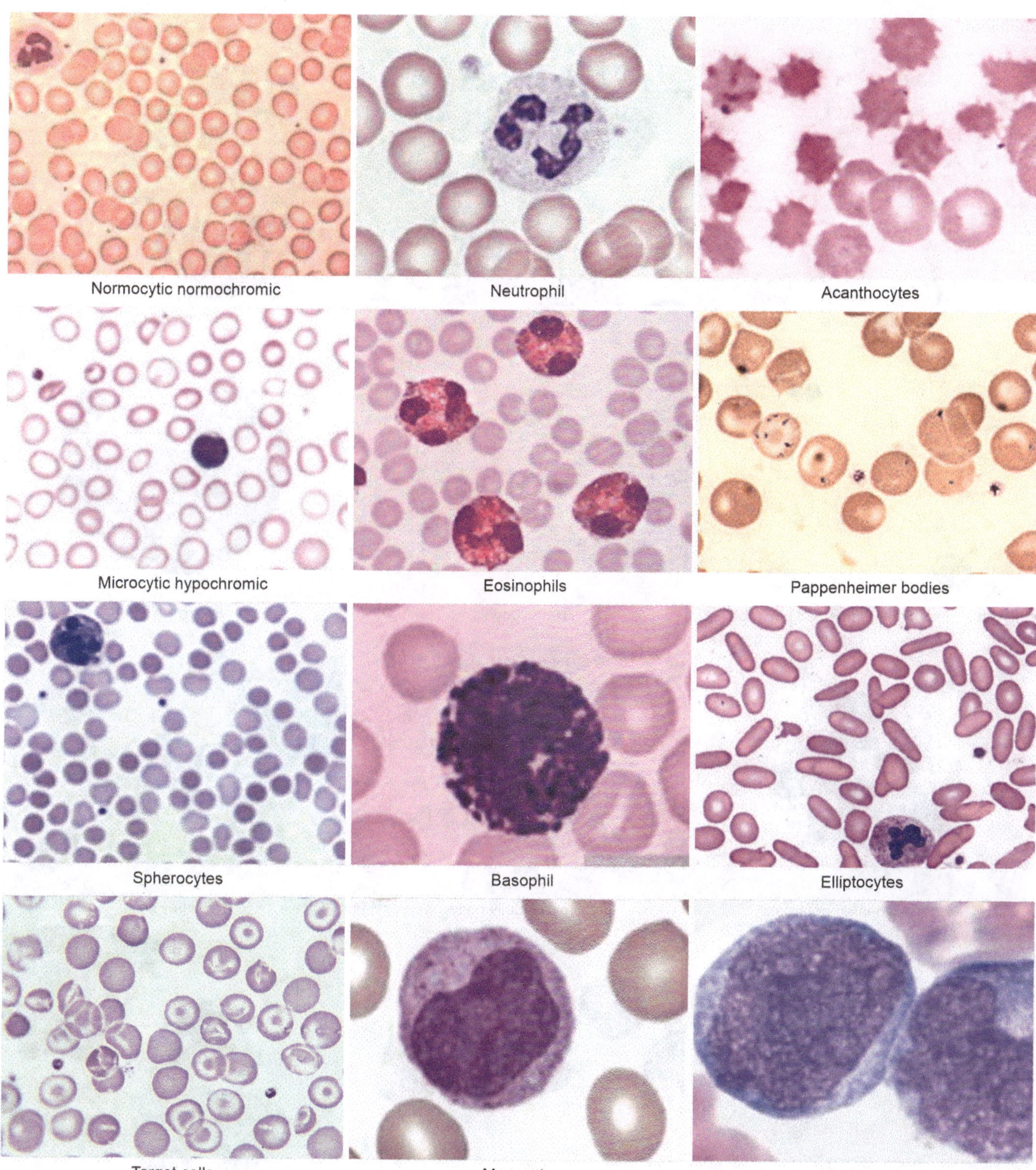

FIG. 3: *Continued*

Continued

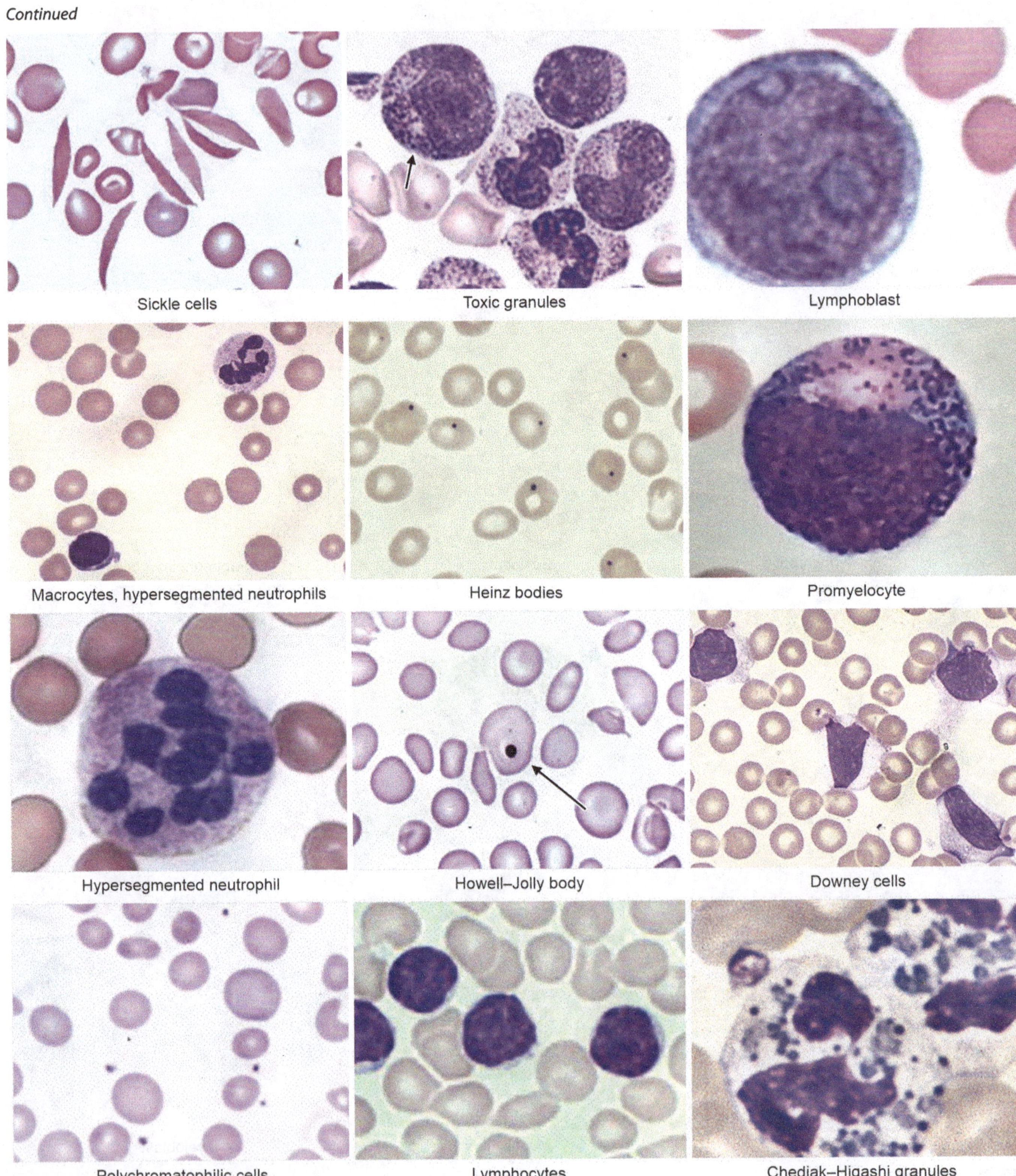

FIG. 3: *Continued*

Continued

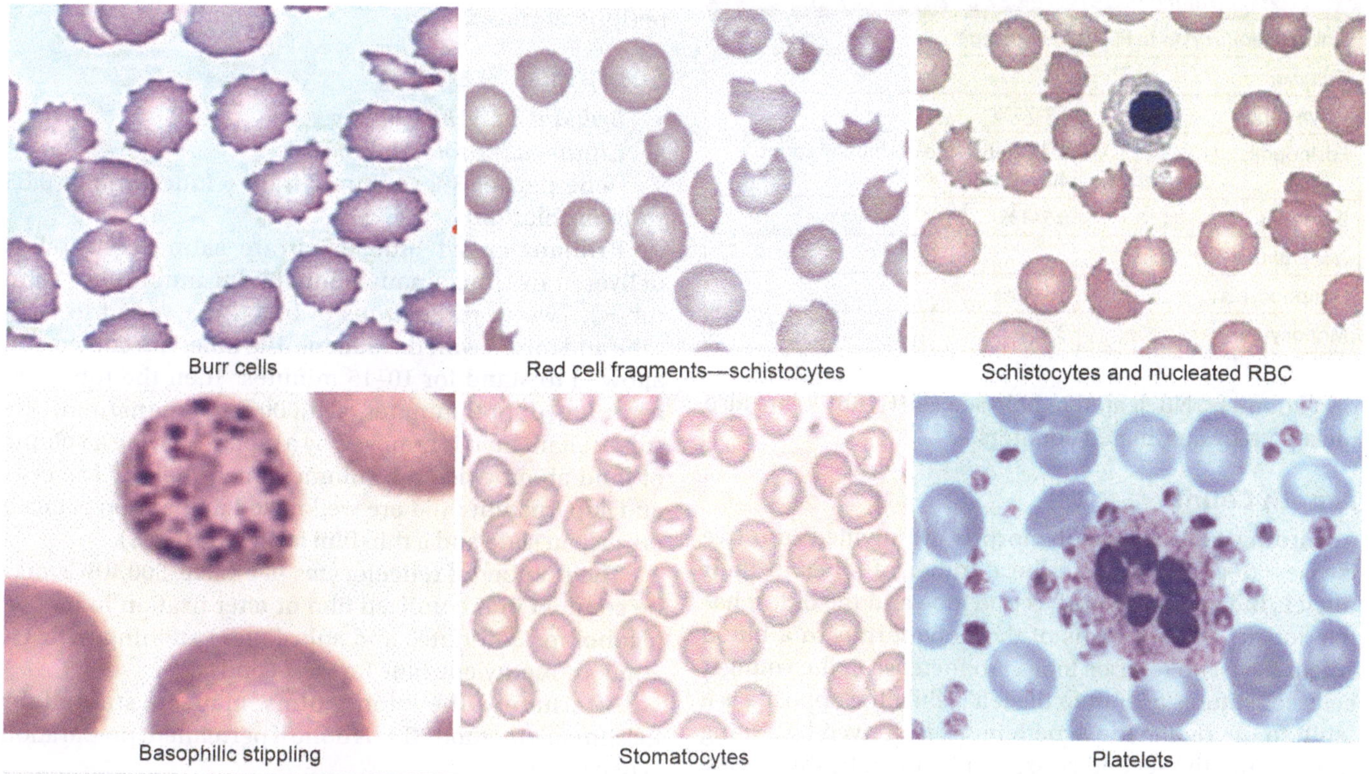

Burr cells

Red cell fragments—schistocytes

Schistocytes and nucleated RBC

Basophilic stippling

Stomatocytes

Platelets

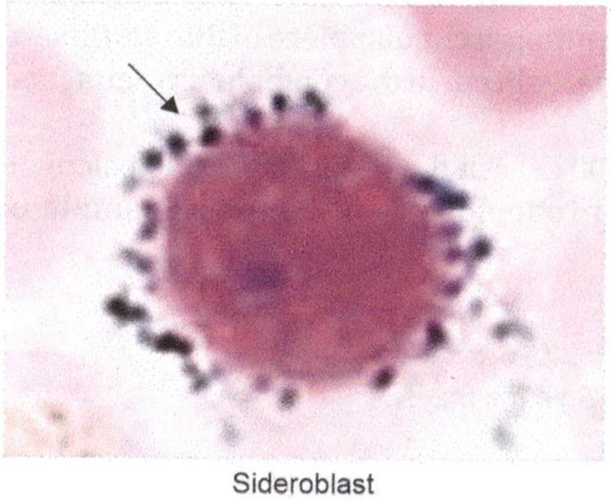

Sideroblast

FIG. 3: Normal and abnormal forms of red cells, white blood cells (WBCs), and platelets as seen in blood films.

Scanning technique for WBC differential count and morphologic evaluation

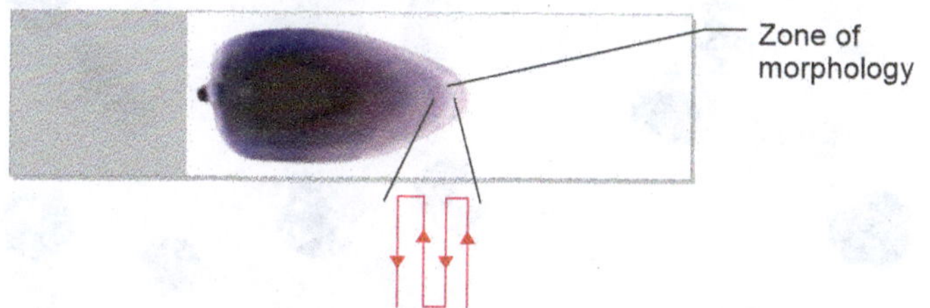

FIG. 4: Peripheral smear to show a method of doing a differential in a zig-zag fashion. The same can be done also in a horizontal fashion.

whole blood in which red cells are lysed or rendered invisible. A three-part differential count assigns cells to categories usually designated as (1) "granulocytes" or "large cells," (2) "lymphocytes" or "small cells," and (3) "monocytes," "mononuclear cells," or "middle cells." Some categories include (2) and (3) in the nongranular series **(Table 1)**. In theory, the granulocyte category includes neutrophils, eosinophils and basophils. Some cell counters can pick up and categorize immature cells or atypical cells or at least tag them. Beckman Coulter Systems and Sysmex are some of the makers of automated three-part and five-

TABLE 1: Normal leukocytes in PS and their percentages.

Normal leukocytes in PS	Percentage
Granular	
Polymorphs	65–75%
Eosinophils	2–5% (absolute eosinophil count 40–440/mL)
Basophils	0.5–1%
Nongranular	
Lymphocytes	20–40%
Monocytes	3–8%

part counters. Nucleated red blood cells (NRBCs) are also picked up by automated counters.

Arneth Count

According to Arneth, polymorphs are divided into five classes, depending upon the number of lobes in their nuclei. The youngest cell has one lobe and the oldest has five lobes. Three-fourths of the polymorphs in a blood smear have two to three lobes. An increase in the younger cells constitutes a "shift to the left" while the opposite is a "shift to the right." The Arneth index is derived by adding the first and the second classes and half of the third class. The normal value is 50–65. A shift to the left occurs when immature cells predominate the peripheral smear.

Schilling's Count

In the course of an ordinary differential count, along with the normal leukocytes, precursors of the white cells—myelocytes, metamyelocytes, and single-lobed polymorphs (stab cells) are noted. This constitutes the Schilling hemogram.

Significance of Arneth's and Schilling's Counts

In normal blood, there are no myelocytes or metamyelocytes. About 3–5% of stab cells are usually found.

A shift to the left with high leukocyte count occurs in acute sepsis, appendicitis, etc. This is a regenerative shift to the left. Metamyelocytes and stab cells appear in the blood. A shift to the right is seen in megaloblastic anemia, where many cells are seen with about five to six lobes.

Reticulocyte Count

Since reticulocytes are premature RBCs and remain in the peripheral blood for a day or two before maturing, a count gives a good indication with regard to the bone marrow response. The normal reticulocyte count is 0.5–2%. A decrease in reticulocyte count occurs in iron deficiency anemia as production is less. When supplements or treatment of anemias is given the reticulocyte count increases which can be used to measure response to therapy.

Method of demonstrating reticulocytes in the peripheral smear.

Supravital Staining

- *Brilliant cresyl blue*: 0.15 g
- *Citrate saline solution*: 100 mL

(One part of 3% sodium citrate + four parts of 0.85 sodium chloride)

Brilliant cresyl blue in citrate saline solution is delivered in 1 mL amounts into 80 × 1 mm tubes (Kahn tubes). Two to three drops of blood are added to each tube and mixed with the diluent. The tubes are corked and allowed to stand for 10–15 minutes. Then the tubes are centrifuged for 2 minutes, at 1,000 revolutions/min. The supernatant fluid is removed by a pipette leaving a volume of fluid about twice the volume of cells below. The cells and supernatant fluid are well mixed and a drop is taken on a clean slide and a thin film is drawn **(Fig. 5)**.

The number of reticulocytes per 1,000/500 RBCs may be counted in the unfixed film or after fixation in methyl alcohol for 3 minutes and subsequent staining with 1% aqueous methylene blue for 30 seconds.

Alternately the blood films may be stained by Leishman's method. This is done if permanent preparation is necessary.

To facilitate counting, a circular piece of thin cardboard or paper with a square slit cut in the center may be attached to the eyepiece.

Count about 500 cells in the unfixed film and calculate the percentage of reticulocytes in the given sample of blood.

Normal values:
- *Infants at birth*: 2.0–6%
- *Children up to 5 years*: 0.2–5%
- *Adults*: 0.2–2%

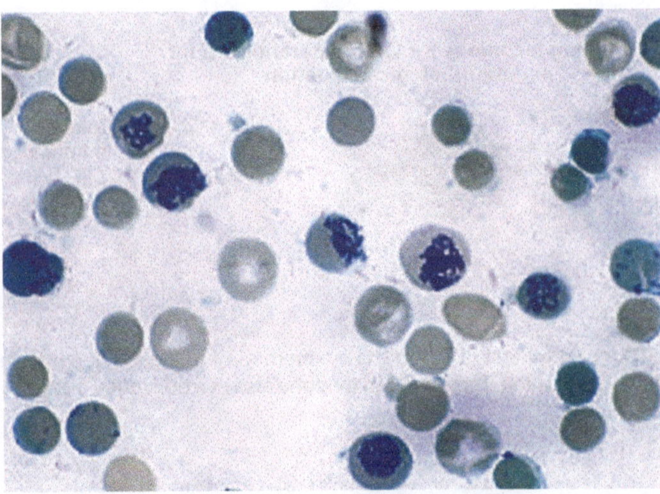

FIG. 5: Supravital staining—methylene blue stain × 1,000.

Interpretation

Reticulocyte counts are low in ineffective erythropoiesis, e.g., myelosclerosis, aplastic anemia, megaloblastic anemia, thalassemia, erythroleukemia, and sideroblastic anemia. Reticulocytosis occurs after blood loss or effective therapy for certain kinds of anemia, e.g., therapy of iron deficiency or megaloblastic macrocytic anemias. Reticulocytosis is also seen in hemolytic anemias.

An increase of 15–20% in reticulocyte count is considered an index of therapeutic efficiency.

CHAPTER 4

Bone Marrow Aspiration and Biopsy

INTRODUCTION

A bone marrow (BM) aspiration is done using a bone marrow aspiration needle. This may be followed by a bone marrow biopsy.

INDICATIONS

For Diagnosis

- High color index anemias—(1) megaloblastic anemias marrow shows typical megaloblastic red-cell formation with the presence of giant metamyelocytes. Such a picture occurs in pernicious anemia, nutritional megaloblastic anemia usually secondary to steatorrhea, megaloblastic anemia of pregnancy, and megaloblastic anemia due to anticonvulsant drugs; (2) hemolytic anemia—suggested by cellular normoblastic marrow; (3) aplastic anemia, few cells mostly lymphocytes, monocytes, and plasma cells are observed; and (4) myxedema and renal failure—hypoplastic marrow with moderate diminution of all cell types.
- Tropical diseases—kala-azar—*Leishmania donovani* (LD) bodies may be readily distinguished within the monocytes
- *Aleukemic leukemia*—50% or more of the cells are primitive leukocytes/blasts through abnormal cells are absent or too few for the diagnosis in peripheral blood.
- Myelomatosis—infiltration with plasma cells.
- *Lymphoma*—marrow shows groups of abnormal lymphoma cells though there may not be a clinical enlargement of lymph glands.
- Malignancy—at times secondary infiltrating cells from malignant tumors occur in marrow smears.
- Gaucher's disease—reticulum cells stuffed with abnormal lipid (cerebroglucoside).

For Prognosis

- Primary form of thrombocytopenic, purpura—if the marrow shows increased activity of normoblasts and megakaryocytes. In this type, the response to therapy is good but not in the secondary type.
- Chronic myeloid leukemia—if myeloblasts are 10% or less, response to treatment is likely to be good, if 50% or more the reverse.

CONTRAINDICATIONS

Hemophilia and allied disorders of coagulation.

Marrow aspiration and trephine biopsy are both complementary to each other and maximum information can be obtained if both techniques are used together. Biopsy alone is inferior to aspirate for identification and study of fine morphological details of individual marrow cells; however, trephine biopsy provides a larger amount of marrow for examination. *Quantitation* of some cell types (e.g., megakaryocytes) is more reliable, and granulomatous lesions and marrow infiltration by lymphoma or carcinoma are also more likely to be detected more clearly in a biopsy.

BONE MARROW BIOPSY NEEDLES

- *Parts*:
    - Wide bore needle:
        - Stylet

- Adjustable guard:
  - Salah's needle—aspiration needle **(Fig. 1A)** (side screw - easy way of identifying salah needle is to remember 'SS' stands for 'Salah' and 'Side screw')
  - Klima needle—aspiration needle **(Fig. 1B)**
  - Jamshidi's needle—both aspiration and biopsy **(Fig. 1C)**
  - Westerman Jensen needle—for both aspiration and biopsy

Sterilization: Autoclaving

Dry sterilization in hot air ovens.

Site of bone marrow biopsy:
- *In infants*: Tibial tuberosity
- *Grown-up children and adults*:
  - Posterior superior iliac spine
  - Anterior surface of sternum
- *Old age*: Spinous process of vertebrae

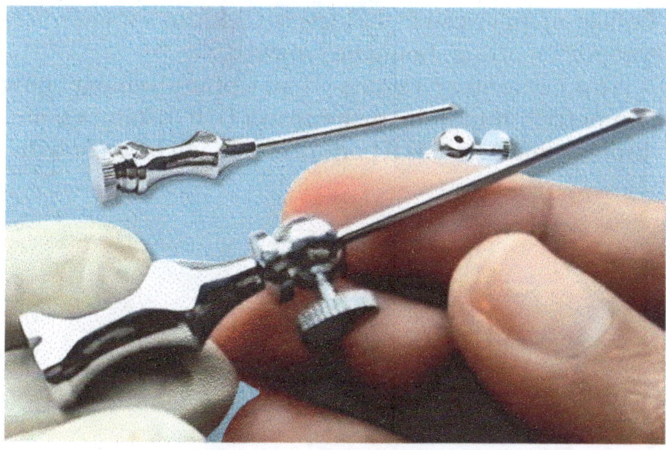

FIG. 1A: Salah's bone marrow aspiration needle with a side screw.

Technique

- Marrow aspiration is done with a marrow aspiration needle. The skin, subcutaneous tissue, and periosteum over the posterior iliac crest (or manubrium sterni) are infiltrated with 2% xylocaine. The marrow needle is pushed through the bone with a boring motion, the guard being kept at a distance of about 1 cm above the surface of the skin. When the needle has entered the marrow, the stylet is withdrawn and a 1 mL syringe is attached, 0.2–0.3 mL of marrow fluid is aspirated. The needle with trocar is removed and the site of aspiration is sealed with benzoin tincture. Marrow fluid drawn is smeared onto glass slides. In selected patients, the residual aspirate is placed in appropriate specimen containers for chromosomal analysis, microbiological culture, cell culture, and electron microscopy.
- *Marrow trephine*: Bone marrow aspiration is usually combined with bone marrow biopsy and both are complimentary to one another. Bone marrow aspiration is often performed with a bone marrow biopsy, one following the other. However, a different needle is used in a bone marrow biopsy to remove a core of solid tissue from the bone marrow. A biopsy is complimentary in the assessment of blood conditions and is of particular use in:
  - Leukopenia, leukocytosis, thrombocytopenia, thrombocytosis, pancytopenia, and polycythemia
  - Carcinomas of the blood or bone marrow, including leukemias, lymphomas, and multiple myeloma
  - Metastatic carcinomas in the bone marrow
  - Hemochromatosis and myelofibrosis
  - Cause of fevers of unknown origin

Immediately upon completion of the aspiration, a trephine biopsy (with a Jamshidi needle) of an adjacent area of bone is performed through the same puncture site.

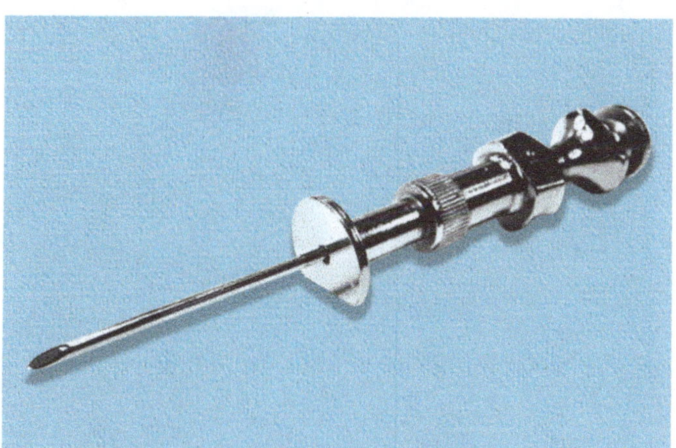

FIG. 1B: Klima's bone marrow aspiration needle.

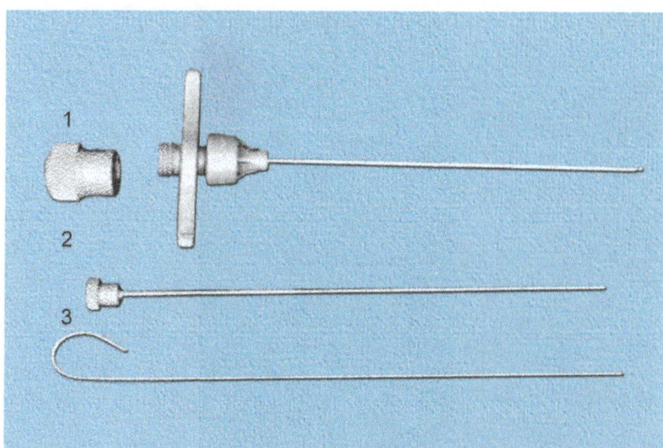

FIG. 1C: Jamshidi bone marrow biopsy needle shows (in the fig. from above down) (1) Hollow needle with bevelled tip; (2) Stylet; and (3) Probe to express biopsy from the needle.

After the expulsion of a 2 cm core of bone and its enclosed marrow, from the needle; the biopsy specimen is smeared gently across three glass slides (touch smears) and then placed in a fixative for subsequent histopathological processing and staining.

Normal Aspiration Marrow

Nucleated cells 20,000–100,000/mm^3 predominant cells—granulocytes of normal types, and few normoblasts, both showing some mitoses. M:E ratio is 3-4:1. Megakaryocytes are present, but other cells are few. No abnormal cells.

Reporting of bone marrow smear:

- Cellularity
- M:E ratio
- Erythropoiesis
- Granulopoiesis
- Megakaryocytes
- Abnormal cells
- Iron stores

Cause of a "Dry" or "Bloody Tap"

- *In cases of hypercellular marrow*:
  - Acute myeloblasts of lymphoblastic leukemia (preleukemia stage)
  - Acute promyelocytes leukemia
  - Hairy cell leukemia
  - Malignant infiltration of marrow
  - Refractory anemia with cellular marrow
- *In cases of marrow fibrosis*: Idiopathic myelosclerosis
- *Hypocellular marrow*: Aplastic anemia

Bone Marrow Biopsy

The site is usually the post iliac crest, done bilaterally and collected in separate bottles in fixative (10% of formalin); then sent for routine paraffin processing. The sternum is another site where a biopsy may be performed. The patient is asked to discontinue any blood thinners which he may be on.

Reporting of Bone Marrow Biopsy

Bone marrow pathology reports are highly variable, with diagnostic statements ranging from a one-line diagnosis to lengthy narratives with the term acute leukemia buried in extensive textual paragraphs. The significant variability in the reporting of bone marrow specimens may result in incomplete information or misleading information.

For a consensus and uniformity of reporting the 'College of American Pathologists (CAP) 2019 's' criteria of synoptic reporting should be followed.

Supplementary results of peripheral smear, flow cytometry, immunohistochemistry (IHC) staining, and chromosomal analysis if performed should be included.

CHAPTER 5

Anemia, Microcytic, and Macrocytic Anemias

ANEMIA

Anemia is usually defined as decreased levels of hemoglobin and/or a decreased packed cell volume (hematocrit), and/or a decreased red blood cell (RBC) count. In its broadest sense, anemia is a functional inability of the blood to supply the tissue with adequate O_2 for a proper metabolic function.

Anemia is not a disease, but rather the expression of an underlying disorder or disease. Anemia may develop when RBC loss or destruction exceeds the maximal capacity of bone marrow RBC production or when bone marrow production is impaired.

Classification of Anemia

Classification of anemia according to the underlying mechanism (etiological classification of anemias):

- *Blood loss*: Acute or chronic
- Increased red cell destruction (hemolysis)
- Decreased red cell production

Increased Red Cell Destruction

Inherited Genetic Defects

- *Red cell membrane disorders*: Hereditary spherocytosis and elliptocytosis
- *Enzyme deficiencies*:
  - Hexose monophosphate shunt enzyme deficiencies—glucose-6-phosphate dehydrogenase (G6PD) deficiency and glutathione synthetase deficiency
  - Glycolytic enzyme deficiencies—pyruvate kinase deficiency and hexokinase deficiency
- *Hemoglobin abnormalities*:
  - Deficient globin synthesis: Thalassemia syndromes
  - Structurally abnormal globin-(hemoglobinopathies): Sickle cell
  - Disease and unstable hemoglobins

Acquired Genetic Defects

Deficiency of phosphatidylinositol-linked glycoproteins—paroxysmal nocturnal hemoglobinuria.

Antibody-mediated Destruction

Hemolytic disease of the newborn (Rh disease), transfusion reactions, drug-induced, and autoimmune disorders.

Mechanical Trauma

- *Microangiopathic hemolytic anemias*: Hemolytic uremic syndrome (HUS), disseminated intravascular coagulation (DIC), and thrombotic thrombocytopenic purpura (TTP)
- *Cardiac traumatic hemolysis*: Defective cardiac valves
- *Repetitive physical trauma*: Marathon running and karate chopping

Infections of Red Cells

Malaria and babesiosis

Toxic or Chemical Injury

Snake venom, lead poisoning, and clostridial sepsis

Sequestration

Hypersplenism

Decreased Red Cell Production

Nutritional Deficiencies

- Deficiencies affecting deoxyribonucleic acid (DNA) synthesis—B_{12} and folate deficiencies
- Deficiencies affecting hemoglobin synthesis—iron deficiency anemia (IDA)

Erythropoietin Deficiency

Renal failure and anemia of chronic disease

Immune-mediated

Aplastic anemia and pure red cell aplasia

CLINICAL FEATURES OF ANEMIAS

- Tiredness
- Muscle fatigue and weakness
- Headache and vertigo (dizziness)
- Dyspnea (difficult or labored breathing) from exertion
- Gastrointestinal (GI) problems
- Overt signs of blood loss such as hematuria (blood in urine) or black stools

Physical Examination

Hepato or splenomegaly, heart abnormalities, and skin pallor

A specific diagnosis is made by:

- Patient history
- Patient physical exam
- Signs and symptoms exhibited by the patient
- Hematologic lab findings
- Identification of the cause of anemia is important so that appropriate therapy is used to treat the anemia

Laboratory Investigations

A complete blood count (CBC), will include the following and will be variant depending on the severity and type of anemia.

Red Blood Cell Count

- At birth the normal range is $3.9–5.9 \times 10^6$/uL (10^{12}/L)
- The normal range for males is $4.5–5.9 \times 10^6$/uL
- The normal range for females is $3.8–5.2 \times 10^6$/uL

Hematocrit or Packed Cell Volume in Percentage

- At birth the normal range is 42–60% (42–60)
- The normal range for males is 41–53% (41–53)
- The normal range for females is 38–46% (38–46)

Red Cell Indices

Mean Corpuscular Volume (MCV)

It is the average volume/RBC in femtoliters (10^{-15} L)

- At birth the normal range is 98–123
- In adults the normal range is 80–100

The MCV is used to classify RBCs as:

- Normocytic (80–100)
- Microcytic (<80)
- Macrocytic (>100)

Mean Corpuscular Hemoglobin Concentration (MCHC)

It is the average concentration of hemoglobin in g/dL (or %):

- At birth the normal range is 30–36 g/dL
- In adults the normal range is 31–37g/dL
- The MCHC is used to classify RBCs as:
  - Normochromic (31–37)
  - Hypochromic (<31)

Mean Corpuscular Hemoglobin (MCH)

It is the average weight of hemoglobin/cell in picograms (pg = 10^{-12} g)

- At birth the normal range is 31–37
- In adults the normal range is 26–34

Red Cell Distribution Width (RDW)

It is a measurement of the variation in RBC cell size, i.e., standard deviation/mean MCV × 100

- The range for normal values is 11.5–14.5%
- A value > 14.5 means that there is increased variation in cell size above the normal amount (anisocytosis)
- A value < 11.5 means that the RBC population is more uniform in size than normal.

Reticulocyte Count

Reticulocyte count gives an indication of the level of the bone marrow activity. It is done by staining a peripheral blood smear with new methylene blue to help visualize the remaining ribosomes and endoplasmic reticulum (ER). The number of reticulocytes/1,000 RBC is counted and reported as a percentage of the red cells.

- At birth the normal range is 1.8–8%
- The normal range in an adult (i.e., in an individual with no anemia) is 0.5–1.5%.
  Note: This percentage is not normal for anemia where the bone marrow should be working harder and throwing out more reticulocytes per day. In anemia, the reticulocyte count should be elevated above the normal values.

The laboratory investigation may also include:

- *Bone marrow smear and biopsy:* In a bone marrow sample, the following things should be noted:
  - Maturation of RBC and WBC series
  - Ratio of myeloid to erythroid series—normal M:E is 3-4:1
  - Abundance of iron stores (ringed sideroblasts)
  - Presence or absence of granulomas or tumor cells
  - Red to yellow ratio
  - Presence of megakaryocytes
- *Hemoglobin electrophoresis*: It can be used to identify the presence of abnormal hemoglobin as in sickle cell anemia and thalassemias. Different hemoglobins will

move to different regions of the gel and the type of hemoglobin may be identified by its position on the gel after electrophoresis.

- *Antiglobulin testing*: It tests for the presence of an antibody or complement on the surface of the RBC and can be used to support a diagnosis of autoimmune hemolytic anemia.
- *Osmotic fragility test*: This measures the RBC sensitivity to a hypotonic saline solution. Saline concentrations of 0–0.9% are incubated with RBCs at room temperature and the percent of hemolysis as compared to the normal is measured. Patients with spherocytes—membrane defect; have increased osmotic fragility. They have a limited ability to take up water in a hypotonic solution and will; therefore, lyse at a higher sodium concentration than will normal RBCs.
- *Serum iron, iron-binding capacity, and percentage saturation:* It is used to diagnose IDAs.

SPECIFIC ANEMIAS

Iron Deficiency Anemias

It is defined as anemia due to a deficiency of iron with microcytic hypochromic red cells, an MCV < 80 Fl, and MCH < 25 pg. Findings to suspect this are:

- Hemoglobin levels are low and vary depending on whether the anemia is mild, moderate, or severe. It can vary from as low as 3–10 g/dL.
- *PCV*: It is reduced (13–30%)
- *MCV, MCH, and MCHC*: These are reduced with the degree of reduction being proportional to the severity of anemia.
- MCV < 80 fL, MCH < 25 pg, and MCHC < 27 g/dL
- RDW is increased in Fe deficiency anemia while it is normal in thalassemia the closest differential at morphology of blood picture. A combination of low MCV and high RDW is a good screening test for Fe deficiency anemia.
- *Reticulocyte count*: It is low, normal, or only mildly increased, unless on the treatment when it may go up.
- *Bone marrow examination*: Erythropoiesis is micro-normoblastic. The granulocytic and megakaryocytic lines are normal.

Investigations Specific to Iron Deficiency Anemia

- *Peripheral blood smear*: Depending on the severity there is a moderate degree of anisopoikilocytosis. RBCs are microcytic hypochromic with varied shapes. Occasional pencil-shaped cells and target cells are seen. Ring forms (pessary cells) are seen in severe cases where the central pallor is marked and beyond the normal one-third. Occasional nucleated (late normoblasts) red cells may be detected. WBCs and platelets were normal **(Fig. 1)**.
    - Differential diagnosis of microcytic hypochromic blood picture: The closest differential of a microcytic hypochromic blood picture is (1) thalassemia and (2) sickle cell anemia. Thalassemia is diagnosed by hemoglobin electrophoresis which shows either HbF or HbA2. A normal RDW is seen in thalassemia.

Sickle cell anemia/trait shows sickled erythrocytes in the peripheral smear in addition to the microcytic hypochromic picture. It is confirmed by Hb electrophoresis and sickling phenomenon.

- *Reticulocyte count*: Normal to a slight increase (2–5%) in the early stages and low later on. An increase is seen in treatment.
- *Bone marrow*:
    - Cellularity—increased (erythroid progenitors)
    - M:E ratio—4:1
    - Erythropoiesis—polychromatic normoblasts are predominant, micronormoblastic **(Fig. 2)**
    - Cytoplasm is decreased and stains irregularly.
    - Cytoplasmic maturation lags behind the condensation of nuclear chromatin
    - Perls stain—the disappearance of iron from macrophages

Bone marrow staining for iron on the aspirated bone marrow particles gives a good idea as to the presence of iron in the marrow. A minimum of seven particles must be examined to establish the absence of stainable iron and to conclude that iron stores are reduced, normal, or increased. A special stain for iron called *Perl's Prussian blue reaction* shows markedly reduced or the absence of

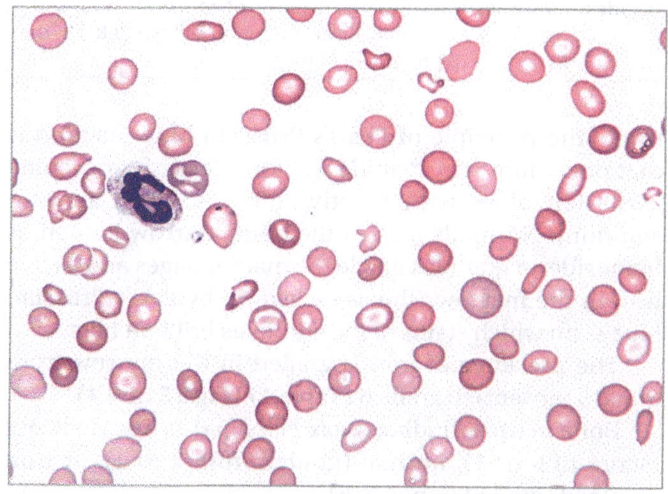

FIG. 1: Peripheral smear in iron deficiency anemia—shows microcytes (anisocytosis), pencil-shaped cells, and pessary cells (poikylocytosis).

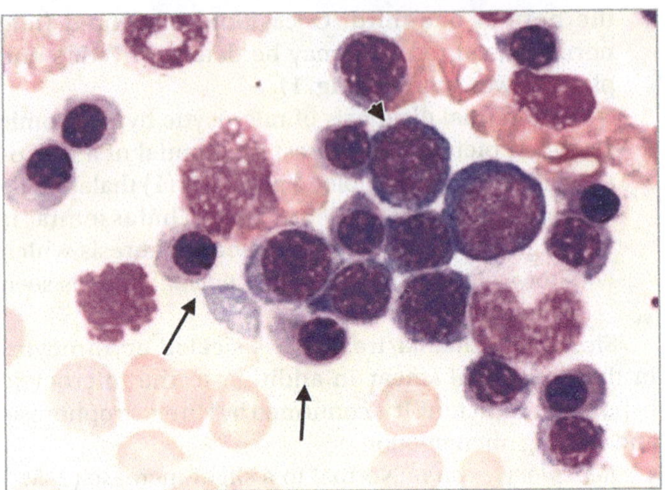

FIG. 2: Microerythroblasts in bone marrow aspiration of iron deficiency anemia (IDA) (blue arrows).

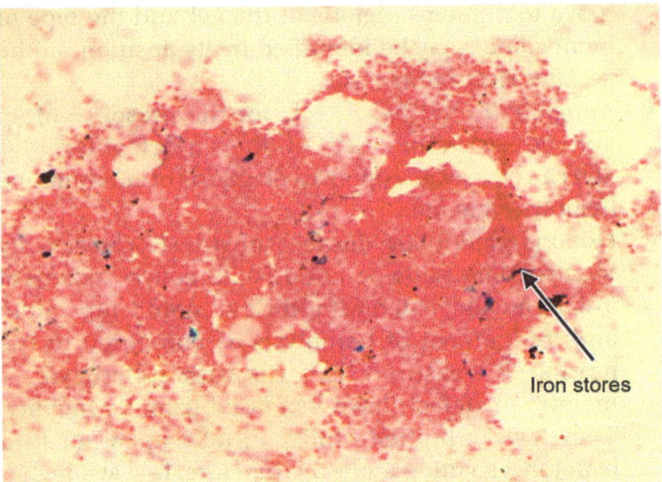

FIG. 3: Dark blue color indicating the presence of iron (Gale's grade 3). Perl's with hematoxylin and eosin (H&E) ×100.

TABLE 1: Gale's grading system iron in the bone marrow.

Grade 0	None	No visible iron under high power magnification (×1,000)
Grade 1	Very slight	Small iron particles just visible in a few reticulum cells under high power magnification (×1,000)
Grade 2	Slight	Small, sparsely distributed iron particles just visible under low power magnification (×100)
Grade 3	Moderate	Numerous small iron particles present in reticulum cells throughout the marrow fragment (×100)
Grade 4	Moderate	Larger iron particles throughout the fragment with a tendency
	Heavy	To aggregate into clumps (×100)
Grade 5	Heavy	Dense, large clumps of iron throughout the fragment (×100)
Grade 6	Very heavy	Very large deposits of iron, both intra- and extracellular, obscuring cellular detail in the fragment (×100)

iron. [The principle of Pearl's Prussian blue reaction is that potassium ferrocyanide will form ferric ferrocyanide (Prussian blue) with reactive ferric salts in an acid solution]. Normally iron in the bone marrow is seen as hemosiderin granules inside the macrophages and as free iron in the marrow. This is picked up by Perl's Prussian blue stain which stains hemosiderin as brilliant blue.

The presence of iron is graded in the marrow from grade 0 (absent) to grade 6 **(Table 1) (Figs. 3 and 4)**.

Bone marrow findings were classified as iron deficient (score of 0 or 1), normal (graded from 2 to 3), or iron overload (graded from 4 to 6).

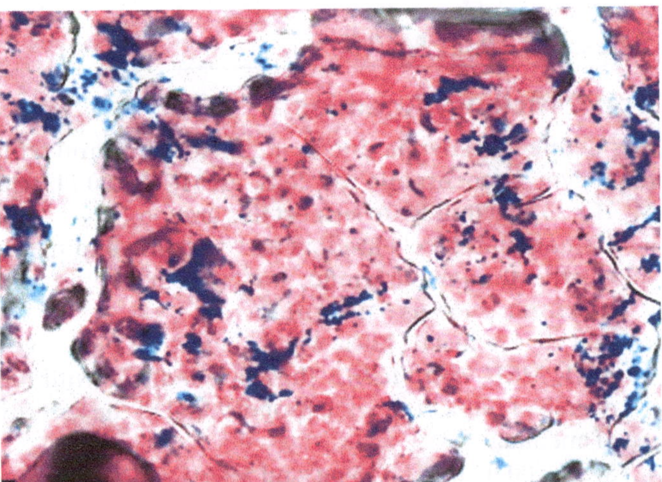

FIG. 4: Bone marrow iron Gales grade 4. Perl's stain ×400.

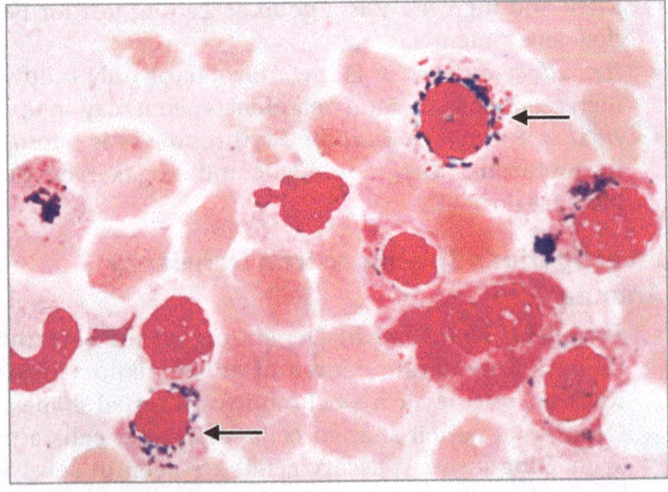

FIG. 5: Sideroblasts in bone marrow.

Perl's reaction is also useful in picking up sideroblasts in sideroblastic anemia **(Fig. 5)**.

Biochemical Findings

- *Serum iron*: Normal values are 50–150 μg/L; values drop to about 10–15 μg/L.
- *Serum ferritin*: It measures the stored form of iron. Serum ferritin levels are low. Estimation of serum ferritin is a reflection of storage iron. Normal levels of serum ferritin vary between 15 and 300 μg/L. There is a direct correlation between the amount of storage iron and serum ferritin. In IDA < 12 μg/L (normal 15–300 μg/L) values below 12 μg/L strongly indicate a lack of storage of Fe. It is a sensitive and specific test for Fe deficiency. It should be known that serum ferritin is also an acute phase reactant and a nonspecific increase occurs in inflammation, neoplastic disorders, and liver disease. In the presence of these, it should not be relied on as it may give normal values despite Fe depletion.
- *Total iron-binding capacity (TIBC)*: TIBC and transferrin is a measure of the blood's ability to bind to iron and transport it around the body. When iron stores are low, transferrin levels increase, while transferrin is low when there is too much iron. Usually about one-third of the transferrin is being used to transport iron. Normal is about 250–340 μm/dL; it goes up in Fe deficiency anemia to more than about 350–450 μg/dL.
- *Unsaturated iron-binding capacity (UIBC):* The UIBC is calculated by subtracting the serum iron from the TIBC.
- *Transferrin saturation*: This is determined by the amount of iron that is bound to transferrin circulating in the blood. The average normal is 30% (range 20–55%) saturation. Transferrin saturation is measured as a percentage, which is the ratio of serum iron and TIBC. Transferrin saturation is a more useful indicator of iron status in the body than just iron or TIBC alone. In iron deficiency, the iron level is low, but the TIBC is increased, thus transferrin saturation in iron deficiency becomes very low, <15%; (it is increased in hemochromatosis).

$$\text{Transferrin saturation} = \frac{\text{Serum Fe} \times 100}{\text{TIBC}}$$

- *Serum transferrin receptor assay*: The test is a measure of increased RBC production, and these receptors are released by the erythroid precursors into blood, and levels are increased in Fe deficiency anemia (normal values 4–8 μg/L).
- *Free erythrocyte protoporphyrin (FEP):* FEP is a combination of protoporphyrin with iron to form heme occurs in the mitochondria of erythroid precursors. This combination fails to occur in IDA and the level of FEP increases.
    - Treatment: Most anemias respond to iron supplements to restore iron deficiency in the body. The most commonly prescribed supplement is ferrous sulfate, taken orally (by mouth) two or three times a day, and treatment is monitored by the reticulocyte count done a week or 10 days after starting of therapy. Fe supplements should be given up to 5–6 months after the Hb values are normalized in order to replenish the iron stores.

Sideroblastic Anemias

Sideroblastic anemia is a type of anemia characterized by an impaired ability of the bone marrow to produce normal RBCs. In this condition, though adequate is present it is inadequately used to make hemoglobin. As a result, iron accumulates in the RBCs, giving a ringed appearance to the nucleus (ringed sideroblast).

Causes of sideroblastic anemia can be categorized into three groups: (1) Congenital sideroblastic anemia, (2) acquired clonal sideroblastic anemia, and (3) acquired reversible sideroblastic anemia. All of them involve dysfunctional heme synthesis. This leads to a granular deposition of iron in the mitochondria of cells that form a ring around the nucleus of the developing erythrocyte. Congenital forms often present with normocytic or microcytic anemia while acquired forms of sideroblastic anemia are often normocytic or macrocytic.

Ringed sideroblasts are seen in which anemia?
The most common form of inherited SA is known as X-linked sideroblastic anemia. It is caused by a mutation, or change, in a gene that disrupts normal hemoglobin production. Ringed sideroblasts on a bone marrow biopsy are pathognomic. Serum iron, ferritin, and transferrin are typically increased.

Macrocytic Anemias

Investigations

- *Hemoglobin values* are in the range of 5–10 g/dL
- *Hematocrit*: Decreased
- *Red cell indices*:
    - MCV is characteristically increased to >100 fL
    - MCHC remains normal as the hemoglobin content in the red cell is proportionately increased
    - MCH is increased
- *Peripheral smear:* The majority of cells are macrocytes and oval in shape (macroovalocytes; whereas, nonmegaloblastic macrocytes are more round in

shape). Macrocytes are larger in size, thickness, and volume. Because they are thick, the central pallor of normal RBCs is not visible. Anisopoikilocytosis is seen. Also seen is evidence of dyserythropoiesis such as basophilic stippling [blue-black cytoplasmic inclusions representing ribosomal ribonucleic acid (rRNA)], Cabot rings (nonhemoglobin iron); Howell-Jolly bodies (nuclear remnants). The WBCs are decreased (leukopenia) and show characteristic hypersegmented neutrophils with 5-6 nuclear lobes. Platelets are reduced.

- *Reticulocyte count*: It is normal or low.
- *Bone marrow*: It is hypercellular due to proliferating erythroid precursors. Erythropoiesis is of the megaloblastic type. These are large abnormal counterparts of normoblasts and they have open, stippled, and lacy chromatin basophilic, polychromatic, and orthochromatic megaloblasts. They are larger than erythroblasts, with an increase in both nuclear and cytoplasmic size at every stage of development. Myeloid precursors are decreased and the M:E ratio is altered. The characteristic feature is the presence of large, atypical granulocytes which are seen at all stages, particularly at the metamyelocyte stage. Megakaryocytes are normal or increased in number and may have bizarre multilobate nuclei.

Vitamin B_{12} Deficiency Confirmation

In addition to the features outlined above, the diagnosis is confirmed by:

- Serum vitamin B_{12} levels are decreased. Done by radioisotope technique or microbiologic assay. Normal levels are 160–900 ng/L. In B_{12} deficiency they range from 5 to 100 ng/L.
- Serum methyl malonic acid levels are increased. In vitamin B_{12} deficiency methyl malonyl CoA is not converted to succinyl malonyl CoA and therefore accumulates and is excreted in the urine as methylmalonic acid.
- Urinary excretion of methylmalonic acid is increased.
- *Schilling's test for vitamin B_{12} absorption*: Radioactive vitamin B_{12} (cyanocobalamin) is used to assess the status of intrinsic factor (IF) and vitamin B_{12} and helps to identify megaloblastic anemia due to intrinsic factor deficiency (pernicious anemia) from other causes of vitamin B_{12} deficiency. It is diagnostic of pernicious anemia.
    - Procedure: An oral dose of 1 µg radioactive vitamin B_{12} is administered to a fasting person followed 2 hours later by a large 1,000 µg parenteral injection of unlabeled B_{12}. This injection flushes out about one-third of the absorbed radioactive B_{12} into the urine in the next 24 hours. Normal persons excrete about 10% of the 1 µg dose in their urine. Patients with pernicious anemia excrete < 5%.

Other tests for intrinsic factor insufficiency: Anti-intrinsic factor (anti-IF) antibody is a type of anti-IF antibody (specific to pernicious anemia). Serum antibodies to intrinsic factors are highly specific for pernicious anemia. (Antibodies against parietal cells are also detected in pernicious anemia but are not specific for diagnosis.)

The intrinsic factor antibody can reduce or stop intrinsic factor production. The intrinsic factor antibody prevents the intrinsic factor from binding to cobalamin or prevents cells from absorbing the IF-complex with the cobalamin (Cbl) complex.

Chromosome 11 location: It controls gene expression for intrinsic factor synthesis. If both chromosome alleles of this *gastric intrinsic factor (GIF)* gene are damaged, less, or no intrinsic factor is produced.

There are two types of intrinsic factor antibody tests that can be performed:

- Type 1 intrinsic factor blocking antibody
- Type 2 intrinsic factor blocking antibody (also called precipitating antibody type 2)

B_{12} is prevented from binding to intrinsic factors in the ileum by a type 1 intrinsic factor-blocking antibody. This type of IF deficiency is responsible for the majority of cases of pernicious anemia.

Folic acid deficiency confirmation: It has all the features of megaloblastic anemia and is diagnosed by the following tests:

- *Serum folic acid levels*: They are decreased. They are done by the radioisotope method and microbiologic assay method.
- *Formiminoglutamic acid (FIGLu) test (in urine)*: Formiminoglutamate is an intermediary product in the conversion of histidine to glutamate and is excessively excreted. Normally FIGLu combines with tetrahydrofolate to form glutamate, this reaction does not occur in folic acid deficiency.
- *Serum homocysteine levels*: They are increased in folic acid deficiency.

Applied aspects

Treatment: Vitamin B_{12} administration results in (1) reversal of erythropoiesis from megaloblastic to normoblastic and peripheral smear reverts to normal (2) healing of glossitis, and (3) some improvement of neurological symptoms.

Folic acid administration: (1) Reversal of megaloblastic erythropoiesis to normal, (2) improvement in anemia to a large extent, (3) glossitis (due to vitamin B_{12} deficiency) may improve initially but recurs after some time, and (4) neurological symptoms worsen and therefore it is dangerous to give folic acid in vitamin B_{12} deficiency. Both B_{12} and folic acid may be administered together as the former protects the spinal cord from damage.

Nonmegaloblastic Macrocytic Anemias

In some diseases, macrocytic anemia occurs with a normoblastic bone marrow. These are called *macrocytic anemia* in which the MCV is increased. MCV in excess of 100 fL is abnormal. So macrocytic anemias can be classified into megaloblastic macrocytic anemias and normoblastic macrocytic anemias. These differ in etiology, prognosis, and response to treatment.

The normoblastic macrocytic anemias usually occur in the following conditions:
- Hemolytic anemias
- Posthemorrhagic anemias
- Alcoholism
- Adult leukemias
- Liver disease
- Aplastic anemias
- Sideroblastic anemias
- Drug therapy
- Hypothyroidism scurvy

These conditions usually are associated with a normocytic blood picture but rarely with a macrocytic blood picture. These anemias are not cured by the administration of either vitamin B_{12} or folic acid. The specific disorder has to be corrected in order to correct this anemia.

Macrocytic anemia is either due to the presence of more number of reticulocytes or in the marrow of such cases nucleated macronormoblastic maturation occurs. This may be as a result of an increase in the rate of erythropoiesis as occurs in macrocytosis of hemolytic and posthemorrhagic anemias which are most commonly associated with macrocytes; or due to an abnormality of marrow function as in aplastic anemia, sideroblastic anemia, leukemia, and liver disease.

CHAPTER 6

Special Tests for Hemolytic Anemias

GENERAL FEATURES OF HEMOLYSIS/ INVESTIGATIONS IN A CASE OF HEMOLYTIC ANEMIA

- *Complete blood counts*: This helps to determine the red blood cell (RBC) count, size, and hematocrit levels.
- *Peripheral blood smear*: This is done to study the morphology of RBCs and picks up spherocytes, stomatocytes, Heinz bodies, etc., indicating evidence of hemolysis.
- *Reticulocyte count*: This increases in hemolytic anemias; and is used to check for erythropoiesis and see whether the bone marrow compensates for the premature destruction of red cells
- *Serum bilirubin*: High unconjugated serum bilirubin levels can indicate hemolysis.
- *Lactic dehydrogenase (LDH)*: High serum LDH also indicates RBCs are undergoing hemolysis.
- *Serum haptoglobin*: This protein binds to hemoglobin (Hb) when RBCs die. When too much Hb is in the circulation due to hemolysis, haptoglobin levels drop.
- *Coombs test*: This helps identify serum antibodies that may be responsible for immune hemolytic anemias.
- *Hb electrophoresis*: This identifies the abnormal Hb which may undergo premature hemolysis.
- A rapid onset of anemia or significant hyperbilirubinemia in the newborn should prompt consideration of the presence of hemolytic disease in the newborn.

OSMOTIC FRAGILITY TEST

- To test osmotic fragility, RBCs are added to solutions with different salt concentrations. Normal blood cells are better able to remain intact at low salt solutions than the more fragile blood cells of spherocytosis.
- If the RBCs are more fragile than normal, the test is considered positive.
- Entire curve may be "shifted to the right," **(Fig. 1)**, or most of it may be within the normal range but with a "tail" of fragile cells. The curve within the normal range is seen only in 10–20% of cases.
- *Principle*: The osmotic fragility of freshly taken red cells reflects their ability to take up a certain amount of water before lysing. This is determined by their volume-to-surface area ratio. The ability of the normal red cell to withstand hypotonicity results from its biconcave shape, which allows the cell to increase its volume by about 70% before the surface membrane is stretched; once this limit is reached lysis occurs. Spherocytes have an increased volume-to-surface area ratio; their ability to take in water before stretching the surface membrane is thus more limited than normal,

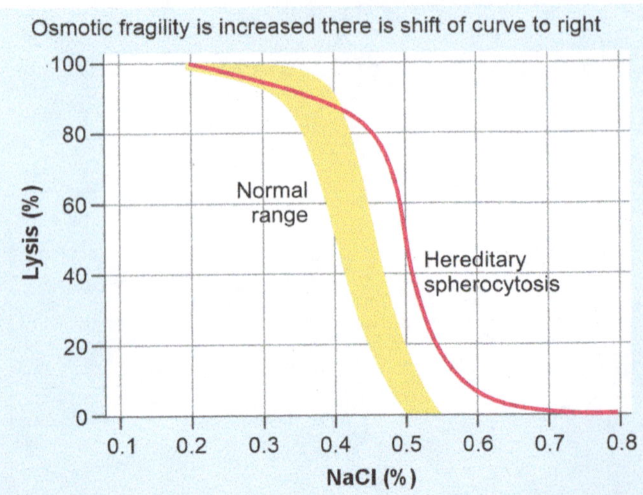

FIG. 1: After incubation for 24 hours, abnormalities are usually more marked, abnormality usually correlates with the severity of the disease.

and they are therefore particularly susceptible to osmotic lysis. The increase in osmotic fragility is a property of the spheroidal shape of the cell and is independent of the cause of the spherocytosis.

- *Procedure*:
  - In preparing hypotonic solutions for use, it is convenient to make first a 10 g/L solution from the 100 g/L NaCl stock solution by dilution with water.
  - Dilutions equivalent to 9.0, 7.5, 6.5, 6.0, 5.5, 5.0, 4.0, 3.5, 3.0, 2.0, and 1.0 g/L are convenient concentrations. (intermediate concentrations such as 4.75 and 5.25 g/L are useful in critical work and an additional 12.0 g/L dilution should be used for incubated samples). It is convenient to make up 50 mL of each dilution. The solutions should be kept at 4°C.
  - Heparinized venous blood or defibrinated blood is used; oxalated or citrated blood is not suitable because of the additional salts added to it.
  - The test should be carried out within 2 hours of the collection with blood kept at room temperature or within 6 hours if the blood has been kept at 4°C.
  - Deliver 5.0 mL of each of the 11 saline solutions into 12 × 75 mm test tubes. Add 5.0 mL of water to the 12th tube.
  - To each tube add 50 µL of well-mixed blood and invert the tubes several times, avoiding foam, so as to mix.
  - Leave for 30 minutes at room temperature.
  - Mix again and then centrifuge for 5 minutes at 1,200 g.
  - Remove the supernatants and estimate the amount of lysis in each using a spectrometer at a wavelength setting of 540 nm or a photoelectric colorimeter provided with a yellow-green (e.g., Ilford 625) filter.
  - Plot a graph with NaCl concentration on the X-axis and the percentage of lysis on the Y-axis **(Fig. 1)**. The hemolytic curve is seen to shift to the right of the normal.

COOMB'S TEST

Coomb's test is performed to detect *incomplete antibodies* on red cell surfaces [direct Coombs' test (DCT)] or antibodies in the sera of patients (indirect test). This has a major application and indications in autoimmune hemolytic anemia (AIHA), in Rh incompatibility, and also in transfusion medicine.

- *Complete antibody*: This (such as anti-A) appears to react with two cells at the same time clumping them together (agglutinating them). This can be identified in the microscope (and by a slide test).
- *Incomplete antibodies*: These [such as anti-Rh (D)] appear to be able to react with only one cell at a time. They coat the cell but have no way of reacting simultaneously with a second cell. The antigen-antibody reaction has occurred, but we cannot tell as we cannot see this under the microscope. The cells are coated with antibodies but since they do not clump we cannot see the reaction. *The Coomb's test detects these incomplete antibodies.*
- *Coomb's serum also called antihuman globulin reagent*: This is prepared by injecting human serum into rabbits. The rabbits make antibodies against human globulin antibodies, i.e., against all human antibodies. A positive direct antiglobulin test (DAT) confirms the presence of immunoglobulins [most often of the immunoglobulin G (IgG) class, sometimes immunoglobulin M (IgM) and immunoglobulin A (IgA) and/or complement usually C3d] attached to erythrocytes which are globulins.

Direct Coomb's Test (also called Direct Antiglobulin Test)

Tests incomplete antibodies coated on the red cell surface **(Fig. 2)**.

Method

Wash the cells to be tested (fetal cells in Rh incompatibility or patient's cells in transfusion cases) three times in saline to remove any trace of serum and then make a 5% suspension of the cells in saline. Incubate with Coomb's serum at 37° for 10 minutes. Centrifuge slowly for 1 minute. Examine for agglutination both macroscopically and microscopically.

Applications

- AIHA, to detect coated antibodies on red cells
- Hemolytic transfusions (patient's cells in transfusion)
- Rh incompatibility (fetal cells coated with antibodies)

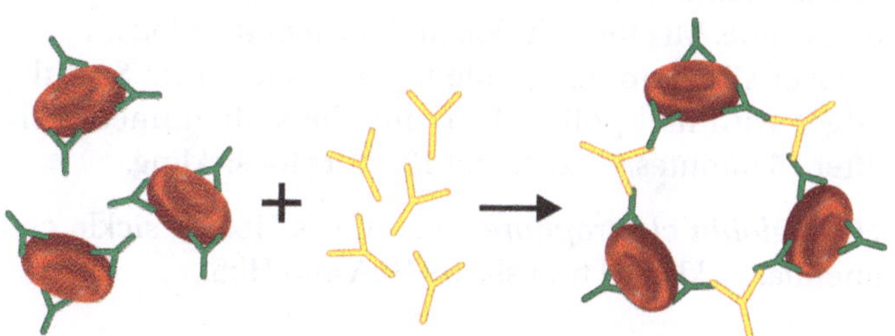

FIG. 2: Direct antiglobulin test, demonstrating the presence of autoantibodies (shown here) or complement on the surface of the red blood cell.

Indirect Coomb's Test

This is done on serum. This detects the presence of Rh antibodies in Rh-negative persons who have been exposed to Rh (D) antigen and thus may have become sensitized. It is also used in investigations of other types of hemolytic anemia and transfusions.

Method

Take control O +ve cells and wash them three times in saline. Make a 5% suspension. Test serum is taken in a tube. Add four drops of 5% saline suspension of the O cells to the tube. Incubate for one hour at 37% centigrade. (If incomplete antibodies are present, they will coat the O cell surface). Wash cells three times in saline. Add one drop of Coomb's serum (antihuman globulin reagent). Stand at room temperature for 10 minutes and then centrifuge slowly for 1 minute. Examine for agglutination both macroscopically and microscopically.

Applications

- Mother's serum in Rh incompatibility
- Coomb's cross-matching to detect incomplete antibodies in sera.
- Hemolytic transfusion reactions
- Detection of atypical antibodies, such as Kell, Duffy, Kidd, and Bombay blood group.

SICKLING PHENOMENON

It has applications in hemoglobinopathies, such as sickle cell anemia and trait. The time taken for sickling to develop depends on the amount of hemoglobin; in sickle cell disease, the sickling develops within half an hour due to the presence of HbS while in a trait it is generally demonstrated within 4 hours.

Method

A drop of 2% sodium metabisulphite solution is taken on two separate slides one marked test and the other control. Add less than a drop of the patient's blood to the first slide and the same quantity of normal blood (as control) to the other slide. Mix the solution and the blood added and put a cover slip onto each slide to cover the mixer. Seal the edges with nail polish. Examine the slide immediately after 15 minutes, ½, 2, 4, and 12 hours for sickling.

Hemoglobin electrophoresis: It shows HbS in sickle cell anemia. Sickle cell trait shows HbA and HbS.

TYPES OF HEMOGLOBIN

In the newborn, fetal hemoglobin (HbF) is about 60–80% and reduces to 1–2% by the end of year 1.

In adults 95–98% of the Hb is adult type HbA. HbA2 is 2–3%.

Fetal hemoglobin level is increased in hemoglobinopathies, such as thalassemia. Hb electrophoresis demonstrates bands of both HbA and HbF in beta-thalassemia (β+/β+ or β+/β0). The Hb composition is 92–95% HbA, >3.8% HbA2, and variable amounts of HbF amounting to 0.5–4%.

In β0 thalassemia, since no beta chains are formed there is no HbA. The major Hb is HbF with normal or low HbA2.

HEMOGLOBIN ELECTROPHORESIS

Principle

The process of electrophoresis passes an electrical current through the Hb in the blood sample. This causes the different types of Hb to separate into different bands. The blood sample is then compared to a control healthy sample to determine which types of Hb are present.

CELLULOSE ACETATE ELECTROPHORESIS

The electrophoresis on cellulose acetate membrane is most widely used because of its simplicity and is without the use of any sophisticated instrument other than the electrophoresis apparatus and the cellulose acetate strip.

Electrophoresis is typically performed at pH 8.6 using cellulose acetate as the support medium. At this pH, the overall Hb molecule is negatively charged and when placed in an electric field, will move toward the positive terminal (anode). This procedure is based on the fact that if an amino acid substitution alters the overall charge of the molecule, then the mobility of the variant Hb will be different from that of HbA.

Procedure

- The cellulose acetate membrane strip is soaked in a mixture of buffer A and buffer B together with saponin (0–1%). This is most easily prepared by adding 1 mL of 10% saponin to 100 mL of a 50–50 mixture of buffer A and buffer B.
- The strip is blotted dry and applied to the bridge of the tank. A thin line of whole blood (or even hemolysate in which case saponin is not needed) is applied at the midpoint (between the anode and cathode) of the strip. (Blood anticoagulated with EDTA is taken.) The sample is best applied with an artist's fine camel hair brush (for good results only a trace of blood is needed).
- Because the cellulose acetate membrane should not be allowed to come into direct contact with the buffer, two

filter paper wicks (e.g., 20 × 10 cm) are used to maintain electrical contact between the membrane and the tank. The wicks are immersed in buffer solution.

- Bridge gaps of 5–6 cm are adequate.
- The apparatus is covered, and the samples are allowed to soak into the cellulose acetate membrane strip.
- After 3–5 minutes the current is switched on (9–14 mA at 200 V).
- The Hb bands move to the anode. Half an hour is enough to distinguish the presence of abnormal bands, and the run may be continued for up to 2 hours.
- At the end of the separation, remove the membrane and either dry it in an oven at 80–100°C or fix it in a fixing bath accordingly. The Hb bands are clearly seen without staining. Alternatively staining by Ponceau S for 5 minutes may be done.

(*Preparing hemolysate*: Dilute 20 μL of the packed red cells of the sample with 150 μL of the hemolyzing reagent. Mix gently and leave for at least 5 minutes. If purified hemolysates are used, dilute 40 μL of 100 g/L hemolysate with 150 μL of lysing reagent.)

Buffer A (anode):

- Tris (hydroxymethyl-aminomethane) 25.2 g
- EDTA (ethylene diamine tetra-acetic acid) 2.5 g
- Boric acid 1.9 g
- Water to 1,000 mL

Buffer B (cathode):

- Sodium diethyl barbiturate 5.15 g
- Diethyl barbituric acid 0.92 g
- Water to 1,000 mL

Interpretation and Comments

Hemoglobin S moves faster than HbA and [**Fig. 3** depicting mobilities of Hb in cord blood **(Fig. 3A)**, thalassemia **(Fig. 3B)**, and sickle cell trait and sickle cell disease **(Fig. 3C)**] the mobility of HbF is in between the two. HbA2 level is estimated by elution of the separated bands rather than scanning.

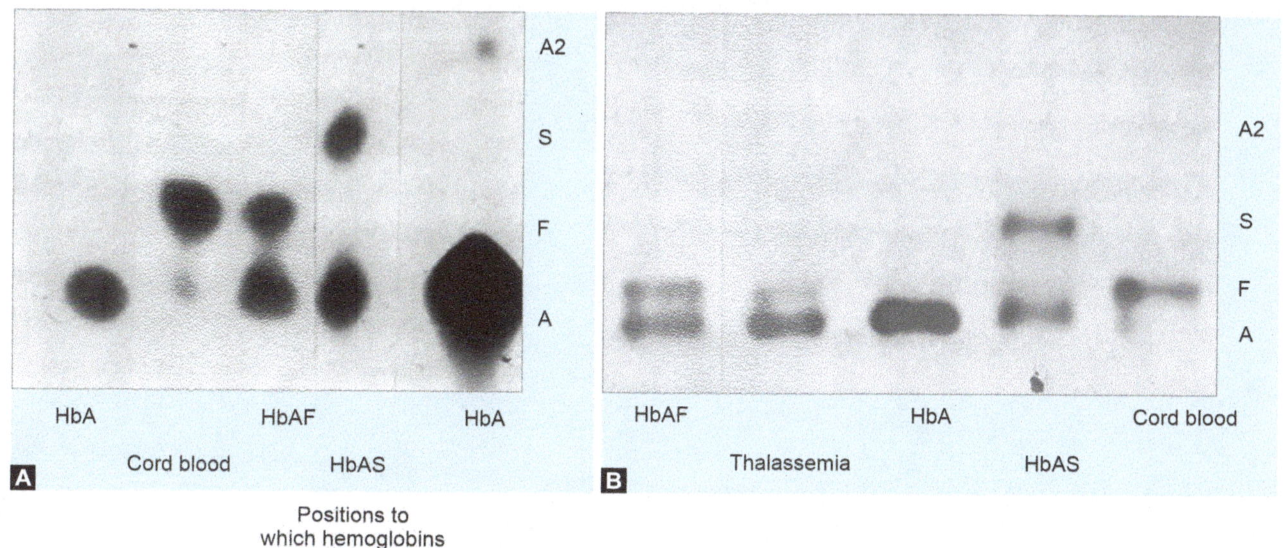

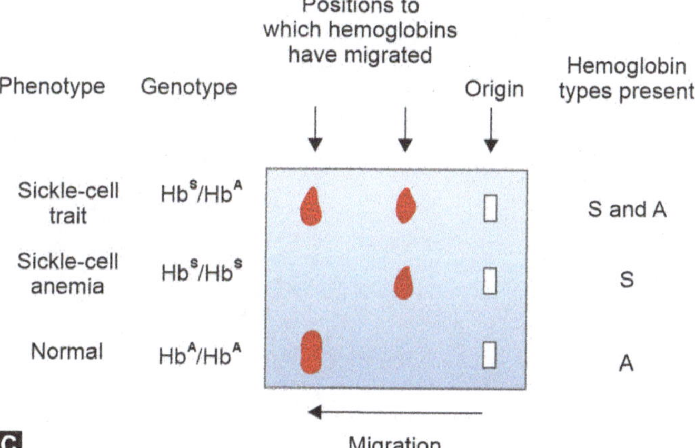

FIGS. 3A TO C: (A) Mobilities of hemoglobin in cord blood; (B) Thalassemia; and (C) Sickle cell trait and sickle cell disease.
Source: J Kohn. Separation of haemoglobin on cellulose acetate. Biology, Medicine. Journal of Clinical Pathology, 1969.

The α thalassemias are characterized electrophoretically by the presence of the fast-moving variants, Hb Bart's (γ4) and HbH (β4), which are most obvious in neonatal samples. In hydrops fetalis owing to homozygous α0 thalassemia, Hb Bart's predominates and is found in smaller amounts in other α thalassemia syndromes in the neonatal period. Hemoglobin H may also be detected by staining for HbH inclusion bodies.

Other Methods

Other methods are more complicated and are agar gel, starch, or polyacrylamide.

HIGH PERFORMANCE LIQUID CHROMATOGRAPHY

- High-performance liquid chromatography (HPLC) is a technic that has recently been applied in the diagnosis of hemoglobinopathies and thalassemias. It has an advantage over other methods due to it is increased sensitivity, resolution, simplicity of performance, and speed.
- HPLC was formerly referred to as *high-pressure liquid chromatography* and is used to separate, identify, and quantify each component in a liquid mixture. It relies on pumps that pass through a pressurized liquid solvent containing the sample mixture, through a column filled with a solid adsorbent material. Each component in the liquid sample interacts differently with the adsorbent solid material, causing different flow rates for the different components and leading to the separation of these, as they flow out of the column.
- HPLC performed on *fresh lysates* is now the standard test for identification of thalassemia provided the facility is available.
- Samples in the form of dried blood spot(s) (DBS) can also be mailed to distant laboratories for the test.

CHAPTER 7

Coagulation Time and Bleeding Time

COAGULATION TIME

Coagulation of blood involves two mechanisms, i.e., (1) intrinsic and (2) extrinsic. **Figure 1** depicts a schematic representation of the same.

CAPILLARY TUBE METHOD

Clean a finger and puncture deeply so as to obtain a spontaneous free flow of blood. Allow two capillary tubes of 4 inches to fill with blood to give about 3 inches continuous column of blood. Place the tubes on the table. At the end of minutes and then at every half-minute intervals break off 1 cm length of tubing. The onset of coagulation is indicated by the development of fibrin bridging the two broken ends. The time of the appearance of fibrin threads is the coagulation time.

Normal range: 4–7 minutes

SLIDE METHOD

Place several drops of blood on a clean slide from a deep finger puncture. At 30-second intervals, draw a needle

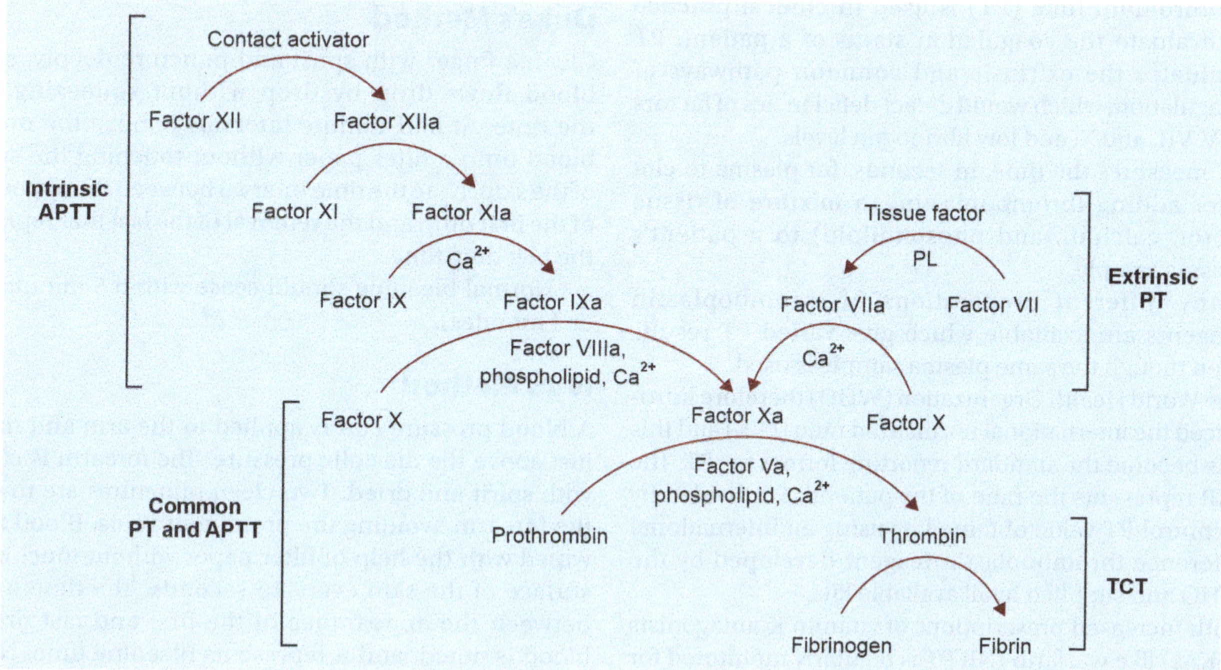

FIG. 1: Mechanism of coagulation—intrinsic and extrinsic.
(APTT: activated partial thromboplastin time; PT: prothrombin time; TCT: thrombin clot time)

through one of the drops. As soon as the needle picks up fibrin threads and drags them along, coagulation takes place. Note the time. The time interval between the placing of the drop on the slide and the formation of fibrin threads is the coagulation time. Normal time is 2–8 minutes.

LEE AND WHITE METHOD

For about 5 mL of blood is drawn into a siliconized syringe aseptically and 1 mL of blood is placed into each of three clean 13 × 100 mm test tubes previously rinsed with physiological saline and drained. The blood is allowed to flow down the sides of the test tubes after removing the needle. The tubes are kept in a water bath at 37°C. The third tube is gently tilted every 30 seconds until the blood in it clots; the second tube is then done in the same manner; last, the first tube is tilted until no flow of blood is observed on tilting. Coagulation time is recorded as the time interval between the appearance of blood in the syringe and the time at which blood no longer flows on the complete inversion of the last tube.

Normal values 5–11 minutes (6–9 minutes usually).

The coagulation time is increased in the following conditions:

- Hemophilia
- Christmas disease
- Presence of circulating inhibitors

PROTHROMBIN TIME

- Prothrombin time (PT) is used in clinical practice to evaluate the coagulation status of a patient. PT evaluates the extrinsic and common pathways of coagulation, which would detect deficiencies of factors II, V, VII, and X, and low fibrinogen levels.
- PT measures the time, in seconds, for plasma to clot after adding thromboplastin, (a mixture of tissue factor, calcium, and phospholipid) to a patient's plasma sample.
- Many different preparations of thromboplastin reagents are available which give varied PT results even though the same plasma sample is used.
- The World Health Organization (WHO) therefore introduced the international normalized ratio (INR) and this has become the standard reporting format for PT. The INR represents the ratio of the patient's PT divided by a control PT value obtained by using an international reference thromboplastin reagent developed by the WHO and supplied in all available kits.
- With increased prescriptions of vitamin K-antagonists (VKAs) like warfarin INR PT is regularly monitored for patients.
- Coagulation tests must be performed using plasma samples and not serum as clotting factors get removed in serum preparations. Standard percutaneous phlebotomy is the recommended method used to collect venous blood samples.
- PT/INR use is typically in conjunction with activated partial thromboplastin time (aPTT), which evaluates the intrinsic and common pathways of coagulation. PT/INR and aPTT results together can help in diagnosing various hematologic disorders.

Procedure

Phlebotomists collect venous blood samples in plastic tubes with a light blue top that contains 3.2% sodium citrate. Sodium citrate serves to chelate the calcium in the blood sample and prevents the activation of the coagulation cascade. This chelation keeps the blood sample in stasis until ready to be tested. Tube filling must be within 90% of the full collection volume with a blood-to-sodium citrate ratio of 9:1. The tube is then gently inverted a few times to mix the sodium citrate solution with the blood. The tube should not be shaken to avoid hemolysis which would lead to inaccurate results. Once the blood sample is ready to be tested, calcium chloride is then added to restore the calcium required for coagulation activation. Clot formation can then be detected mechanically or optically depending on the instrumentation used.

BLEEDING TIME

Duke's Method

Clean a finger with spirit and puncture deeply, so that blood flows drop by drop without squeezing. Note the time. At half-minute intervals remove the drops of blood onto a filter paper without touching the surface of the skin. Note the time interval between the appearance of the first drop and the removal of the last that represents the bleeding time.

Normal bleeding should cease within 5 minutes (1–3 or 4 minutes).

Ivy's Method

A blood pressure cuff is applied to the arm and inflated just above the diastolic pressure. The forearm is cleaned with spirit and dried. Two clean punctures are made on the forearm avoiding the prominent veins. Blood flow is wiped with the help of filter paper without touching the surface of the skin every 15 seconds. The time interval between the appearance of the first and last drops of blood is noted, and it represents bleeding time. Normal 3–5 minutes.

CHAPTER 8

Blood Collection and Anticoagulants

INTRODUCTION

The blood should preferably be collected early in the morning before the patient has eaten and stored in a chemically clean and sterile container in order to avoid bacterial contamination.

CAPILLARY BLOOD

It is collected by pricking the fingertip or ear lobe in adults and the heel or great toe in children. The preferred site in an adult is the distal digit of the third or fourth finger on its palmar surface. Sterile needles, disposable lancets, spring lancets, or capillary glass prickers can be used for pricking. The part should be sterilized with spirit and the surrounding area gently pressed to produce venostasis. A free-flowing, large drop of blood should be obtained.

The capillary blood is used for the following tests:

- Estimation of Hb%, red blood cell (RBC), white blood cell (WBC), and platelet counts
- Preparation of peripheral smears
- Blood grouping
- Estimation of blood glucose level by Somogyi's micromethod

VENOUS BLOOD

This is collected by using a dry, sterile syringe and needle. Antecubital vein in adults and dorsal veins of the hand in children are the usual sites of venepuncture. Blood should be drawn by a neat, clean puncture in order to minimize hemolysis. Blood should be stored in a chemically clean container with or without the anticoagulant as the case may be.

Venous blood is necessary for the following tests:

- Estimation of erythrocyte sedimentation rate (ESR), packed cell volume (PCV), etc.
- Estimation of blood constituents, such as sugar and urea
- Bacteriological and serological examinations
- Blood grouping and cross-matching

ARTERIAL BLOOD

Sometimes it may be impossible to collect blood from veins. In such cases, arterial puncture can be attempted. The brachial artery and radial artery are the usual sites. Sometimes arterial blood gives positive culture results when venous blood is negative as in the case of subacute bacterial endocarditis.

ANTICOAGULANTS

The blood has to be kept in a fluid state for many of the hematological and chemical examinations. In order to achieve this, anticoagulants have to be added in appropriate proportions. Various anticoagulants commonly used are discussed further.

Oxalates

These salts unite with the calcium in the blood to form insoluble compounds and thereby deplete the blood of its calcium which is necessary for the coagulation of blood.

- *Dried potassium oxalate*: 2 mg/mL of blood
    - Disadvantages—causes shrinkage and destruction of cells.
- *Lithium oxalate*: Used in the case of estimation of blood constituents since it does not introduce an

element that may be tested for, in the blood. About 2 mg of dried salt is sufficient for 1 mL of blood.

- *Double oxalate or Wintrobe's salt*: Combination of ammonium and potassium oxalates (1.2 and 8 g of these salts respectively and distilled water added to 100 mL) 1 mL of this solution dried in a container at 80°C. is sufficient for 10 mL of blood.
    - Advantages: Ammonium oxalate causes swelling of the cells whereas potassium oxalate shrinks. The action of both these salts is counterbalanced and thereby the cells retain their original shape and size.
    - Uses: Used in the estimation of ESR by Wintrobe's method and PCV.
- *Saturated potassium oxalate*: It is a 20% solution of potassium oxalate. One drop of the supernatant solution is sufficient for 10 mL of blood. It mixes more readily with blood than dry salt.

Citrates

- *Sodium citrate*: One part of a 3.8% solution of the salt and nine parts of blood mixed for coagulation studies. Used in blood transfusion as the salt is relatively nontoxic and the salt is excreted by the kidneys or utilized by the body 3.8% solution ratio with blood used in ESR (Westergren method) (1:4).
- *Acid citrate dextrose (ACD) solution*: Erythrocytes are better preserved in the ACD than in trisodium citrate alone.
    - Trisodium citrate 1.32 g
    - Citrate acid 0.42 g
    - Dextrose 1.40 g
    - Distilled water added to 100 mL
    - 1 mL of ACD is sufficient for 4 mL of blood. This is used in blood transfusion.

Heparin

It has an affinity for blood proteins and acts as an antithrombin and antithromboplastin. About 1 mg of dry heparin or 1,000 IU of liquid heparin suffice for 10 mL of blood. Used in hematocrit studies and blood transfusion especially exchange and rapid transfusion as in the case of thoracic surgery ESR and osmotic fragility test. It lasts for only 3 days.

Ethylene Diamine Tetra Acetate

Its disodium and dipotassium salts are used. They act as a chelating agent and thus separate the calcium ions from the blood. Used for most of the hematological and chemical tests.

VACUTAINER TUBES

A vacuum blood collection tube is a sterile glass or plastic test tube with a "colored rubber stopper" creating a vacuum seal inside of the tube, facilitating the drawing of a predetermined volume of liquid **(Table 1)**. Vacutainer tubes contain anticoagulants designed to preserve the collected specimen before analysis/testing. The color of the rubber stopper indicates the type of anticoagulant in the vial. The tubes are available with a safety-engineered stopper.

When drawing blood, the syringe which comes with the tube is designed to fit the tube and not allow any leakage of the withdrawn blood from the vein. Once the vein is entered blood is drawn into the plastic tube through vacuum suction. These tubes have an expiry date and the vacuum action too reduced over time.

BLOOD COLLECTION AND STORAGE

Single Blood Bag

- For whole blood collection **(Fig. 1)**.
- The bag contains anticoagulant citrate phosphate dextrose adenine (CPDA) solution.
- Available in capacity of 350 and 450 mL
- After collection, the blood units should be stored standing upright in baskets or lying flat on the shelf. The bags should never be packed tightly, nor should they be stored near the freezer compartment/in the door of the refrigerator.

Double Blood Bag

It is designed for the collection and separation of whole blood into two different blood components, i.e., (1) plasma and (2) red cells. This is obtained through the process of centrifugation and extraction. The primary bag contains CPDA-1 anticoagulant solution.

TABLE 1: Color coding for routine investigative purposes.

Light blue	Sodium citrate (anticoagulant)	Coagulation tests, such as PT, PTT, and TT. The tube must be filled 100%
Mint green	Lithium heparin (anticoagulant)	Plasma tube inversions prevent clotting
Lavender ("purple")	EDTA (chelator/ anticoagulant)	*Whole blood*: CBC, ESR, Coombs test, platelet antibodies, flow cytometry, blood levels of tacrolimus, and cyclosporin

(CBC: complete blood count; EDTA: ethylenediaminetetraacetic acid; ESR: erythrocyte sedimentation rate; PT: prothrombin time; PTT: partial thromboplastin time)

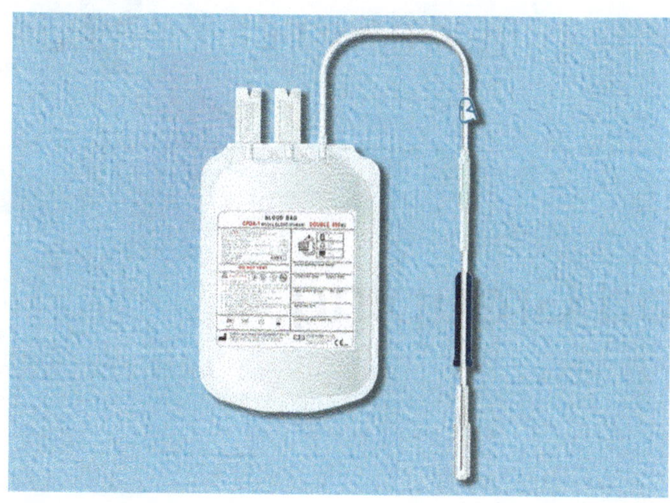

FIG. 1: Single blood bag.

Triple Blood Bag

It is designed to separate whole blood into three blood components, i.e., (1) RBCs, (2) platelets, and (3) plasma (platelet-rich) through the process of centrifugation and extraction. Triple top and bottom blood bags are used to collect and separate three different blood components: (1) Plasma, (2) red cells, and (3) buffy coat (with platelets). Each bag is composed of the following: Anticoagulant additive solution, primary bag, platelets transfer bag for 5-day platelet storage, and a donor needle gauge.

The primary bag contains citrate-phosphate-dextrose (CPD), and one satellite bag contains saline-adenine-glucose-mannitol (SAGM).

CHAPTER 9

Method of Blood Grouping

ANTIGENS

The antigens of significance are A, B, and H.

Two main antigens A and B result in four blood groups, i.e., (1) A, (2) B, (3) AB, and (4) O. These antigens are under the control of *A* and *B* genes. Expression of *A* and *B* genes appears to be dependent on gene "*H*." Most individuals are homozygous for *H* genes (*HH*).

Interaction of *H, A,* and *B* genes leads to:

- The *H* gene leads to the secretion of the basic precursor substance "H."
- H substance is partly converted under the influence of *A* and *B* genes into A/B substance, some of the H substance remains unconverted.
- Since O group individuals do not have *A/B* genes, therefore, no A/B substance is formed, and these have large amounts of H substance.
- A, B, and H antigens (A, B, and H substances) can be found in the saliva of the majority of people—secretors while the rest are nonsecretors.

A, B, and H are detected on red cells even in fetal life. However, these antigens are not fully developed at birth, and attain complete development by 1 year of age.

TABLE 1: Antigen distribution of A, B, and Bombay blood groups with respective antibodies in serum.

Blood type	Antigens present	Antibodies in serum
AB+	ABH, Rh D	None
AB–	ABH	Rh D
A+	AH, Rh D	B
A–	AH	B, Rh D
B+	BH, Rh D	A
B–	BH	A, Rh D
O+	H, Rh D	AB
O–	H	AB, Rh D
Bombay	None	ABH, Rh D

BOMBAY BLOOD GROUP

Some people do not inherit the *H* gene (genotype *HH*) and thus cannot synthesize H substance. Such people may inherit the *A* or *B* gene but cannot express it, as they are unable to produce the H substance. Such individuals are said to have Bombay phenotype or Bombay blood group (i.e., blood group Oh) (the genotype of Bombay phenotype is HH) **(Table 1)**.

The name is derived because it was first detected in persons living in Bombay, India. It has also been described in other populations. This blood group is extremely rare. There is a complete lack of *H* genes.

Their red cell type is group O; however, unlike group O individuals, Oh persons have no H antigen in addition to anti-A and anti-B. On cross-matching, all units are incompatible, therefore, Bombay group persons should be transfused only with Oh blood.

- *Blood group*: O
- *Cross-matching*: Serum incompatible with O cells
- Red cells yield negative reactions with anti-H lectin
- *Method*: Slide and tube method.

SLIDE TECHNIQUE FOR BLOOD GROUPING

- Take a slide and mark it with anti-A, anti-B, and anti-AB. Put one drop of anti-A, anti-B, and anti-AB sera on the marked slide.
- Add one drop of 20% washed red cell suspension to each antiserum.

- Mix each cell-serum mixture separately with applicator stick and rock the slide gently.
- Read for "agglutination" macroscopically within 5 minutes and identify the blood group as per **Figure 1**.

TUBE METHOD FOR BLOOD GROUPING

- Take three test tubes (65 × 10 mm size), labeled anti-A, anti-B, and anti-AB respectively.
- Add one drop of each of the corresponding serums to each tube, i.e., anti-A, anti-B, and anti-AB sera.
- Add one drop of 2% suspension of red cells to the three test tubes and mix the suspension by gently tapping the tubes.
- Leave the tubes at room temperature for 90 minutes or place the tubes in a water bath at 37°C for 30 minutes.
- Transfer one drop of serum-cell suspension mixture onto a glass slide, using a thin bore Pasteur pipette. Spread the cells over an area of 2 × 1 cm, using the pipette as a spreader.
- Examine the slide under a microscope for "agglutination," and interpret the result for the blood group as given in the above table.

The above method is called the "forward typing" of doing the blood group, as it is done on the cells. In order to confirm this "reverse typing" is done on the serum.

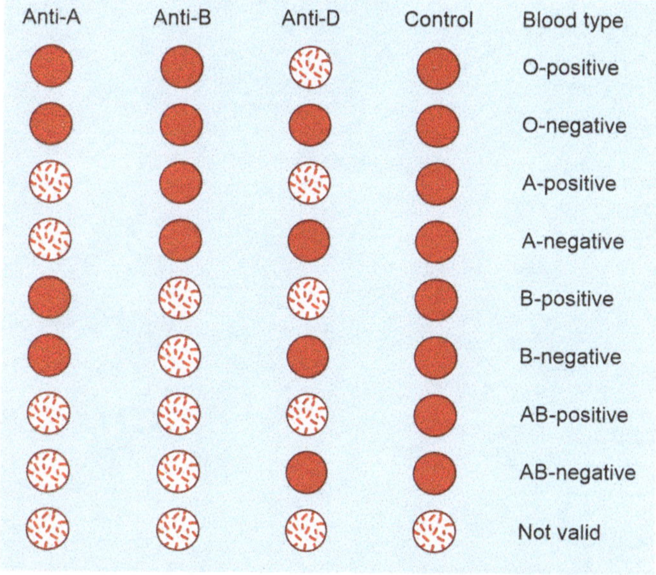

Anti-A Anti-B Anti-D Control Blood type
O-positive
O-negative
A-positive
A-negative
B-positive
B-negative
AB-positive
AB-negative
Not valid

Antibody added	Anti-A	Anti-B	Ani-AB	Result group
Agglutination	–	–	–	O
	+	–	+	A
	–	+	+	B
	+	+	+	AB

FIG. 1: Method of blood grouping in slide technique.

BIBLOGRAPHY

1. Bain BJ, Bates I, Laffan MA, Lewis M. In: Emeritus S (Ed). Dacie and Lewis Practical Haematology, 12th edition. Amsterdam: Elsevier; 2016.
2. Firkin F, Chesterman C, Penington D, Rush B. de Gruchy's Clinical Haematology in Medical Practice, 5th edition. New Jersey: Wiley-Blackwell Publications; 1991.
3. Kohn J. Separation of haemoglobins on cellulose acetate. J Clin Pathol. 1969;22(1):109-11.
4. Shariff S. Essentials of Pathology for Medical Students (As per the Competency-based Medical education Curriculum (NMC) for Indian Medical Graduates, 1st edition. CBS Publishers and Distributors Pvt. Ltd.; 2023.
5. Yang Y, Zubair M, Moosavi L. Prothrombin Time. In: StatPearls [Internet]. Treasure Island (FL): StatPearls Publishing; 2024.

PART 2

Cytology, Histopathology, and Other Techniques

CHAPTER 1

Cytopathology: An Overview

INTRODUCTION

Cytology is the study of cells and gives important insight into disease processes. When the term "cytology" is used it actually refers to "cytopathology;" both terms are used interchangeably to designate pathological changes.

Changes in the nucleus, assessed by its size, shape, and appearance of chromatin, are used to diagnose cancer and precancerous change, i.e., dysplasia which takes years to progress to cancer. George N Papanicolaou introduced exfoliative cytology as a means of detecting cancer/dysplasia in the early 20th century. His far sight in picking up dysplastic changes in exfoliated cells of the cervix led to the acceptance of Papanicolaou smear as a means for screening for cancer cervix; this has resulted in a reduction in the incidence of cervical cancer across the world.

BRANCHES OF CYTOLOGY

The principle of exfoliation of diseased cells from epithelial surfaces into body fluids (fluid cytology) is the basis for the examination of sputum, urine, and other body fluids for presence of disease and is called *"exfoliative cytology"*. Inflammations, infections, and neoplastic changes can be picked up.

The other method of study of exfoliation is *"brush cytology"*, i.e., forced exfoliation of cells from suspected diseased lesions. Endoscopy as an advanced diagnostic tool allows the visualization of and simultaneous brushing of abnormal mucosae, obtaining specimens as well as mucosal biopsy samples for pathologic evaluation.

Fine needle aspiration cytology/biopsy (FNAC/FNAB), a method of removing cells by a fine needle, is presently accepted as a simple, noninvasive diagnostic technique and a first-line diagnosis in diseases of several organ systems. Endoscopic ultrasound-FNA (EUS-FNA) has revolutionized the practice of gastrointestinal pathology and is rapidly becoming the technique of choice for sampling lesions that were previously accessible only by laparotomy and surgery. Such advances have brought pathologists to the forefront in the diagnosis by noninvasive techniques.

Fine needle aspiration cytology coupled with ancillary supportive measures, such as flow cytometry, immunohistochemistry, and molecular techniques has to a large extent replaced excision biopsy not only in the diagnosis but also staging of disease. The method is applicable to superficial as well as deep lesions with the help of imaging guidance.

ADVANCES

The branches of cytology have expanded to include *intraoperative cytology*, *imprint cytology*, and *conjunctival smears*. Such advances as various prongs of diagnostic cytology pose a challenge for the reporting cytologist.

Besides, the growing advances in automation and computerization have made it possible to analyze several samples simultaneously, thus reducing fatigue factor. Telecytology has enabled interinstitutional discussions and consultations across the globe making cytopathology an important contributor to disease management.

QUALITY CONTROL AND QUALITY ASSURANCE

The accuracy of the cytologic examination from any body site depends greatly on the quality of collection of specimens, processing and preparation, staining, and interpretation of the material. Inadequacy in any of these steps will adversely affect the quality of reporting and thereby the predictive value of a positive report. The practice of diagnostic cytology therefore needs uniformity and streamlining at all steps—in the collection and preservation of samples, training of personnel in processing procedures, staining, and competent persons for interpretation. This is quality control and quality assurance and plays an important role in the standardization and outcome of cytology results. There is a growing need for good quality control and assurance measures to be implemented. Standard internationally accepted terminology for reporting, documentation, and archiving, interinstitutional comparisons of results, correlation between cytology and histopathology and molecular techniques is the hour of the need.

RECEIPT OF SAMPLES

It is the duty of the technician/junior doctor to check that a request for performance of the cytological examination accompanies each specimen with the name of the requesting clinician, name of patient/age/sex/hospital/department/unit, and signature of the clinician. An adequate clinical history and reference biopsy number of any previous biopsies performed on the patient and the diagnosis made should be entered in the request form. The technician should also make sure that gynecology smears are delivered in coplin jars with adequate amount of fixatives; and fresh cytology samples are immediately attended to and taken for centrifugation as per the special operational procedures (SOPs) and formalities for sample receiving and fixation of the same. The technician receiving the sample should sign the request form after checking all parameters.

All specimens received should be given a laboratory accession number which runs in serial order for the type of specimen received for that particular year. The labeling depends on the practice of the laboratory, e.g., FNAC serial numbering for all fine needle aspiration samples would be FNA-01/2020 which means for the year 2020 the fine needle aspiration sample was the first sample for the year. The last sample for the year would be FNA 1800/2020 if that particular laboratory had 1,800 specimens of FNAC for that particular year. This number would hold valid for all slides prepared on this specimen including any special stain, with the name of the special stain beneath it. Most laboratories separate gynecology cytology to read as Gyn 01/2020 and other body fluids as F01/2020. A cell block preparation on any cytology sample will carry the same number as the smear.

CONCLUSION

All cytopathology laboratories receive specimens in various numbers as per the laboratory turnover. The duty of every cytologist in the laboratory is to receive these and deliver a written and typed report to the patient/clinician with accuracy and precision within a reasonable specified and acceptable time period. In order to achieve this, the pathologist has to adhere to certain criteria and norms. The objective should be to produce a quality report within a certain period of time (turnaround time) to the clinician requesting it.

CHAPTER 2

Serous Effusions

INTRODUCTION

The most important goal of effusion cytology is in the recognition or ruling out of malignancy. Effusions that are commonly sent to a laboratory for diagnostic purposes are pleural fluid, ascitic fluid, pericardial fluid, hydrocele fluid, and synovial fluid. Besides these fluids, the other body fluids are the cerebrospinal fluid (CSF) and urine.

METHODS OF SPECIMEN COLLECTION

All paracenteses are done by the clinician under aseptic precautions keeping in mind the timing of the tap (to be done in the morning hours when laboratory personnel are around) in order to get the best result; and to see that the specimen reaches the laboratory immediately after the procedure. At least 10 mL of fluid must be available for proper assessment.

- A *pleural tap or thoracentesis* is collecting the fluid accumulated in the pleural cavity. The patient is made to sit up and bend slightly forward. Under aseptic precautions a wide bore needle is inserted into the pleural space just above the rib margin in the 8th, 9th, or 10th intercostal space (at least 2 inches below the scapula tip) **(Figs. 1A and B)**.
- An *ascitic tap* or paracentesis of the abdomen is removal of fluid from the abdominal cavity. More than 200 mL of fluid collects before the ascites becomes clinically evident. With the patient lying supine the needle is usually inserted in the right iliac fossa a little lateral to the midpoint of a line drawn from the umbilicus to the anterior superior iliac spine. Ultrasound may be used to guide the location of the fluid.
- Usually in case of effusions about 150–200 mL is collected for examination at any one time. *Fluid should*

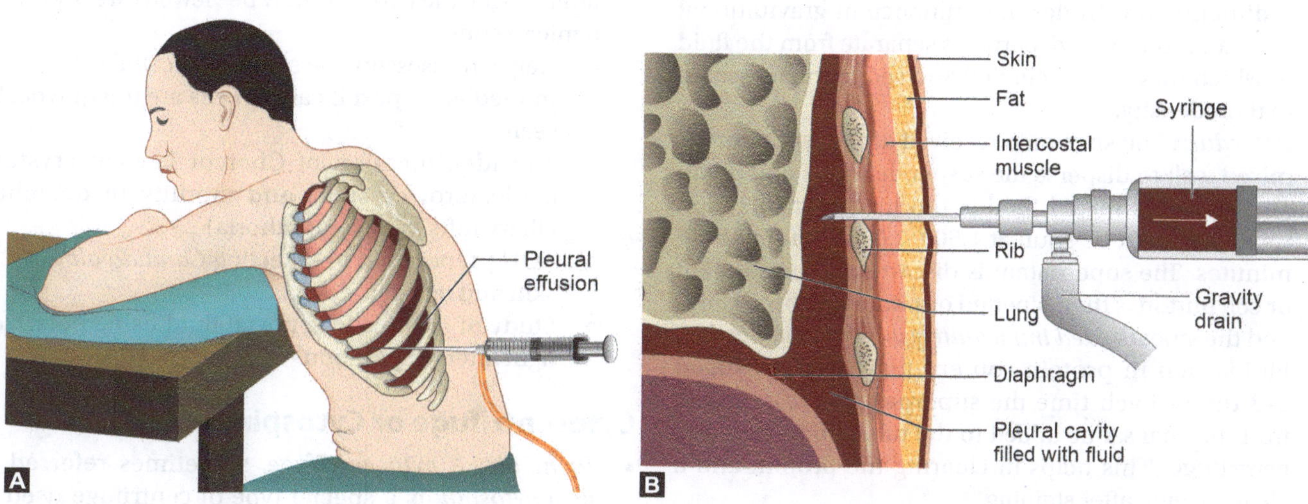

FIGS. 1A AND B: Thoracentesis with the left side showing position of patient and right side the needle tip in the pleural space.

not be taken for cytological examination from a drainage bottle wherein cell morphology is compromised due to autolysis and cells tend to sediment down and may be missed if the supernatant fluid is collected.

IMMEDIATE PROCESSING

- All laboratories should aim at processing fluids as soon as they are brought to the laboratory.
- If fresh specimens cannot be brought directly to the laboratory the specimen should be refrigerated. Pleural, peritoneal, or pericardial fluids can be preserved for 24–48 hours with refrigeration. (The protein content of these fluids acts as a culture media for survival of cells.)
- Prefixation of fluids, i.e., the addition of alcohol (the ideal fixative for fluids) or alcohol-ether mixture is not recommended as a routine practice as alcohol is a protein coagulant and interferes with staining. It may only be undertaken if the hospital is located away from the laboratory.

METHODS OF PROCESSING[1-4]

Before fluids can be taken for processing, a visual examination of all fluids should be performed by a doctor and the relevant details noted with regard to quantity, color, appearance, etc.

A variety of methods of processing fluids exist and each has its advantages and disadvantages depending upon the type of fluid that one is dealing with.

Centrifugation

It is the most popular, cost-effective, and simplistic method practiced routinely by all laboratories.

- *Principle*: Centrifugation works on the principle of sedimentation. Under the influence of gravitational force and rotor speed, particles separate from the fluid in which they are suspended and sediment according to their density.
- *Procedure*: The specimen received at the laboratory is mixed well to disperse the suspended cells and about 10 mL of this mixed fluid is put in a centrifugation tube and the tube spun at 1,500–2,000 rpm for 10–15 minutes. The supernatant is discarded; the sediment or cell button is then pipetted out, smeared onto slides and the smears *fixed immediately while wet in alcohol.*
- Fluids rich in protein content may be centrifuged 2–3 times. Each time the supernatant is discarded, fresh normal saline added to the tube, tilt to mix, and centrifuge. This helps in clearing the protein and a clear viewing after staining.
- Any excess sediment may be taken for special stains and as a paraffin block for processing. Addition of albumin flakes gives body to the cell button for smearing or cellblock preparation.
- To concentrate more cells in thin watery or serous fluid, pour off the supernatant after the first centrifugation, and add more of the sample to the same tube and recentrifuge. This procedure repeated twice or thrice collects most of the cells which may then be smeared.
- *Bloody aspirates:* Bloody aspirates show much red blood cells (RBCs) in the background obscuring morphology. Such fluids are treated with either (1) a few drops of 10% glacial acetic acid or (2) 0.1 N HCl, or (3) Carnoy's fluid each, to about 50 mL of the sample. (4) Distilled water also causes hemolysis. Newer methods, using proprietary commercial agents, are available; these not only lyse the RBCs but also fix the other cellular elements—CytoRich Red and CytoLyte solutions.
- 1 mL of this fixative is added to 25–50 mL of the sample. After letting the sample sit for few minutes, it is centrifuged and the slides prepared from the sediment.
- *Advantages*:
    - Simplicity of usage. Does not require great technical expertise.
    - Routinely practiced in all laboratories
    - Wet mounts can be prepared from sediment
- *Disadvantages*:
    - Aerosol during spinning may lead to risk of contamination and infection to the performer
    - Cell loss during pipetting of cell button
- *Wet preparation:* Besides the permanent stains, a wet preparation of this centrifuged sample may be done for a quick viewing of the sample. A drop of the sediment is taken and layered onto a slide with or without a drop of toluidine blue stain on it. Coverslip the preparation after mixing the two. This may be viewed directly under a microscope.
    - Helps in assessing the sample for cellularity
    - Immediate report if cancer cells are unequivocally seen.
    - The identification of Charcot Leyden crystals, cholesterol crystals, and motility in detached ciliary tufts (ciliocytophthoria)
    - KOH preparation in detecting *Candida albicans* in skin and other infections
    - Study of crystals in synovial fluid using polarized light after preparation

Cytocentrifuge or Cytospin

- *Principle*: A *cytocentrifuge*, sometimes referred to as a *cytospin*, is a special type of centrifuge used to concentrate cells in small quantities of fluid specimens directly onto a microscope slide by to centrifugal forces. It is an instrument used to concentrate cells suspended in small-volume specimens like the CSF. Two such instruments in use are the Shandon Cytospin-Cytocentrifuge and the Sakura Auto Smear.

- *Procedure*:
  - A funnel assembly is attached to the front of a microscope slide. The surface of the funnel assembly that is in contact with the slide is lined with filter paper to absorb excess fluid.
  - The well mixed sample (from few drops in cellular aspirates to about 1 mL in hypocellular aspirates) is placed in the funnel and spun in the especially designed centrifuge at varying speeds (800–2,500 rpm) for about 2–5 minutes (speed and time can be adjusted).
  - Centrifugal force enables the fluid sample and the suspended cells to reach the glass surface of the slide and stick to it.
  - The smaller the sample quantity the better it is absorbed by the filter card.
- *Advantages:*
  - Results are a monolayer of well-preserved and well-displayed cells within a 6-mm area on the slide. The machine can prepare 12 slides simultaneously.
  - Cell yield is good particularly in low yield specimens like CSF and urine.
  - The method can be used on many different types of specimens including fine needle aspirates, CSF, serous and synovial fluid, and urine.
  - Results are reproducible under identical conditions.
  - The sealed head of the tube prevents aerosol of infected samples during spinning and the instrument can be easily sterilized after use.
- *Disadvantages:* Loss of cells though minimal due to absorption into the filter paper.

Millipore Filters

- *Principle*: Membrane filters utilize pressure in order to force carrier fluid through a porous or semipermeable membrane (pore size of 0.45–5 μm) which retains the cells due to the pore size. This process of filtration separates the particulate matter (cells) from the soluble and fluid components. The filters used are cellulose acetate in nature. Gelman, Millipore, and Nuclepore are some of the filters available with a filtering pore diameter of 5 μm.
- *Procedure:*
  - Specimens should be filtered as soon they reach the laboratory.
  - The filter is marked with marking ink and suspended in a Petri dish filled with 95% ethyl alcohol for 10–15 seconds.
  - Wet the grid of the filter after setting it up with balanced salt solution
  - Lay the wet expanded filter onto the grid
  - The funnel is placed on top of the filter. Add 15–20 mL of balanced salt solution to the funnel and apply the clamp.
  - Add 1–2 drops of the cell sediment from the sample to the solution in the funnel.
  - Vacuum is applied—up to 100 mm Hg for Millipore and Gelman filters and up to 20 mm Hg for Nuclepore filters. As the specimen filters, balanced salt solution is added from a squeeze bottle to the filter paper so as to rinse it well. The surface of filter should always be covered with excess fluid and not merely moist or wet looking. About 20–30 mL of 95% ethanol may be added to fix cells in situ.
  - After filtration the funnel is unclamped and the wet filter is removed and it is placed, cell side up in a Petri dish with 95% ethanol for half an hour for fixation, then transferred onto a glass slide.
  - The slide containing the cytology specimen is stained by the Papanicolaou method and examined under a light microscope.
- *Advantages:*
  - This technique provides the added advantage of a clearer background with the cells of interest confined to a demarcated area on the slide
  - Infiltration of microorganisms. Membranes with a pore size of 0.1–10 μm perform microfiltration; this removes all bacteria.
- *Disadvantages:* Fluids used in these preparations should be fresh as prefixation coagulates proteins which may then clog the filters and harden cells into spherical shapes and prevent flattening of the cells on the membrane surface.

Slow Sedimentation Technique[4,5]

- *Principle*: Spontaneous sedimentation of cells occurs in fluid set up in a vertical cylinder open at both ends (at 4°C) on a glass slide placed beneath the cylinder as the liquid part of it slowly seeps out and is absorbed by a filter paper. The cells settle gently like snowflakes due to gravitational force undergoing minimal physical change.
- *Slow sedimentation apparatus:* Various apparatus have been devised for this including the sedimentation cylinder with brass rings devised by Blonk and Arentz (1977) and the sedimentation technique of Bots et al. (1964) using adjustable weights. An apparatus made

of Perspex sheets and designed by Shariff and Thomas (1985) consists of a series of cylinders with an open base mounted on a stage.

- *Procedure*: Setting up of slow sedimentation apparatus-sequential steps **(Figs. 2A to F)**.

a. Clean glass slide coated with egg albumin.
b. Slide with filter paper over it.
c. Slide with filter paper placed on to the stage of apparatus.
d. Slide with cylinders of the apparatus over it.

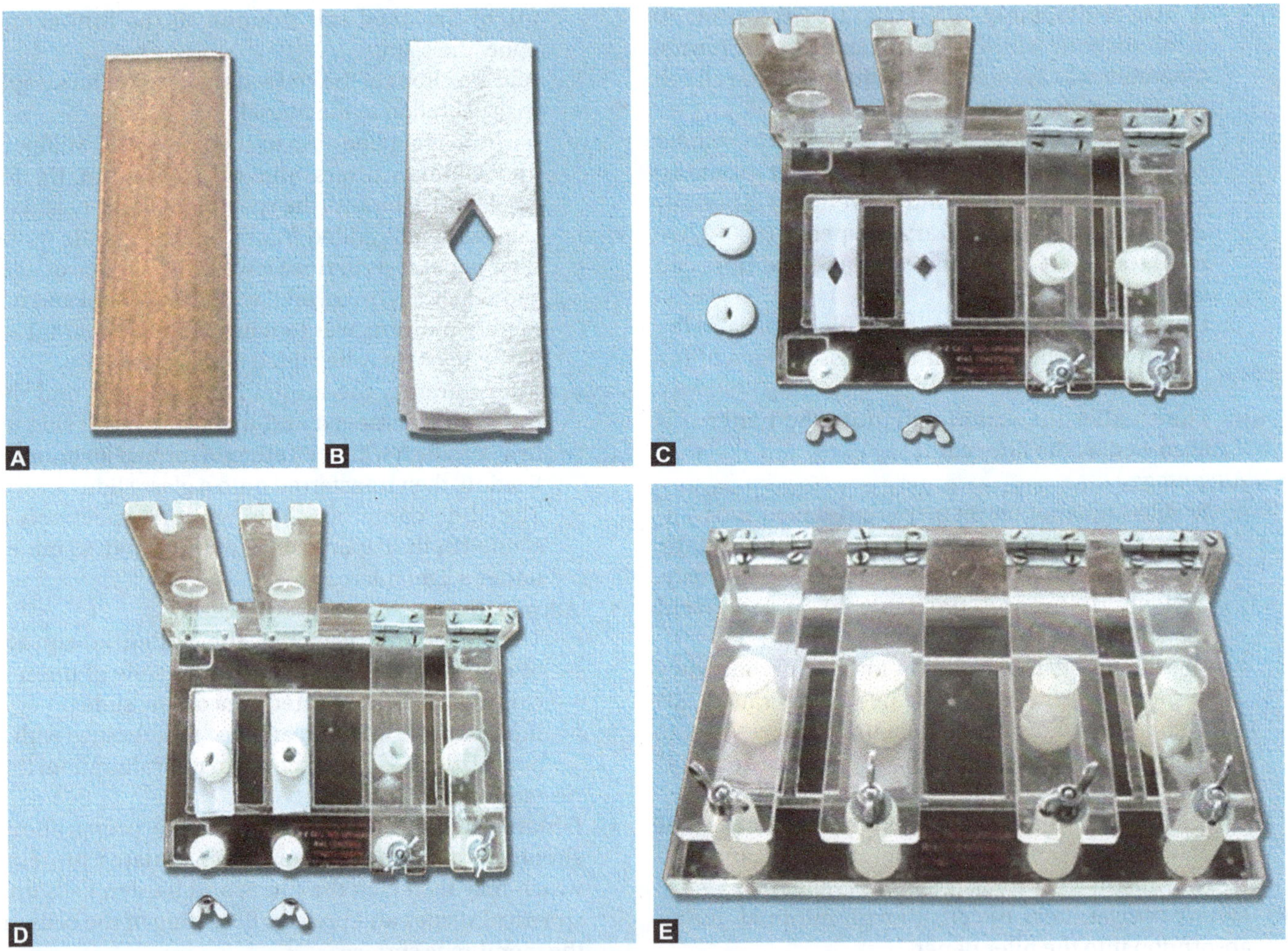

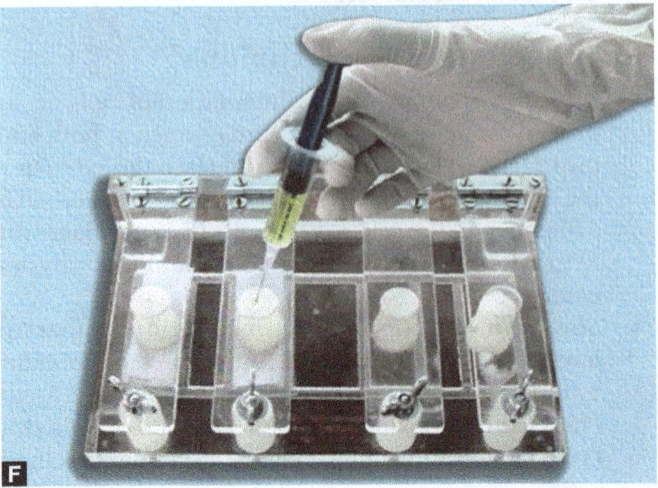

FIGS. 2A TO F: (A) Filter paper with hole cut into it; (B) Place filter paper on top of a slide and place it on the apparatus as shown; (C) Place cylinder over blotting paper and slide; (D and E) Lower hood on cylinders and tighten the screws; and (F) Inserting test sample into cylinder through the hole on top.

e. Screws tightened and cylinders mounted on to the stage so that base of cylinder coincides with the hole in the filter paper. The screws are tightened to the maximum so that the cylinders sit snugly on the filter papers. The tightness of the screws facilitates the rate of liquid seepage.
f. Loading of sample (about 2 mL) with the help of a disposable syringe into the cylinder. The same sample can be loaded in more than one cylinder and removed at different timings.
   - The apparatus is placed aside for 1–2 or 6 hours at 4° in the lower compartment of the fridge or kept overnight for cells to sediment onto the slides. Overnight sedimentation is generally used when the fluid is fed into the apparatus in the evenings and the instrument kept in the lower compartment of the fridge.
   - After the specified time of sedimentation, the screws are loosened and the hoods with the cylinders gently lifted up. The filter papers were gently lifted off the slides. The sediment corresponded to the circular hole cut in the filter paper.
   - The smears are taken out, gently lowered in a container with 95% alcohol for fixation and stained with hematoxylin and eosin (H&E) stain/Papanicolaou stain after 20 minutes of fixation **(Fig. 3)**.
   - If the cellularity at the end of 2 hours is inadequate, the slide at the end of 6 hours with more cellularity is used for interpretation. Times of sedimentation can vary depending on the type of fluid (shorter times for protein-rich fluids).

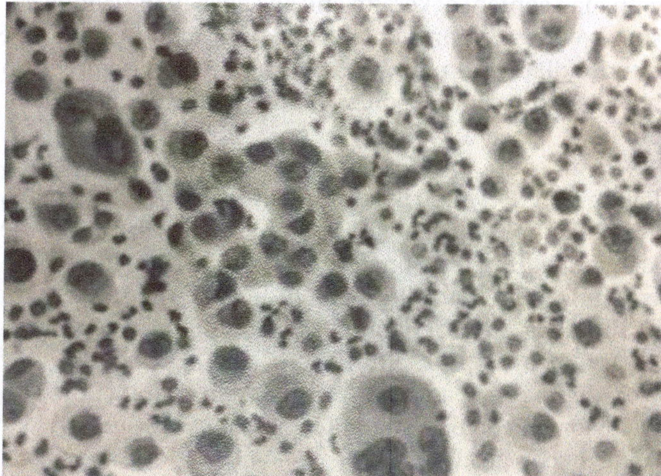

FIG. 3: Ascitic fluid processed by the slow sedimentation technique. Adequate cellularity with good morphology for interpretation (H&E × 400).

- *Advantages:* Minimal cell distortion as the cells settle by their own weight and force of gravity and excellent cell morphology is obtained. The procedure is ideal for clear fluids and has been used to advantage in urine, CSF, and low-protein effusions.
- *Disadvantage*: It takes time, practice, and care in loading the sample in the various cylinders.

Cellblock Technique

This technique is used on any cellular and excess sample obtained by any of the above procedures and can be used on all sites. Cellblock material provides valuable diagnostic information on architectural pattern that cannot be identified on smears and can be used on tissue fragments that may not be processed by cytological techniques. It is of particular use in sputum, bronchial washings, and material from gastrointestinal tract and FNAC material and may also be used for processing all residual material like cell sediments, after completion of smear preparation.

There are different methods of cellblock preparation.

- *Procedure*: Where tissue fragments are readily obtained, wrap material in a piece of filter paper and place in a tissue capsule after which it may be processed as for regular paraffin processing.
- Where material is not adequate as in cell sediments after centrifugation, then to the sediment add egg albumin flakes and some ethyl alcohol and centrifuge. Take the sediment in a filter paper as above. The ethyl alcohol coagulates the protein of the egg albumin which forms the matrix to hold the cells.
- Modified technique using acetyl alcohol formalin fixative (95% ethyl alcohol 34 mL + formalin 4 mL + glacial acetic acid 2 mL).

  The cell pellet remaining after preparing smears (with one or two drops of the supernatant fluid) is mixed with thrice the volume of acetyl alcohol formalin fixative and centrifuged for 10 minutes at 2,000 rpm.

  Discard the supernatant. Set aside the centrifuge tube for 4–6 hours. This allows the coagulum to form a gel.

  Scrape out the cell button and wrap in lens paper and process in tissue processor.

FIXATIVES USED ON SMEARS

Cytological Fixatives

Fixation of smears is necessary to preserve cytologic details of cells spread on a glass slide. Fixation means prevention of degeneration of cells by the autolytic enzymes present in the cells and preservation of cells as close as possible to the living state. To achieve this smear are placed as soon as they are made (before drying) in the fixative solutions for specific periods of time before the staining procedure is started. Fixatives do not excessively shrink or swell cells thereby maintaining morphology of cell components. They have a bactericidal effect and also improve optical differentiation and enhance staining.

Fixation by Immersion

The process of submerging of freshly prepared smears immediately in a liquid fixative is called wet fixation. This is the ideal method for fixing all gynecological and nongynecological smears and any of the alcohols are used. All alcohol fixatives should be discarded or if necessary for reuse; filtered (Whatman No. 1 filter paper) after each use.

- *95% ethyl alcohol (ethanol):* This is the ideal fixative recommended in most of the laboratories for cytological specimens. Most alcohol fixatives fix by dehydration. Other cytological fixatives are *absolute (100%) ethanol, ether-alcohol mixture (50–50), 100% methanol*, and *80% propanol and isopropanol* (cause more cell shrinkage).
- *Time of fixation:* Minimum 15–20 minutes of smear fixation prior to staining is essential. Prolonged fixation for days or weeks will not affect the morphology of cells. If smears are to be preserved over a long period of time they may be removed from the fixative after fixation, left to dry, wrapped in paper, and transported or preserved.
- *Acetone fixation*: It should be short (1 h) at 4°C and used only on small specimens/smears. Acetone produces excessive shrinkage and hardening and results in microscopic distortion. It is good for immunohistochemistry (IHC) staining and enzyme studies in smears as it facilitates entry of large molecules of antibody reagents in IHC studies.
- *Compound alcoholic fixatives*: Like Clarke's, Newcomers, and Carnoy's fixative are alcoholic fixatives used in histology as well as cytology (See **Appendix 1** for constituents).

Coating Fixative

Coating fixatives are substitutes for wet fixatives. They are aerosols applied by spraying the smear immediately after spreading of the cellular contents. They are composed of an alcohol base, which fixes the cells; and a wax-like substance, which forms a thin protective coating over the cells, e.g., Carbowax (polyethylene glycol).

The distance from which the slides with smears are sprayed with an aerosol fixative affects the cytology details and a distance of 10–12 inches (25–30 cm) is the optimum distance recommended for aerosol fixation. Aerosol sprays are not recommended for bloody smears, because they cause clumping of erythrocytes.

Prefixation of Fluids

Prefixation of cytologic material may preserve specimens for days without deterioration. It is generally not recommended unless needed as it results in precipitation of proteins, hardening of cells in spherical shapes, and condensation of nuclear chromatin. Fresh processing and smear making is always preferable.

The most common solutions used for this purpose are:

- Ethyl alcohol (50–95% solution; or ether-alcohol mixture)
- Mucolex (a commercial mucus-liquifing preservative for the collection of mucoid and fluid specimens).
- Albuminized slides should be used to prepare smears from prefixed samples as cells may not fix well to slides after prefixation.

STAINS USED IN CYTOLOGY[4,6]

Papanicolaou Stain

It is a routine staining procedure used in all laboratories for cytology specimens. Named after George Papanicolaou who discovered the stain in 1942, it is a combination of eosin A [eosin azure (EA)] and OG-6 (orange gelb 6) with hematoxylin as the nuclear stain. This multicolored staining technique provides excellent cytoplasmic staining of gynecological and nongynecological samples. The wide range of combinations available allows the user to vary the color intensities and hues. In a well-stained preparation, the cell nuclei are crisp blue to black. The Pap stain emphasizes nuclear detail and chromatin granularity, allowing better identification of malignant cells. The details are made out even on superimposition of cells; therefore, it is called the transparent stain. Cells with high content of keratin and glycogen in the cytoplasm stain yellow. Superficial cells stain orange to pink and intermediate and parabasal cells are turquoise green to blue. Metaplastic cells often stain both green and pink at once.

Eosin azure is composed of three dyes, i.e., eosin Y, light green SF yellowish, and Bismarck brown Y in 95% ethyl alcohol with a small amount of phosphotungstic acid and lithium carbonate. This solution, designated EA, is followed by a number which denotes the proportion of the dyes and their ratios; formulations include EA-36, EA-50, and EA-65. The time of staining may also vary with these. EA-36 and EA-50 are used in conjunction with OG-6 for gynecologic staining. EA-65 is used with OG-6 for nongynecological staining.

- *Stain components*:
  - EA-50 (or EA-36):
    - Light green SF (yellowish) 0.1% solution in 95% ethyl alcohol

  - Bismarck brown 0.5% solution in 95% ethyl alcohol
  - Eosin (yellowish) 0.5% solution in 95% ethyl alcohol
  - Phosphotungstic acid lithium carbonate [saturated aqueous solution, (about 2 g saturates)] 10 drops.
- EA-65: The formula is similar to the formula for EA-50 but the amount of light green SF (yellowish) is halved. For this reason, it is preferred to EA-36 for staining nongynecological smears.
- Orange G (OG-6): Orange G stock solution (0.5% ethyl alcohol 100 mL and phosphotungstic acid 0.015 g)

  OG is a monochromatic stain. "O" stands for *orange* and "G" stands for *gelb*, a German word for "yellow". The dye has a relatively small molecule which enables the stain to rapidly penetrate the cytoplasm. It stains keratin brilliant orange.

Principle of Papanicolaou Stain

- *Nuclear staining*: Usually Harris hematoxylin is used as a regressive stain, in which the smears are overstained with hematoxylin and the excess stain removed by using a differentiating solution such as acid alcohol (0.05% HCl in 70% ethyl alcohol) or 0.05% aqueous solution of HCl alone. After the excess hematoxylin is removed—"blueing" is done, i.e., the stained slide is brought from an acidic to alkaline pH, changing the color from brown pink to blue. Running tap water which is slightly alkaline (pH 8) can be used as a blueing solution or Scott's tap water or ammonium hydroxide solution can be used.
- This is followed by cytoplasmic staining, dehydration, clearing, and mounting.
- The mounting media must be miscible with the clearing agent.
- All solutions and stains should be filtered daily after use, to keep them free of sediment.

Papanicolaou Staining Procedure

Various reagents (in separate containers) in which the slide has to dipped and the time exposure has been given in **Table 1**.

Results: Nuclei-stain blue; cytoplasm in varying shades of pink to orange in varied intensities, and blue.

Rapid Papanicolaou Staining

The principle is to combine OG and EA, hence reducing the time of staining and the number of rinses. Results are not comparable to the conventional technique but resorted to in circumstances when the situation demands an immediate cytology review/report as at a surgical intraoperative procedure.

Many commercial stains composed of rapid Pap-nuclear stains and rapid Pap-cytoplasmic stains as well as dehydrants are available.

TABLE 1: Reagents (separate containers) and time of exposure during procedure of Papanicolaou staining.

90% ethanol (fixation)	15 minutes
80% ethanol	2 minutes
50% ethanol	2 minutes
Distilled water	5 dips
Distilled water	5 dips
Hematoxylin stain	2 minutes
0.05% HCl solution	10 seconds, if necessary regressive stain
Running tap water (bluing)	10 minutes
50% ethanol	2 minutes
80% ethanol	2 minutes
80% ethanol	2 minutes
95% ethanol	2 minutes
OG-6 stain	2 minutes
95% ethanol	2 minutes
95% ethanol	2 minutes
95% ethanol	2 minutes
EA-36 stain	2 minutes
95% ethanol	2 minutes
95% ethanol	2 minutes
95% ethanol	2 minutes
95% ethanol	2 minutes
Absolute ethanol	2 minutes
Absolute ethanol	2 minutes
Absolute ethanol + Xylene (1:1)	2 minutes
Xylene	5 minutes
Xylene	5 minutes
Xylene	Till clear
Mount in a drop of DPX	Tilt the coverslip gently on the slide

Hematoxylin and Eosin Staining Method

Some laboratories use routine H&E stain for nongynecological smears, e.g., for fluids and for staining FNAC material as comparison to histological sections is closer. However, it is unacceptable for cervical smears and cancer screening as the nuclear detail does not match the Pap results.

May–Grünwald–Giemsa Staining Method

It is a Romanowsky stain:

- *Principle of Romanowsky stain*: The "neutral" dyes combine with the basic dye methylene blue and the acid dye eosin, giving a wide range of hues. The pH of the staining *solution* is critical and ideally should be adjusted for different fixatives. Cytoplasmic details are well preserved in this method. Colloid, mucin, endocrine cytoplasmic granules, etc., are better brought out in air-dried preparations. Paravacuolar granules in the thyroid cells stain excellently. It is also ideal for morphology in hematological malignancies like lymphoma or leukemia.

  Many laboratories use only May-Grünwald-Giemsa (MGG) for FNA samples; others use Pap as well as MGG; and yet others H&E in addition to this. The combination of all these stains increases the efficiency of microscopic interpretations. MGG stain is performed on air-dried aspirates or fluids.

Staining Procedure (as per Sigma-Aldrich Protocol)[6]

- *Procedure*: May-Grünwald Giemsa
  - Dilute Giemsa stain 1:20 with deionized water. For bluer coloration, water buffered at pH 7.2 may be used in place of deionized water.
  - Place slides in May-Grünwald stain for 5 minutes.
  - Place slides in working phosphate buffer or Trizma® Buffer (20–70 mmol/L). pH 7.2 for 1.5 minutes.
  - Place slides in dilute Giemsa solution from step 1 for 15–20 minutes
  - Rinse slides *briefly* in *deionized* water
  - Air dry and evaluate
- *Results*: Nuclei will be varying shades of purple. Cytoplasmic staining will be varying shades of blue to light pink. Fine reddish to lilac granules may be present in cytoplasm of some cell types. Basophils will demonstrate dark blue-black granules in the cytoplasm. Eosinophils will demonstrate bright orange granules in the cytoplasm. RBCs should be pink to orange.

Stain Components: Giemsa Stain

- Giemsa stain, modified, 0.4% weight/volume (w/v), in a methanol solution, pH 6.9, with stabilizers.
- *May-Grünwald stain*: May-Grünwald stain, 0.25% w/v, in methanol.
- Phosphate buffer pH 7.2 at 25°C (a mixture of sodium phosphate and potassium phosphate)
  - Store Giemsa and May-Grünwald solutions at room temperature (18–26°C)

Deterioration: Discard Giemsa and May-Grünwald solutions if a precipitate develops. Discard the working phosphate buffer if turbidity or visible bacterial growth is present.

Preparation: Giemsa and May-Grünwald solutions are supplied ready to use, although the Giemsa solution may be diluted 1:20 before use in either deionized water or in phosphate buffer solutions. Prepare working phosphate buffer by diluting contents of one vial phosphate buffer pH 7.2 at 25°C to 3.8 L or 1 gal with water. Mix well to dissolve.

SEROUS EFFUSIONS: GUIDELINES FOR INTERPRETATION[3]

Fluids occurring in body spaces and between membranes lining organs in the body are called serous fluids. The organs lined by serous membranes are the heart, lungs, and the peritoneal cavity. A serous cavity has a visceral layer surrounding the organ and a parietal layer lining the outer layer. Normally, the fluid within these cavities is minimal and acts as a lubricant (50–100 mL). In pathological conditions and diseases affecting these organs excessive accumulation occurs. Such excessive fluid collection is called a serous effusion. It could be an active effusion with increased proteins and cells within as a result of increased capillary permeability as occurs in inflammation/malignancy (exudate) or passive effusion as a result of a block in the circulation and exudation of fluid through the membranes (transudate). The latter occurs in congestive heart failure and cirrhosis. An exudate is rich in cells and proteins (>3 g/100 mL) with a specific gravity of >1.015.

The examination of such collections gives evidence to pinpoint the diagnosis in diseases and is routinely done in the cytology laboratories. The following features may be noted:

- Accurate clinical details must be obtained before reporting.
- An excess volume of fluid sent repeatedly in half liter and 1 L quantities invariably denotes malignancy; bloody aspirates also indicate malignancy.
- All effusions associated with cancer need not always contain malignant cells as effusions may also result due to indirect mechanisms like venous obstruction caused by the neoplasm and may be associated with a transudate-type effusion.
- Few or no cells would be seen in effusions when the neoplastic process is limited to the submesothelial tissues; however, a protein content of <3 g% is rarely seen in cancerous cases.

- A cytological diagnosis of cancer should be avoided if the morphology of cells is not clear; no obvious structural nuclear abnormalities are present; there is evidence of an inflammatory process with numerous polymorphonuclear leukocytes, macrophages, and cell necrosis with no obvious evidence of malignancy.
- A second tap yields better morphology than the first one and should be resorted to in doubtful cases.
- Clots of fibrin or blood or solid mucus particles may be identified at the bottom of the sample bottle and should be taken for cellblock preparations. These may have cellularity and contribute toward diagnosis.
- Pus in the fluid gives it a homogenous milky appearance and indicates a pyogenic etiology, empyema, etc. Chylous effusions are also milky.
- Coagulation in fluid and yellow color indicates excess of protein and invariably an exudate
- Watery fluids usually indicate transudates
- It should be noted that errors are made on technically inadequate material, such as thick overstained smears, poorly prepared and stained filter preparations, and inadequate specimens.

Cell Types in Effusions

Mesothelial cells: Free-floating mesothelial cells in fluids appear singly and in clusters. Single mesothelial cell in body fluids is round or oval and measure between 9 and 60 (average 20–40) μm in diameter. The cyanophilic or eosinophilic cytoplasm is opaque and homogenous and sharply demarcated. Most often the cell membrane shows a "brush border appearance" and where this is not clearly discernible, it is represented at light microscopy by a clear zone surrounding the cell membrane, seen as a window between two cells and better appreciated on electron microscopic preparations [may represent surface structures (microvilli or blebs) observed by scanning electron microscopy]. The nuclei are large and occupy about half the cell diameter and are centrally or eccentrically located. The nuclear membrane is prominent. The chromatin network is fine with one or two small nucleoli.

Reactive mesothelial cells in fluids occur more commonly in clusters. The clusters may more often be made up of a small number of cells. These clusters are usually flat and consist of a single layer of uniform cells adherent to each other. The uniformity of the nuclei speaks strongly in favor of their mesothelial origin. Cells often display a molding of the cell surfaces. Sometimes adjacent molded mesothelial cells appear to be separated from each other by a narrow, regular, and slit-like clear space (already referred to) called the "window" **(Fig. 4)**. Multinucleation is a common feature and when it occurs there are usually two nuclei which are very similar to each other. One cell "grasping" an adjacent cell (cell cannibalism) is an often seen feature of mesothelial cells. Large clusters of mesothelial cells have a "knobby" counter due to individual cells protruding at the periphery. It is the presence of these "peripheral knobs" which is one of the hallmarks of mesothelial cells, differentiating them from adenocarcinoma cell clusters which in contrast have a smooth periphery.

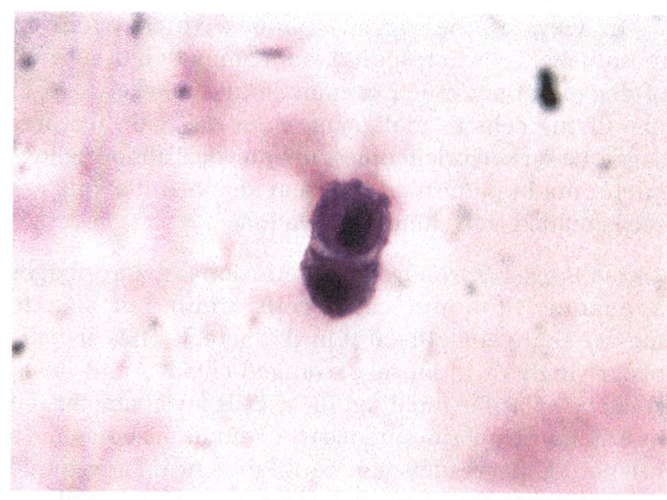

FIG. 4: Two mesothelial cells with a clear space in-between called the "window" (Giemsa stain × 400).

Inflammation: It shows considerable reactive changes in mesothelial cells. A size variation may occur from cells which measure 9 μ to giant forms >60 μ. Multinucleation increases in frequency and the number of nuclei in the multinucleated cells also increases. Mitotic figures are more frequently seen and do not always imply malignancy. Individual nuclei may show an increase in size and may have a more coarsely granular but still uniform chromatin pattern. Nucleoli may also enlarge and become more prominent and occasionally multiple nucleoli are seen. In benign cells, however, the nuclei retain a smooth outline, a uniform chromatin pattern with rounded nucleoli, and an adequate amount of cytoplasm.

Degeneration: Degenerative changes in mesothelial cells cause alterations in both cytoplasm and nuclei. The cytoplasm may be completely lost and the denuded nuclei may appear suspicious. Cytoplasmic vacuoles may also be observed either as small or large vacuoles pushing the nuclei to one side as in a signet ring malignant cell. However, the uniform round or oval nuclear outlines, normal chromatin pattern, appearance of single or small loosely arranged groups in contrast to the compact clusters of tumor cells, establish their benign nature.

In view of the varied changes which occur in mesothelial cells in response to inflammation or a result of degeneration, much caution should be exercised in identifying cells as malignant when the main features suggest a serosal origin unless unequivocal abnormalities of chromatin pattern and nuclear shape and atypia are seen coupled with clinical correlation.

Macrophages (histiocytes): In effusions, macrophages appear as mononucleated cells similar in size to mesothelial cells (10–20 μ in diameter). They usually occur singly or in loosely arranged clusters and never show cytoplasmic molding. These cells are characterized by a foamy cytoplasm studded with minute vacuoles and a cell border that readily blends with the smear background in contrast to the sharply demarcated mesothelial cell outline or brush border. The cytoplasm of macrophages sometimes becomes markedly distended with large vacuoles. The nuclei are usually peripheral in location and oval or kidney-shaped. Binucleated and multinucleated macrophages may also be observed. Phagocytic activity of macrophages may be used to advantage in the identification of these cells from mesothelial cells. Stains for enzymes such as acid phosphatase and supravital staining with neutral red or Janus green are other methods for identifying macrophages.

Macrophages appear in effusions not only as a consequence of inflammation but also in the presence of cancer and under other circumstances as well.

Leukocytes: These commonly occur in effusions and may predominate in long-standing effusions. Lymphocytes may be the chief cells in tuberculosis, lymphocytic leukemia, or lymphoma.

Polymorphonuclear neutrophilic leukocytes: Invariably indicate an inflammatory process. Such a process may also be associated with neoplasms. Eosinophilic leukocytes may also be seen in eosinophilic pleural effusion (EPE) and in variety of inflammatory processes. They are rarely seen in cases of Hodgkin's disease.

Neoplastic cells in effusions: It is well-recognized that the diagnosis of neoplastic cells in the effusion does not depend upon any single morphological criteria or constellation of criteria. A very useful method to identify cancer cells is by attempting to recognize cells that are alien to the nature of the specimen. Metastatic tumor cell appearance varies according to the tumor type. The cells may be classified according to size into three groups—(1) large, (2) small, and (3) medium.

Large cells are significantly larger than mesothelial cells. Metastatic epidermoid and adenocarcinoma, anaplastic carcinomas, malignant melanomas, and sarcomas belong to this group. The identification of such tumor cells is easy. Small cells tumors are made up of cells much smaller than mesothelial cells. Malignant lymphomas are small cell neoplasms, such as neuroblastomas, Wilms tumors, or even oat-cell carcinoma belong to this category. Close attention should be paid to nuclear features which are small and dark staining. Medium cells are approximately of the same size as mesothelial cells. A variety of carcinomas—of mammary, gastric, pancreatic, or of lung origin belong to this group. This is perhaps the most important area of diagnostic error due to similarities to reactive mesothelial cells.

Certain important aspects and hints at picking up neoplastic features are nuclear clear zones, nuclear holes, i.e., cytoplasmic invagination in nuclei, are observed in a variety of cancer cells, such as cells of papillary thyroid carcinoma, metastatic melanomas, pulmonary adenocarcinomas, breast, and liver; bizarre spindle-shaped cells always suggest a metastatic sarcomas; other cell configurations are columnar cells resembling bronchial lining cells in bronchogenic carcinoma; aggregate composed of papillary projections or glandular structures are helpful in identifying features to suggest adenocarcinoma; cell products, such as mucin, melanin pigment, psammoma bodies, cytoplasmic cross-striations, and keratin invariably suggest primaries from various sites. Special stains may demonstrate these better on smears or on cellblock preparations. Melanoma effusion may be dark brown, cells show brown to black pigment. A Masson's Fontana stain helps where pigment is sparse. Bile may be identified in polygonal small or large cells from a hepatocellular carcinoma. Glycogen may be observed in vacuolated cells from squamous cell carcinoma.

Immunohistochemistry detects minute quantities of the above cell products which may be missed on routine staining.

Malignant mesotheliomas: They are characterized by massive effusions which reaccumulate rapidly even on repeated drainage and sometimes may be hemorrhagic. The cells retain the characteristics of benign mesothelial cells particularly in well-differentiated tumors. They are characterized by an eccentric nucleus, frayed margin, cannibalism, and knob-like periphery in morulae of tumor cells and vacuolation of cytoplasm. Binucleation and multinucleation is also common. Accompanying profuse exfoliation of atypical mesothelial cells together with medium sized and small differentiated and undifferentiated malignant cells helps in clinching the diagnosis **(Fig. 5)**.

Tables 2 and 3 show lists of the differences between *an adenocarcinoma and malignant mesothelioma in any effusion*.

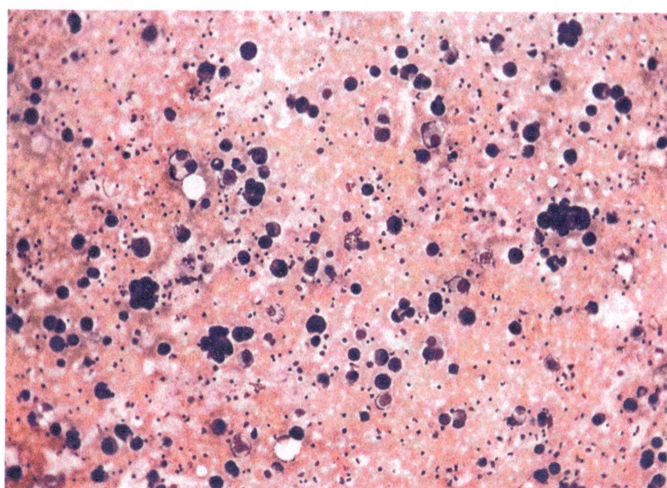

FIG. 5: Low-power view of malignant mesothelioma with increased cellularity; knobby periphery to cytoplasmic groups, and cannibalism.

TABLE 2: Differences between an adenocarcinoma and malignant mesothelioma.

Adenocarcinoma	Mesothelioma
Clinical features—mass, localized thickening, and pleural effusion	Clinical features—pleura studded with nodules on imaging, massive pleural effusion, and reaccumulates rapidly on tapping
Gross	
• Periphery of lung • Involvement of lung and pleura • More commonly localized • Nodules are large • Cut surface gray white	• Along pleura—visceral or parietal • Involvement of pleura—may infiltrate lung • Diffuse • Fine to large nodules 1 mm to a few centimeters • Cut surface gray white with well demonstrable slit-like spaces
Microscopy	
• Glands ++ • Sheets of cells in poorly differentiated forms	• Glands ++ in epithelial variant. Poorly formed basement. Lining cells seemingly rest directly on stroma • Glands and stroma in mixed variant • Only stroma in sarcomatoid variant
Mucin	
Neutral mucin (PAS and mucicarmine +ve)	Acid mucin—hyaluronic acid (alcian blue +ve at pH 2.5 digested by hyaluronidase) Very rare cases of glycogen-rich mesothelioma may be PAS +ve

(PAS: periodic acid–Schiff)

TABLE 3: Differences between adenocarcinoma and mesothelioma [immunohistochemistry (IHC) markers below].

	Immunohistochemistry
Calretinin –ve	(sometimes +ve) +ve
Cytokeratin 5/6 –ve	+ve*
WT1 –ve	+ve
Thrombomodulin -ve	+ve
Vimentin -ve	+ve
CEA +ve	-ve
B72.3 +ve	-ve
Ber Ep4 +ve	-ve
MOC-31 +ve	-ve
TTF +ve	-ve
Pan keratin +ve	+ve
EMA +ve	+ve
Basement membrane component +ve	+ve
D2-40 -ve	+ve

*Also +ve in SCC and transitional CC.

Note: Calretinin, cytokeratin 5/6, and WT1 at present are the best +ve markers for mesothelioma and CEA; B72.3 and MOC-31 are the best -ve markers. A panel of four markers—calretinin, cytokeratin 5/6 (or WT1), CEA, and MOC-31 (or B72.3) enables a correct diagnosis in most cases.

(CEA: carcinoembryonic antigen; EMA: epithelial membrane antigen; TTF: thyroid transcription factor; WT1: Wilms' tumor 1)

Source: Ordóñez NG. The immunohistochemical diagnosis of mesothelioma: a comparative study of epithelioid mesothelioma and lung adenocarcinoma. Am J Surg Pathol. 2003;27:1031-51.

Malignancies of lymphoreticular system: Serous effusions are a common complication of lymphomas and leukemias. In most cases, diagnosis of such malignancies is already made much before the occurrence of effusion. It is very rare for a diagnosis of this condition to depend on cytological interpretation and cytology in such conditions is done to only confirm the presence of neoplastic lymphoid cells.

Hodgkin's disease is characterized by lymphocytes and plasma cells and eosinophils in effusions. Reed-Sternberg cells are rarely identified.

Nonmalignant serous effusions: They occur in several conditions—hypoproteinemia, generally associated with anasarca which is a transudate with low protein and low cell count and poses no diagnostic problems; congestive cardiac failure is one of the most common causes of chronic pleural effusion, is associated commonly with a right-sided effusion, and is classically a transudate; acute inflammatory processes—acute bacterial pneumonias, lung abscesses, acute pleurisy, and postsurgical states are often associated with pleural effusions of the exudative type, containing numerous polymorphonuclear leukocytes and nuclear material; in viral pneumonias, a predominance of lymphocytes and macrophages is generally seen; cirrhosis shows a transudate; tuberculosis effusion is an example of a chronic pleural effusion and characterized by a lymphocytic predominance with only a few mesothelial cells (due to covering of the pleural surface by fibrin). A specific diagnosis of tuberculosis cannot be made on fluid cytology alone in the presence of an occasional Langhans type of giant cell unless acid fast-bacilli are identified. Only a pleural biopsy and/or microbiological studies can establish a specific diagnosis as the finding of epithelioid cells is a rarity in effusions. An EPE is ill-defined and heterogeneous and there are as such no definite universally agreed criteria to define EPE. A finding of >10% eosinophils (Koss 1979) or 50% eosinophils (Robertson 1954) in the fluid has been suggested as a prerequisite for diagnosis by these authors. An EPE may be secondary to ingestion of drugs, hypersensitivity, parasitic infections, or in the absence of all this may be an idiopathic eosinophilic effusion.

Curschmann's spirals: They are rarely seen in pleural and peritoneal effusions, but when seen tend to be shorter and less spiral than those seen in sputum and cervical smears. They are thought to be derived from mucus and/or submesothelial mucosubstances and are seen in a variety of conditions ranging from serous to mucinous carcinomas.

Ferruginous bodies: They are rarely encountered in pleural effusions in cases of asbestosis and are better enhanced with an iron stain.

HYDROCELE FLUID[3,4]

A hydrocele in the scrotum occurs when fluid collects between the visceral and parietal layers of the tunica vaginalis. Hydrocele fluid examination for cytology is a rare procedure in the laboratory diagnostic set-up. Although aspiration of fluids accumulating in the hydrocele sac is a common procedure in the wards, a cytological examination is rarely requested for.

The hydrocele fluid is usually hypocellular but occasionally may show several mesothelial cells. When this occurs, these reactive mesothelial cells may constitute an important source of diagnostic error.

Malignant mesothelioma of the tunica vaginalis is a rare occurrence, but when this occurs, the cytology is a very similar to those of mesotheliomas occurring in the pleural cavity.

Testicular neoplasm: Very rarely malignant cells from testicular neoplasm may be encountered in the hydrocele fluid in which case the morphology of the cells is similar to that of the primary neoplasm. Seminomas rarely exfoliate as they are confined to the tunica vaginalis; however, embryonal carcinoma and other high-grade tumors may exfoliate cells into the fluid.

CONCLUSION

A cytological examination of any effusion is a routine laboratory investigation done in all laboratories, its main value lies in picking up malignant effusions or ruling it out. In several cases, it gives valuable information with regard to the site of primary.

REFERENCES

1. Lynch MJ, Raphael SS. Lynch's Medical Laboratory Technology, 3rd edition. Philadelphia, London, Toronto. Igaku Shion Ltd. Tokyo: WB Saunders Company; 1976.
2. Carson FL, Hladik C. Histotechnology: A Self-Instructional Text, 3 edition. Hong Kong: American Society for Clinical Pathology Press; 2009. pp. 361-3363.
3. Koss LG, Melamed MR. Koss' Diagnostic Cytology and Its Histopathologic Bases. Philadelphia: Lippincott Williams and Wilkins; 2006.
4. Shariff S, Kaler AK. Principles and Interpretation of Laboratory Practices in Surgical Pathology. New Delhi: Jaypee Brothers Medical Publishers (P) Ltd.; 2016.
5. Shariff S, Thomas JA. Slow sedimentation technique for fluid cytology. J Cytol. 1989;6:42-4.
6. Sigmaaldrich.com. Giemsa stain. [online]. Available from https://www.sigmaaldrich.com/deepweb/assets/sigmaaldrich/product/documents/315/931/gs10.pdf [Last accessed March, 2024].

CHAPTER 3

Semen Analysis

INTRODUCTION

Semen analysis is a routine test carried out in most laboratories and performed as an important diagnostic tool for the evaluation of male fertility. The test is done in individuals wanting to conceive or for purpose of verification in the success of vasectomy and prior to donation in artificial insemination.

SEMEN ANALYSIS[1,2]

Semen is collected by the patient in a clean dry bottle and brought to the laboratory within 30 minutes of collection. The patient should be instructed to avoid ejaculation 24–72 hours before collection. Once collected, it cannot be examined immediately as the highly Viscous fluid should liquefy which it does in 15–30 minutes and subsequently should be examined without delay.

According to recent World Health Organization (WHO) criteria,[1] an ejaculate is normal if at least 1.5 mL of ejaculate shows >15 million sperms/mL of semen. Of these, at least 32% of sperms should swim in a forward direction, and at least 4% should have a normal shape. These criteria classify a man as being fertile.

Gross Examination

- *Volume*: 3.5–5 mL (<1.5 is abnormal)
- *Viscosity*:
  - Normally, it should fall drop by drop
  - Increased viscosity affects sperm motility

Liquefaction

It should liquify within 30 minutes on incubation at 37°C.

Microscopic Examination

- *Sperm count*:
  - Diluting fluid:
    - Sodium carbonate: 5 g
    - Formalin neutral: 1 mL
    - Distilled water: 100 mL

      Count with white blood cell (WBC) pipette and counting chamber, count 4 mm^2 and multiply by 50,000

      Dilution: 1:20

Normal count: 60–120 million/mL

- *Oligospermia*: Reduced count
- *Azoospermia*: No sperms present
- *Necrozoospermia*: Only dead sperms seen

Abnormal sperm counts of significance are seen in:

- Primary testicular abnormalities like bilateral orchitis during younger age lead to reduced count or infertility.
- Age-related testicular degeneration
- Systemic illness may reduce the ability for healthy sperm production. If resolved the count may be restored.

Motility

Normal semen contains >80% actively motile sperms with at least 32% swimming in the forward direction. 20% may be sluggish. Movement should be observed at 3, 6, and 12 hours. There should be no reduction of motility up to 3 hours, normally. A score of 3–4 on a scale of 0–4 represents good movement. Alternatively WHO classifies the grades of motility as follows:

- *Motility IV or grade A*: Sperms that fall in this category are the ones with progressive motility; they move fast in a straight line and are the strongest.

- *Motility III or grade B*: These sperms move in a nonlinear direction, they do move forward but in a curved or crooked motion.
- *Motility II or grade C*: These sperms move in a nonprogressive manner, which means they do move their tails but do not progress forward.
- *Motility I or grade D*: Sperms in this category fail to move at all and are labeled immotile.

Sperm Morphology

Sperm morphology should be studied after a thin smear is made after liquefaction and stained by the Leishman's stain. A note should be made of normal or abnormal sperms. Abnormal sperms are those with double heads, double tails, constricted head, acute tapering form, pin head, and giant head. At least 4% of the sperms should have a normal shape.

Note and report the percentage of dead sperms (necrospermia). Up to 30% of dead sperms is considered within normal limits.

Fructose Level

Fructose is a carbohydrate moiety produced by seminal vesicles; it provides energy to the sperms. The normal value of the semen fructose level is 13 mmol per sample. Defective seminal vesicle secretion results in lower levels of fructose.

Testicular Biopsy

If indicated in low counts and infertility, it is done. Needle/ wedge biopsy/or even fine needle aspiration cytology (FNAC) is often resorted to in these cases.

Abnormalities seen at histopathology are varying degrees of cytoplasmic vacuolization, increased fibrous tissue around seminiferous tubules, and loss of normal tubular architecture. The number of germ cells may be reduced, and in severe cases, may be absent, leaving only the sertoli cells and the supporting tissues. A "Johnson's score" is done to assess spermatogenesis and maturation; 60% or more of tubules at cross sections should score at 10.

Johnson's score (1980) for spermatogenesis:[3] A score of 1–10 is given for each tubule cross section examined according to the following criteria:

10—complete spermatogenesis and perfect tubules
9—many spermatozoa present but disorganized spermatogenesis
8—only a few spermatozoa present
7—no spermatozoa but many spermatids present
6—only a few spermatids present
5—no spermatozoa or spermatids present but many spermatocytes present
4—only a few spermatocytes present
3—only spermatogonia present
2—no germ cells present
1—no germ cells or sertoli cells present

In a normal adult testicle, the mean score count should be at least 8.90, with an average of 9.38, and 60% or more of tubules should score at 10.

Germ cell: Sertoli cell ratio—count at least 30 tubule cross sections. Ratio is relatively constant in healthy males and is 13:1.

- An average of 12 sertoli cells per tubular cross section is considered normal and half the germ cell elements should be in the spermatid stage.
- Any obvious syndromes such as sertoli cell only syndrome should be mentioned with a note to perform cytogenetic studies.
- Any specific inflammation and pathology such as tuberculosis should be looked for.
- Biopsy specimens from infertile men with total lack of spermatozoa (azoospermia) usually fall into one of the following categories:
    - Germ cell aplasia (sertoli cell only syndrome) (29%): In this, the tubules are populated by only sertoli cells; measure 100–150 μ in diameter and may show some thickening of the tubular basement membrane; germ cells are completely absent; Leydig cells are usually normal but on occasion are found to be reduced in size and number.
    - Spermatocytic arrest (26%): Halt of maturation sequence may occur early or late. An early arrest is seen at the stage of primary spermatocyte (presumably at the end of meiotic phase at late pachytene); no spermatids or spermatozoa are present despite the presence of abundant cells in division (Leydig cells are normal).
      A late maturation arrest—stops at the stage of spermatids, which are seen in plenty but no spermatozoa.
    - Generalized fibrosis (18%): It is due to any etiology
    - Normal spermatogenesis (27%): It suggests obstructive azoospermia and implies bilateral obstruction or absence of some part of the duct system. This is a primary indication for performing an FNAC procedure on the testis. A combination of this obstruction and pulmonary infection is Young's syndrome. Diagnostic features of obstruction are—tubular diameter is normal or slightly reduced; all stages of spermatogenesis are present but the normal orderly arrangement is lost; and central lumen is absent. Half or more of the tubules should show these features.

- *Hypospermatogenesis:* It is characterized by spermatogenesis in some tubules with a reduced population of germ cells and improper arrangement of the germ cells.
- *Klinefelter's syndrome*: Fibrosis of tubules, prominent thickening of the basement membrane, and Leydig cell hyperplasia (XXY).

CONCLUSION

Semen analysis is the cornerstone of a case of male fertility. The sperm preparation techniques and procedural standardization are an important parameter for the success of the examination.

REFERENCES

1. Australian Concept Infertility Medical Center. (1998). WHO standards of semen analysis. [online]. Available from https://acimc.org/doctor/dr-syed-sajjad/ [Last accessed March, 2024].
2. Biggers A, Johnson S. (2017). Semen Analysis and Test Results. [online]. Available from https://www.healthline.com/health/semen-analysis#_noHeaderPrefixedContent [Last accessed March, 2024].
3. Goldblum JR, Lamps LW, McKenney JK. Rosai and Ackerman's Surgical Pathology, 11th edition. Philadelphia: Elsevier Health Sciences; 2017.

CHAPTER 4

Joint Effusions

INTRODUCTION

Synovial fluid (SF) is a jelly-like viscous, non-Newtonian fluid, presents in the joint spaces **(Fig. 1)** of all movable joints. It is present within the joint cavity bounded and lined by epithelial cells called synovial cells, these cells secrete the fluid. Its main function is lubrication of the joint allowing for easy mobility, shock absorption, and supply of nutrients to the joint. The main component of the SF is hyaluronic acid secreted by synoviocyte type B cells. Hyaluronic acid is a nonsulfated mucopolysaccaride which is responsible for the elasticity of the articular cartilage; lubricin, a proteoglycan secreted by the chondrocytes, contributes to lubrication.

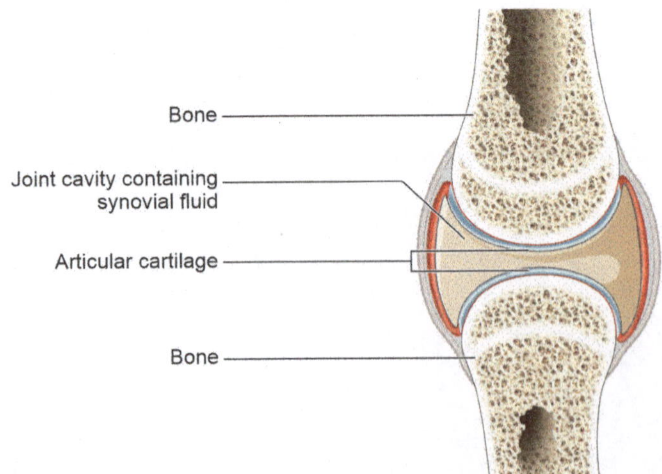

FIG. 1: Joint space containing synovial fluid.

SYNOVIAL FLUID EXAMINATION[1]

Characteristics of Normal Synovial Fluid

The amount of SF in normal joint is quite limited and varies from 0.1 to 3.5 mL. It is crystal clear to pale yellow making it possible to read print through it. The white cell count ranges from 0 to 200/mm^3, most of these being mononuclear cells. The total protein content averages 1.8 g/dL. The fluid fails to clot even in the presence of blood because of the presence of plasminogen activator.

In disease conditions, increased secretion of SF occurs and this increased amount can be assessed clinically by the bulge test.

Indications for Aspiration of Synovial Fluid

Aspiration of SF is done in disease states of the joints, e.g., rheumatoid arthritis (RA), gout, or systemic diseases which involve joints, e.g., systemic lupus erythematosus. A SF examination has to be a correlation between gross appearances, wet mount, and stained film examination with the complete clinical picture as well as chemical and immunological results. At times, a synovial membrane biopsy may be coupled with fluid aspiration, e.g., tuberculosis and RA.

Aspiration

A *synovial tap* yields fluid from the joint space. Joint aspiration should be performed under aseptic precautions only by an experienced operator. Almost any joint can be aspirated. It is usually performed on the extensor aspect of the joint where the synovial pouch is superficial and free of nerves and blood vessels **(Fig. 2)**.

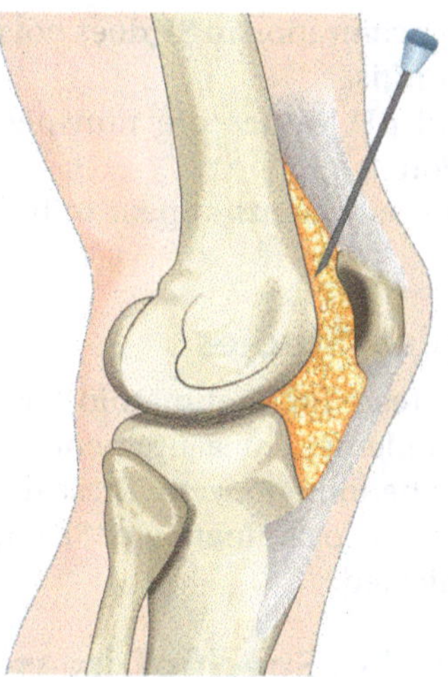

FIG. 2: Needle within the joint space on the extensor aspect of the knee joint where synovial pouch is most approachable.

Synovial fluid removed from the joint space is collected in various tubes for the following purposes:

- A heparinized sample for gross examination, cell counts, mucin clot test, and crystals.
- Nonsterile tube for cytology
- Nonsterile tube for chemistry and immunology
- Sterile tube for microbiological culture studies

Macroscopic Examination

Volume, color and clarity, inclusions, viscosity, and Mucin clot test are to be done.

- *Volume*: Increases in inflammation
- *Color*:
  - Bloody aspirate—traumatic arthritis
  - Turbid—elevated cell counts (leukocytes), crystals, cartilage debris, etc.
  - Xanthochromia—trauma into joint and degenerative joint diseases
  - Milky—gout and pseudogout
- *Viscosity*: Take a drop of fluid onto a glass slide and pull out a string from it with the help of a gloved finger. A length of a few inches of string is normally obtained. Alternatively drop by drop of the fluid can be ejected with a syringe and the length of the string between two drops noted. An Ostwald viscometer can also be used to compare the viscosity of SF to water.
- *Mucin clot test*: Addition of dilute acetic acid (5%) dropwise to a test tube containing SF forms a clot. This is shaken after 1 minute to determine the friability of the same. The consistency of the clot varies with different diseased conditions.
- *Firm, hard, ropy, nonfriable clot (high mucin content)*: It is seen in normal SF.

Microscopic Examination

- *Cell counts*: Cell counts are performed using a saline solution as diluent; using methylene blue as a nuclear staining.

  Normal: Up to 200 cells/mm^3, 25% of these being polymorphs. Leukocytosis occurs in inflammation. The differential leukocyte count is helpful in determining the degree of inflammation, since a predominant neutrophilic response is seen in inflammatory fluids, most notably septic arthritis. Eosinophils are a rare finding and may be seen in allergic reactions to intra-articular injections and parasitic infections.
- *Wet mount preparations*: It is needed for the identification of formed elements such as crystals, cartilage fibrils, and "special cells". A drop of fresh SF is taken onto a slide and cover slipped for viewing. If crystals are seen, this is followed by polarized light microscopic examination to identify the type of crystals or by the insertion of polarized disks into the ocular and condenser of a standard light microscope.

  A polarizing microscope has a retardation plate which is placed between the polarizer (filter which is placed between the substage condenser) and analyzer (filter which is placed between the objective and the eye-piece); the crystals will then appear yellow or blue depending on their direction in relation to the direction of the slow ray of the retardation plate.

  Urate crystals are termed negatively birefringent since their color is yellow when their long axis is parallel to that of the slow ray of the retardation plate whereas calcium pyrophosphate crystals are positively birefringent and blue when aligned in the same direction.

  Synovial fluid for this purpose should not be collected with double oxalate as the calcium in the SF combines with the oxalate and may cause confusion with urate and calcium pyrophosphate crystals.

  Five types of crystals can be identified in various types of arthritis.[2,3] However differentiating between two of them, i.e., urate crystals and calcium pyrophosphate dihydrate is of immense clinical importance for management purposes. This is done by a polarized microscope where a yellow or negative birefringence is seen in the urate crystals and a blue or positive birefringence is seen in the calcium pyrophosphate dihydrate crystals.
- *Urate crystals* are crystals which appear as needle-shaped negatively birefringent crystals varying in length from 2 to 20 µm. With negative birefringence, the crystals appear yellow in parallel light and blue with perpendicular light. They are diagnostic of gout.

- *Calcium pyrophosphate dihydrate crystals* are rod-shaped or rhomboids varying in length from 2 to 20 µm with positive birefringence (blue with parallel light and yellow with perpendicular light). They are seen in chondrocalcinosis or pseudogout.
- The report should state whether the crystals, especially urate and calcium pyrophosphate are lying free in the SF or have been ingested by polymorphs. An intracellular location of crystals suggests that these are responsible for acute arthritis and if found extracellularly in the fluid, it is unlikely that they are responsible for the acute attack.
- Apatite crystals sometimes considered as a cause of synovitis and appear as shiny crystals; cholesterol crystals are large, flat, and plate-like with sharp corners and seen as multicolored forms; talcum crystals are small and seen as maltese crosses; steroid crystals are pleomorphic or needle like and either positively or negatively birefringent. They usually occur after steroid injections.

  Fragments of cartilage may appear birefringent and needle like and are seen due to damage to the cartilage in osteoarthritis or traumatic arthritis; and may be mistaken for crystals.
- *Examination of stained smear*: It is examined after centrifugation at 500–1,500 rpm for 5–10 minutes.

  It is done for the presence of polymorphs, lymphocytes, monocytes, and other cells like synovial lining cells type A and B and abnormal cells such as rhagocytes. Presence of synovial cells is of nondiagnostic value. However, with sudan black staining, type A synoviocytes (phagocytic cells) are stained positive and type B synoviocytes (hyluran secreting cells) are stained negative.

Chemical Examination[1]

- An adjuvant chemical examination of SF is of great help in diagnosis.
- Glucose in normal SF is slightly less than plasma glucose as equilibration between blood and SF glucose is slow. Samples of blood and SF should be obtained to note the difference between the two. In noninflammatory arthritis, the blood-SF glucose difference is about 10 mg/dL. In inflammatory arthritis (e.g., septic, rheumatoid, or tuberculosis), the glucose difference is about 25 mg/dL.
- Protein in SF is about 2 g/dL. The concentration of it in SF also depends on plasma levels. It is markedly increased in RA.
- Uric acid concentration in SF does not play a role even in gouty arthritis.
- Lactate and pH values are nonspecific indices of inflammation.
- Enzyme measurements appear to have little clinical value.

Immunological Studies

These include tests for rheumatoid factor, antinuclear antibodies, complement measurements, lupus erythematosus (LE) cell phenomenon, etc. These tests, however, are not a part of routine examination of SF and are done only if clinically indicated.

Synovial Fluid in Specific Diseases

Septic Arthritis

- *Color*: Turbid; purulent, and opaque
- *Volume*: May be increased
- *Viscosity*: Low, like water
- *Mucin clot test*: Poor, i.e., loose, friable, and flocculent precipitate
- *Cell counts*: Predominantly neutrophils >75%; 80–20,000 WBCs/mm^3
- *Gram stain*: *Staphylococcus* +/=/-, *Streptococcus* ±, and *Neisseria* depending on etiology
- *Culture*: Positive
- *Glucose level*: Low
- *Clinical*: Trauma, history of surgery, fever, swollen, and red joint.

Tuberculous Arthritis

- *Color*: Turbid and yellow; rice bodies may be seen.
- *Volume*: May be increased
- *Viscosity*: Low
- *Mucin clot test*: Poor
- *Cell counts*: About 25,000/mm^3; about 50% lymphocytes
- *Synovial biopsy*: It shows tubercles with epithelioid cells and Langhans type of giant cells.
- *Clinical*: Evening rise of temperature and monoarticular usually knee or hip joint.

Noninflammatory Arthritis: Osteoarthritis/Traumatic

- *Color*: Yellow, clear, and bloody in traumatic; rice bodies may be seen in osteoarthritis (evidence of wear and tear)
- *Volume*: Not increased
- *Viscosity*: High

- *Mucin clot test*: Good, i.e., firm, hard ropy, and nonfriable
- *Cell counts*: <2,000 WBCs/mm^3; <25% are polymorphs
- *Microscopy*: Fragments of cartilage in osteoarthritis
- *Clinical*: Painful joints, swollen, age related in osteoarthritis

Rheumatoid Arthritis

- *Color*: Turbid and yellow greenish
- *Volume*: Equivocal/Increased
- *Viscosity*: Low
- *Mucin clot test*: Poor
- *Cell counts*: <15,000–20,000 WBCs/mm^3; 75% polymorphs
- *Protein*: Markedly elevated
- *Microscopy*: Hypersegmented nuclei and a marked vacuolated cytoplasm
- Intracytoplasmic globules of deoxyribonucleic acid (DNA) identified by Feulgen stain representing ingested nuclear debris from degenerative leukocytes
- *Rheumatoid arthritis cells or rhagocytes or inclusion body cells*: In an unstained wet preparation and with an ordinary microscope, the SF show intracytoplasmic inclusions in polymorphs ranging from 0.5 to 2 μ in size. These are proteinaceous masses composed of immunoglobulin G (IgG), IgM, and complement components. Immunofluorescent stains have shown the inclusions to be the result of neutrophils taking up immune complexes from the fluid.
- *Cholesterol crystals*: Positive
- *Immunology*: RA factor Positive

Gout

- *Color*: Yellow to milky; turbid
- *Volume*: Equivocal/Increased
- *Viscosity*: Low
- *Mucin clot test*: Poor
- *Cell counts*: 10,000–12,000 WBCs/mm^3; 60–70% polymorphs
- *Microscopy*: Urate crystals, short rods with rounded ends, and needle like (yellow color on polarization—negative birefringence)
- *Clinical*: Joints are red and swollen.

Pseudogout

- *Color*: Yellow; slightly cloudy
- *Volume*: Equivocal/Increased
- *Viscosity*: Low
- *Mucin clot test*: Good to poor
- *Cell counts*: 10,000–12,000 WBCs/mm^3; 25–50% polymorphs
- *Microscopy*: Calcium pyrophosphate dihydrate crystals which are rhomboid shaped with sharp corners (blue color on polarization-positive birefringence)
- *Clinical*: Similar to gout—swollen painful joints

Systemic Lupus Erythematosus

- *Color*: Yellow to slightly turbid
- *Volume*: Not increased
- *Viscosity*: High
- *Mucin clot test*: Good
- *Cell counts*: 5,000 WBCs/mm^3; <10% polymorphs
- *Immunology*: Antinuclear antibody (ANA) positive; other nuclear antibodies positive; LE cell positive
- *Clinical*: Associated with clinical features of SLE

In conclusion, a careful complete examination of the SF and clinical correlation may help in diagnosing the type of arthritis in question.

CONCLUSION

A SF examination therefore gives information not only as regards to the local condition of the joint but is able to give insight into the systemic/metabolic condition of the patient.

REFERENCES

1. Eisenberg JM, Schumacher HR, Davidson PK, Kaufmann L. Usefulness of synovial fluid analysis in the evaluation of joint effusions. Use of threshold analysis and likelihood ratios to assess a diagnostic test. Arch Intern Med. 1984;144(4):715-9.
2. Dieppe P, Swan A. Identification of crystals in synovial fluid. Ann Rheum Dis. 1999;58(5):261-3.
3. Swan A, Chapman B, Heap P, Seward H, Dieppe P. Submicroscopic crystals in osteoarthritic synovial fluids. Ann Rheum Dis. 1994;53(7):467-70.

CHAPTER 5

Urine Examination

INTRODUCTION

Urine cytology is a common investigation done to exclude urinary tract infection and in symptomatic and suspected cases of urothelial cancer and high-risk patients. High-risk persons for carcinoma are those exposed to alkylating agents, aromatic amines, with schistosomiasis and chronic smokers. It is a noninvasive and inexpensive technique. Old cases of carcinoma of the urinary bladder can be easily followed up. Screening tests for bladder carcinoma include microscopic urinalysis for hematuria and urine cytology. Patients with positive findings are referred to an urologist for further evaluation.

SAMPLE COLLECTION[1]

- All urine samples for examination should be fresh and the patient is asked to void the sample when he comes to the laboratory. A random midstream sample is collected in a clean container and in a sterile bottle for culture.
- In order to negate presence of a carcinoma, three consecutive morning samples (which yield maximum cells) are examined before a negative report is given.
- Catheterized specimen may be taken in bedridden patients.
- Bladder washings
- *Ileal conduit*: Surveillance of ureters and renal pelvis postcystectomy.

PROCESSING AND EXAMINATION[1,2]

Processing methods include simple centrifugation, cytospin, and slow sedimentation preparations. The sample is centrifuged for 10 minutes at 1,500 rpm; one or two drops of sediment are placed on a glass slide, spread as a smear and fixed immediately. The sample can be refrigerated at 2–8° for a couple of hours to preserve it if not being examined immediately.

Urine microscopy consists of examination for epithelial cells, red blood cells (RBCs), leukocytes, and study of casts and other elements such as crystals and abnormal cells. The cells found in normal urine come from either the desquamation of the lining of the urinary tract epithelium or from the circulating blood. Casts on the other hand are formed in renal tubules.

Urine microscopy can be done on unstained and stained preparations. Examination of unstained preparation is done in rapid scanning of the sample.

- *Examination of an unstained preparation*: A drop of the sediment is placed on a slide and cover-slipped. All cellular elements can be visualized in an unstained preparation—leukocytes, histiocytes, epithelial and neoplastic cells as well as casts by lowering the condenser and using the fine adjustment. Better delineation between various cells and elements (casts) is done by phase contrast microscopy. The interference of the diffracted rays by the specimen provides a darker image contrast which helps in revealing details within the cells. *Phase contrast microscopy* shows details where stained slides are unavailable. By these methods, the red cells appear as refractile gray biconcave disks, while the white cells appear granular with lobulated nuclei. The name "glitter cells" is given to neutrophils with many cytoplasmic particles, as a result of their appearance at phase contrast; characteristic of chronic pyelonephritis. When stained with gentian violet, these appear pale blue and contain refractile granules that exhibit "Brownian movement". Epithelial cells can be differentiated because of their round nucleus.

Polarizing filters: They are best used to distinguish crystals and fibers from cellular and protein cast material. With the addition of a retardation plate, crystals may be further identified as being positively or negatively birefringent.

- *Stained smears*: The Papanicolaou and hematoxylin and eosin stains are used.

Cytology of Normal Urine

- Occasional red cells, 3–4 WBCs/hpf, and a few renal tubular epithelial cells
- *Urothelial cells*: Intermediate and superficial (umbrella) cells in voided urine, besides these basal cells appear in catheterized urine, squamous cells—vaginal contamination or from trigone of bladder, rarely prostate and seminal vesicle epithelial cells, renal tubular cells and casts, crystals, inflammatory cells, and degenerated intestinal epithelial cells (ileal conduit).
- *Umbrella cells*: Low nuclear/cytoplasmic (N/C) ratio, usually seen as flat or polygonal cells with a convex smooth border which corresponds to the lumen of the urinary bladder. Pale finely granular chromatin, smooth nuclear shapes, multinucleation is common, and cytoplasm is transparent
- *Intermediate and basal cells*: High N/C ratio, chromatin is darker, nuclei smaller than that of superficial cells, nuclei-round, even nuclear spacing.

Cytology in Carcinoma: Urothelial Carcinoma

Changes of carcinoma are reflected mainly in the nucleus as nuclear enlargement and hyperchromasia. Such cells appear intermittently at first and may be shed regularly later. **Box 1** shows the John Hopkin's grading for reporting urinary cytology specimens:

BOX 1 The Johns Hopkins Template for Reporting Urinary Cytology Specimens.[3]

Negative for urothelial atypia or malignancy (NUAM):
- *Urothelial carcinoma (UC)*:
  - High-grade urothelial carcinoma (HGUC)
  - Low-grade urothelial carcinoma (LGUC)
- *Atypical urothelial cells (AUCs)*:
  - Of undetermined significance (AUC-US)
  - Cannot exclude HGUC (AUC-H)
- Other (specify type of cancer)
- Inadequate

In frank carcinomas and undifferentiated tumors (UC and HGUC):
- In specimens that are diagnosed as HGUC, the cells are large; nuclei possess coarsely granular and condensed chromatin; show irregular membranes and/or large nucleoli
- Cells appear in groups and vary in size and shape
- The features of malignant cells arising from a transitional cell carcinoma of the ureter or the renal pelvis are essentially similar to those of malignant cells from a transitional cell carcinoma of the bladder

Atypical urothelial carcinoma, high grade cannot be ruled out (AUC-H):
- Most cases reported as AUC-H prove to be malignant
- The most common morphologic features observed in the AUC-H specimens are single cells with hyperchromasia, irregular nuclear borders, increased N/C ratio, and anisonucleosis
- In AUC-H specimens, the atypical cells are often small with marked hyperchromasia that obscures nuclear detail

Atypical urothelial carcinoma of undetermined significance (AUC-US):
- May or may not prove cancerous and lack the features outlined above for AUC-H
- May show mild nuclear enlargement but no irregularity in nuclear membranes

Low-grade urothelial carcinomas remain a challenge at cytology
- Cell size and nuclei mildly increased but chromatin is fine
- Increased N/C ratio
- Elongated nuclei and cell clusters in loose papillae
- Cells may be numerous, resemble urothelium
- Nuclei eccentric, nucleoli are absent, cytoplasm homogenous
- Nuclear membrane irregularity is seen

The Paris System of Urine Cytology[4-6]

The Paris System Working Group, consisting of cytopathologists, surgical pathologists, and urologists, organized at the 2013 International Congress of Cytology, conceived a standardized platform on which to base cytologic interpretation of urine samples. It is centered around the HGUC. The following are the categories:

- Negative for HGUC
- Atypical urothelial cells
- Suspicious for HGUC
- High-grade urothelial carcinoma
- Low-grade urothelial neoplasm
- Other malignancies, both primary and secondary

Ancillary tests for detection of urothelial carcinoma:[7] Recommended by the Paris system is to detect the expression of altered or abnormally expressed subcellular material (proteins, DNA, etc.) in urothelial neoplasms, which is found in tumor cells and/or the urine specimen when the proteins are either excreted or leaked from degenerating tumor cells. The Food and Drug Administration (FDA) approved test is the UroVysion assay. It is done to detect aneuploidy for chromosomes 3, 7, 17, and loss of the 9p21 locus via fluorescence in situ hybridization (FISH) [UroVysion fluorescent in situ hybridization (U-FISH)] on urine specimens. Briefly this is done as follows:

- The basic principle of this is that in Pap-stained smears pretreatment with protease uncovers target DNA and exposes single-strand target DNA.
- Decolorization is not mandatory since the stain is removed during further phases of FISH procedure (if using the archival slides, remove the coverslip, and mounting medium in xylene).
- Place the slides in 1% acid alcohol (HCl and 70% alcohol) overnight or until decolorized.
- The U-FISH assay can subsequently be conducted either manually or automatically.
- U-FISH probes should be prepared accordingly and applied to the selected area of slide and the area should be cover-slipped and sealed immediately to ensure optimal conditions.
- Hybridization of probes to target DNA sequences follows under appropriate conditions.
- The procedure is finished with posthybridization washes to remove excessive probes.
- Slides should be dried in a dark area.
- The procedure should be validated in each individual laboratory, together with positive and negative controls, to ensure optimal hybridization.
- Afterward the specimen chosen for analysis is stained by DAPI (4′,6-diamidino-2-phenylindole) solution. Slides are cover-slipped and stored at –20°C in the dark until analysis.
- The Duet™ system workstation or the Bioview Duet™ system are the two systems for analysis.

Other tests: Presence of Bard bladder tumor antigen (BTA) test, NMP-22 based on nuclear matrix protein 22—these are increased in urothelial carcinoma, microsatellite analysis, and hyaluronic acid production are some of the advanced markers used to detect urothelial neoplasia as recommended by the Paris system.

Other techniques like ThinPrep[8] for detecting low-grade urothelial neoplasms: Diagnosing LGUC on cytologic specimen is difficult, because of the well-differentiated nature of the tumor cells which display only a slight degree of atypia, and closely resemble normal urothelial cells. Separating them from reactive, regenerative, and reparative changes is not always possible. Increased N/C ratio, irregular nuclear membrane, and cytoplasmic homogeneity were three key features reported by Raab et al. for diagnosing LGUC in cytospin specimens. Xin et al. 2003 have reiterated that ThinPrep provides well-preserved, cleaner specimens without significantly altering the morphology. The three key criteria applied in cytospin specimens to diagnose LGUC were reproducible in ThinPrep specimens.

Cytology in squamous cell carcinoma results from chronic Schistosoma haematobium infection. Exfoliation of cells recognizable as being squamous in origin with hyperchromatic nuclei and elongated, spindled, and fusiform shapes. It has to be differentiated from condyloma acuminatum of the bladder, metastatic squamous cell carcinoma, and extension from the gynecologic tract.

Cytology in primary adenocarcinoma: It is rare in the urinary bladder. Cells tend to occur in groups and clusters and show a vacuolated cytoplasm and hyperchromatic nucleus. Appearances are similar to an adenocarcinoma occurring elsewhere with a tendency to gland formation.

Reasons for False-positive Diagnosis of Malignancy

Chronic urolithiasis gives rise to pleomorphic transitional cells, multinucleation, and mechanical avulsion of pseudopapillary groups of transitional epithelium; radiation therapy with enlargement and bizarre appearance of nuclei; chemotherapy—degenerative changes with frayed cell borders; enlarged hyperchromatic but smudgy nuclei; vacuolated cytoplasm; irregular dark nucleoli; multinucleation; papillary aggregates also occur as a result of instrumentation mimicking low-grade neoplasia and giving a false-positive diagnosis. Seminal vesicle epithelial cells are uncommon but show atypia mistaken for carcinoma. Reactive atypia whatever the cause still shows even distributed chromatin as compared to carcinoma.

Reasons for False-negative Diagnosis of Malignancy

Low-grade neoplasms: In the absence of a tissue pattern which includes a delicate fibrovascular stalk, many papillary transitional cell tumors may differ little from normal that they can hardly be considered as neoplasms; prolonged exposure of cells to urine has detrimental effect on morphology and interpretation due to low pH.

NON-NEOPLASTIC CONDITIONS

- *Viral infections*: Polyoma viruses of the BK and JC strain often infect transitional epithelial cells and the infection lies dormant within these cells. Subtype I of the BK virus is the dominant one and has worldwide distribution. A lowering of the immune status and/or an immunocompromised condition can lead to a reactivation of latent polyomaviruses within the epithelial cells resulting in the shedding of viral particles and infected cells into the urine; these are "decoy cells" with intranuclear viral inclusions. Decoy cells often contain polyoma-BK-viruses and are easily

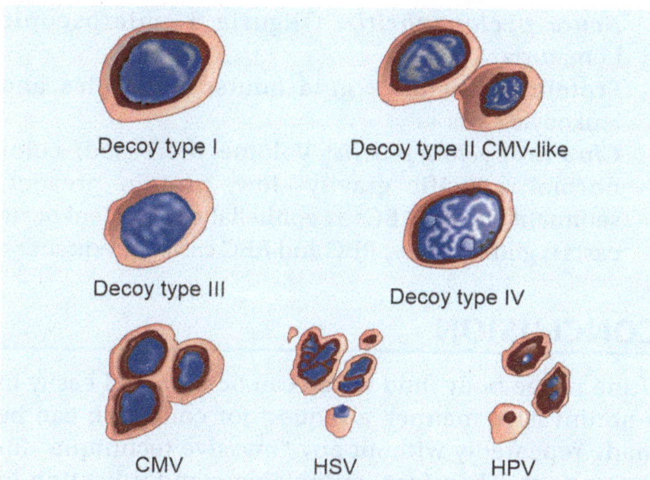

FIG. 1: A diagrammatic representation of the morphology of the cells in various viral infections as outlined in the Table 1.
(CMV: cytomegalovirus; HPV: human papillomavirus; HSV: herpes simplex virus)

identified in the Papanicolaou-stained urine smears. Decoy cells can also be detected in the unstained urinary sediment by phase contrast microscopy. The name "decoy cell" is a descriptive term for epithelial cells with intranuclear viral inclusion bodies that can have different phenotypes (types 1 through 4). Their morphological appearances **(Fig. 1)** as well as features in all viral infections are outlined in the **Table 1**.

Although the BK virus (decoy cells) can mimic HGUC, BK viral changes are observed more commonly in AUC-US (undetermined significance) specimens than in AUC-H specimens.

- *Parasitic infections*: Schistosomiasis—numerous squamous cells. Ova rarely seen.
- *Trichomonas vaginalis*: Organism may rarely be seen in urine of females.
- *Cytology of malakoplakia*: Cells with single or multiple Michaelis-Gutmann bodies. These may vary in size, 5–10 µ and are round laminated and basophilic. These may show calcified cytoplasmic inclusions. Such cells appear in the urine more commonly after a biopsy as malakoplakia is separated from the lumen by normal bladder epithelium.

Cytology of Diseased Urine

- *Casts*: Hyaline (mucoprotein) and granular casts—may occur secondary to dehydration, fever, exercise, etc.
- *Crystals*: It is a common finding of no clinical significance in most cases; but crystal analysis is part of routine urinalysis; uric acid—most common, variable shape; triple phosphate—prism-shaped and resemble coffin lids; ammonium biurate—"thorn apples" (dissolve on addition of acetic acid); calcium oxalate—oval and dumbbell-shaped.
- *Pathologic crystals*: Much less common, bilirubin (brown granules and needles), cholesterol, cystine (colorless, hexagonal plates) seen in cystinuria, soluble in water, resembles uric acid crystals but dissolve in dilute HCl, whereas uric acid does not, and leucine (spheres with radiating striations) similar to fat globules but can be differentiated as they are not soluble in acids and alkalies and tyrosine (slender needles in sheeves). Leucine and tyrosine crystals occur in liver damage; sulfonamide crystals—sheaves of wheat with central binding, petals, needles, etc., seen in drug therapy.
- *Red blood cell casts*: Clear cylinders with RBCs (mucoprotein and red cells), acute glomerulonephritis, and pyelonephritis; on anticoagulants; large doses of aspirin, subacute bacterial endocarditis.
- *WBCs*: "Glitter cells" seen in infections, pyelonephritis, and transplant rejection.

TABLE 1: Cytological features in various viral infections.[9]

Virus	Cytological features Decoy cells
Polyomaviruses	*Type 1*: Classic decoy cells show large, amorphous ground-glass like intranuclear viral inclusion bodies and a condensed rim of chromatin
	Type 2: Granular intranuclear inclusion bodies surrounded by a clear halo, i.e., CMV-like
	Type 3: Decoy cells with granular chromatin and no halo; sometimes multinucleated
	Type 4: Vesicular nuclei with a distinct network of often coarsely clumped chromatin; nucleoli can be found
Adenoviruses	Nuclear features are identical to those seen with polyomaviruses; type 1 decoy cells are most common
Herpes simplex virus	Large multinucleated cells with nuclear molding, well-defined nuclear inclusions of the ground-glass type (Cowdry A)
Cytomegalovirus (CMV)	• Large cells containing prominent intra-nuclear viral inclusion bodies surrounded by clear halos ("owl's eye" appearance) • Additionally, eosinophilic cytoplasmic viral inclusion bodies can be found. Ground-glass appearance of nuclear inclusion bodies is uncommon

Source: Adapted from Madame Curie Bioscience Database [Internet]. Austin (TX): Landes Bioscience; 2000-2013.

- *Renal tubular casts*: In tubular necrosis, heavy doses of analgesics and renal parenchymal disease.
- *Bacteria*: Seen as rods or chains of cocci in infection anywhere along genitourinary tract.
- *Fat bodies*: Oval globules seen in diabetes and nephrotic syndrome
- *Fungal inflammations*: The most common fungus observed in the urinary sediment is *Candida albicans*. In the urine, the organism is observed commonly as fungal spores but pseudohyphae may occasionally be observed.
- *Acute glomerulonephritis*: Oliguria, brown or smoky urine; high specific gravity; proteins <5 g/24 hours; sediment shows numerous red cells and red cell casts.
- *Chronic glomerulonephritis*: Volume increased; color—normal; specific gravity—low and fixed at 1,010; proteins +; red cells ±; granular and waxy casts present in large numbers.
- *Acute pyelonephritis*: Oliguria ±; microscopic hematuria
- Proteins present <2 g/24 hours; leukocytes and leukocyte casts ++
- *Chronic pyelonephritis*: Volume increased; color normal; specific gravity—low; protein present; sediment shows WBCs ±; epithelial casts ±; leukocyte casts+; glitter cells +; RBC and RBC casts infrequent.

CONCLUSION

Urine is one body fluid which can be obtained easily in a noninvasive manner, a request for collection can be made repeatedly without any "invasive technique" for the patient. Therefore, optimizing standardization of reporting can enhance diagnostic accuracy in several urinary as well as systemic diseases.

REFERENCES

1. Shariff S, Kaler AK. Principles and Interpretation of Laboratory Practices in Surgical Pathology. New Delhi: Jaypee Brothers Medical Publishers (P) Ltd.; 2016.
2. VandenBussche CJ, Sathiyamoorthy S, Owens CL, Burroughs FH, Rosenthal DL, Guan H. The Johns Hopkins Hospital template for urologic cytology samples: parts II and III: improving the predictability of indeterminate results in urinary cytologic samples: an outcomes and cytomorphologic study. Cancer Cytopathol. 2013;121(1):21-8.
3. Rosenthal DL, Vandenbussche CJ, Burroughs FH, Sathiyamoorthy S, Guan H, Owens C. The Johns Hopkins Hospital template for urologic cytology samples: part I-creating the template. Cancer Cytopathol. 2013;121(1):15-20.
4. Rosenthal DL, Wojcik EM, Kurtycz DFI (Eds). The Paris System for Reporting Urinary Cytology. Cham, Switzerland: Springer International Publishing; 2016.
5. Barkan GA, Wojcik EM, Nayar R, Savic-Prince S, Quek ML, Kurtycz DF, et al. The Paris System for Reporting Urinary Cytology: The Quest to Develop a Standardized Terminology. Acta Cytol. 2016;60(3):185-97.
6. Bubendorf L, Caraway NP, Fischer AH, Katz RL, Olson MT, Schmitt F, et al. Ancillary studies in urinary cytology. In: Rosenthal DL, Wojcik EM, Kurtycz DFI (Eds). The Paris System for Reporting Urinary Cytology, 1st edition. Cham, Switzerland: Springer International Publishing; 2016.
7. Bonberg N, Taeger D, Gawrych K, Johnen G, Banek S, Schwentner C, et al. Chromosomal instability and bladder cancer: the UroVysion(TM) test in the UroScreen study. BJU Int. 2013;112(4):E372-82.
8. Xin W, Raab SS, Michael CW. Low-grade urothelial carcinoma: reappraisal of the cytologic criteria on ThinPrep. Diagn Cytopathol. 2003;29(3):125-9.
9. Singh HK, Bubendorf L, Mihatsch MJ, Drachenberg C, Nickeleit V. Urine Cytology Findings of Polyomavirus Infections. Madame Curie Bioscience Database [Internet]. Austin (TX): Landes Bioscience; 2000-2013.

CHAPTER 6

Central Nervous System Cytology

CEREBROSPINAL FLUID

INTRODUCTION

Cerebrospinal fluid (CSF) is a clear and watery extracellular fluid that surrounds the brain and the spinal cord. It is an ultrafiltrate of blood plasma and is contained within the subarachnoid space and central canal of the spine. It is produced by the choroid plexus in the lateral ventricles and about 150–250 mL is present in the subarachnoid space.

NORMAL CEREBROSPINAL FLUID

The pH of CSF is close to that of plasma; osmolarity is 295 mOsm/L; protein is 20–40 mg/dL; Na is 14–15 mmol/dL; chloride is 12–13 mmol/dL; and glucose is 50–75 mg/dL. The pressure of CSF is 70–180 mm Hg.

SAMPLE COLLECTION

The sample is obtained by doing a lumbar puncture and is routinely collected in three tubes as follows. Tube 1 is frozen for chemistry and immunology; tube 2 at room temperature is taken for microbiology; and tube 3 sample for cell counts, differential, and cytology. Processing should be immediate but if a delay in processing is anticipated, the sample should be refrigerated.

The main indications for CSF cytology are:

- The diagnosis of intracranial or spinal tumors which are suspected to seed the CSF.
- To confirm or rule out CSF involvement in lymphoma or leukemia and follow up on treatment.
- To determine the nature of cerebral infection

PREPARATION OF MATERIAL

- CSF samples are usually sent in small amounts the lumbar tap being done by the clinician. They have to be handled with care and processed immediately. Urine and CSF preserve only for 1–2 hours on refrigeration.
- Considering the low volume and cellularity, CSF specimen should be processed by using a cytospin or by the slow sedimentation technique.
- Counts are done using 1% toluidine blue as the diluting fluid.
- *Staining*: A Papanicolaou stain is used. Special stains to demonstrate microorganisms are the Gomori's methenamine silver (GMS) and periodic acid-Schiff (PAS) and mucicarmine to demonstrate fungi.
- Air-dried smears are stained with Romanowsky stain such as Leishman or May-Grunwald Giemsa (MGG).

EXAMINATION OF CEREBROSPINAL FLUID[1,2]

Normal cytology: Cerebrospinal fluid is mostly acellular as the blood-brain (BB) barrier prevents the entry of cells except a few mononuclear cells which are mostly lymphocytes and occasional monocytes. Ependymal and meningeal cells are very rarely encountered.

Bacterial meningitis: Cerebrospinal fluid is turbid; pressure is elevated; proteins are elevated; glucose and chloride are reduced; and the cells are increased, mostly polymorphonuclear neutrophils about 1,000–10,000/μL.

Viral meningitis: Clear, pressure is mildly elevated, normal to mild increase in proteins, and glucose and chloride are normal, 0–300 WBCs/μL, mostly lymphocytes.

Tubercular meningitis: Opaque, cobweb formation; pressure may be increased or decreased; cells 100–600 WBCs/μL, mostly lymphocytes; chlorides and glucose are reduced proteins and may vary between 50 and 300 depending on spinal block.

In early stage of tuberculosis meningitis, the CSF is rich in a panorama of cells which includes transformed lymphocytes, plasma cells, activated macrophages, and polymorphonuclear leukocytes. With therapy, the polymorphonuclear leukocytes decreases, lymphocytes persist, and multinucleated giant cells have also been seen.

Fungal meningitis: The most common fungus causing meningitis in the immunocompromised or debilitated patients is *Cryptococcus neoformans*. These are round yeast organisms measuring 4–10 μ with thick mucoid capsules which stain readily with mucicarmine, PAS, or India ink preparations. Cryptococcal antigen from CSF is thought to be the best test for diagnosis of cryptococcal meningitis in terms of sensitivity.

Other fungi, such as *Candida albicans*, *Aspergillus*, and *Mucor* have also been observed in the immnuno-compromised patients.

Reactive changes in cells: Lymphocytes in reactive response may transform to immunoblasts and monocytes to macrophages in chronic inflammation; monocyte may also transform to macrophages and engulf yellow radiopaque material postmyelograms procedures; eosinophils appear in parasitic infections; hemosiderin indicates a past hemorrhagic event. Plasma cells indicate either a chronic inflammatory process or multiple myeloma.

Squamous cells or anucleate squames, bone marrow cells, and cartilage cells originate from the skin or vertebrae due to accidental contamination during the procedure.

Malignant Tumors[3,4]

Medulloblastoma and related tumors are the predominant childhood tumors that are seen seeding the CSF among the primary brain tumors. These tumors are characterized by monotonous small round to oval cells with dark staining nuclei, often arranged in rosettes around a central lumen-like area filled with neurofilaments. These highly malignant tumors are capable of metastasis and are the only tumors of the central nervous system (CNS) which are consistently shed into it. A close differential is lymphoma but this rarely forms rosettes and the cells are rounder than oval. Markers may clinch the diagnosis.

Lymphomas/leukemias occur particularly in a setting of acquired immunodeficiency syndrome (AIDS). Malignant lymphoma with primary CNS involvement is also seen in organ transplant recipients with associated immunosuppression.

In acute leukemia and chronic leukemia showing blast crisis, blast cells are identified in the PAP-stained smears because of their large size (2–4 times that of normal lymphocyte) and the presence of nucleoli and nuclear protrusions. A Romanowsky stain (MGG or Leishman's) highlights the nucleoli more clearly. CSF involvement in chronic myelogenous leukemia as such is very uncommon. Metastasis to brain can occur from any neoplasm but spread to and seeding into the CSF particularly occurs in:

- *Malignant lymphoma*: Cerebromeningeal involvement in non-Hodgkin's lymphoma is sufficiently frequent to warrant examination of CSF. Cells generally lie singly with nuclei showing irregular contours and protrusions in the form of small tongue-shaped structures. Large cell lymphomas have in addition prominent large and irregular nucleoli. Sequential samples of CSF are done to monitor therapy.
- *Plasmacytoma:* A diagnosis of plasma cell myeloma is considered when plasma cells form the sole population of cells in CSF sediment. Isolated plasma cells may, however, be observed in Hodgkin's disease and in chronic inflammatory processes.

Epithelial Tumors

The most common identified metastatic carcinomas in CSF are of mammary and bronchogenic origin.

- *Bronchogenic:* Small cell carcinomas are often shed singly or in clusters. Sometimes the cells are arranged in short chains with nuclear molding resembling a "string of vertebrae". Small cell carcinoma in CSF occurs at an early stage and has led to regimens of aggressive treatment.

  Adenocarcinomas and epidermoid carcinomas shed large tumor cells, often in clusters.
- *Mammary carcinoma:* Ductal type carcinomas are readily recognizable and may show cytoplasmic protrusions. Cells have large nuclei, prominent nucleoli, and sometimes exhibit mitotic activity.

CEREBROSPINAL FLUID BIOMARKERS IN DISEASES[5]

- Biochemical assays and biomarker analysis in the CSF have thrown fresh perspective in the diagnosis of several diseases such as early Alzheimer's disease. The neurodegeneration seen here is reflected by structural magnetic resonance imaging (MRI) changes and the core CSF biomarker proteins Aβ42 and tau. CSF Aβ42 and tau are linked to distinct patterns of atrophy.

Reduced Aβ42 is associated with isolated hippocampal atrophy, elevated tau levels are related to thinning in cortical brain of Alzheimer's disease. The new diagnostic workup for preclinical Alzheimer's disease comprises biomarker-based studies and criteria.

- Other biomarkers in CSF have significance in amyotrophic lateral sclerosis and viral meningo-encephalitis as a result of altered brain metabolism.

SQUASH CYTOLOGY IN CENTRAL NERVOUS SYSTEM[3-6]

Squash cytology is a well-established simple, rapid, and inexpensive intraoperative diagnostic tool. First introduced in 1930, it has dependable accuracy in CNS tumors. The soft CNS tissue is not ideally suited for frozen section diagnosis but amenable to preparing squash smears for interpretation as well as touch cytology, as a rapid means to arrive at a diagnosis in order to proceed further with surgery.

Smear or squash preparation: Procedure—any tissue can be squash prepared but the soft brain tissue lends itself best to this smear making. All cell types are readily identified by this method. A small piece of tissue about 1 mm is placed at one end of a plain glass slide. A second glass slide may be kept perpendicular on it to gently crush the specimen and then drawn across the slide to produce a uniformly spread cellular smear. Following smearing, the slide is immediately fixed in acetic alcohol (95% alcohol + 5% glacial acetic acid).

Staining is done routinely as for other smears. Rapid hematoxylin and eosin (H&E), Diff-Quik Giemsa, and Leishman or aqueous toluidine blue can also be used. The technique is suitable for small pieces of soft tumors, such as gliomas, soft meningiomas, choroid plexus papilloma, hemangioblastomas, and metastatic tumors. Most centers use this as an intraoperative procedure for diagnosis. Intraoperative diagnosis by squash cytology is of utmost importance to neurosurgeons on the table in decision-making and optimizing surgical procedures. The role of squash cytology has increased with the advent of stereotactic biopsies which provide very tiny tissue and in centers where neurosurgical departments are busy. All pathologists/cytologists should familiarize themselves in the interpretation of such smears. The application of squash preparations, frozen section, and imprint cytology can be used as an intraoperative procedure adding new dimensions to morphological interpretation. Tissue if remaining should be taken for formalin fixation and paraffin embedding and other techniques. In correlation with MRI findings, squash cytology has high sensitivity and specificity in diagnosing CNS lesions.

TOUCH/IMPRINT PREPARATIONS

Touch smears in CNS cytology are invaluable. They may be complementary to squash preparations or even biopsy.

- Touch the surface of the tissue with a clean glass slide
- Air dry the smears and stain it with Giemsa
- The technique is valuable in the case of lymphomas and metastatic carcinomas for rapid diagnosis. Morphology is excellent with minimal artifacts.

CONCLUSION

The cytological examination on CSF should be done with utmost care as it is a specimen which cannot be obtained easily, preservation alters morphology and immediate cytological examination yields optimal results. It is a low-volume sample which needs to be processed by cytospin or slow sedimentation preparations.

REFERENCES

1. Seehusen DA, Reeves MM, Fomin DA. Cerebrospinal fluid analysis. Am Fam Physician. 2003;68(6):1103-8.
2. Kennedy PGE, Quan PL, Lipkin WI. Viral Encephalitis of Unknown Cause: Current Perspective and Recent Advances. Viruses. 2017;9(6):138.
3. Patil SS, Kudrimoti JK, Agarwal RD, Jadhav MV, Chuge A. Utility of squash smear cytology in intraoperative diagnosis of central nervous system tumors. J Cytol. 2016;33(4):205-9.
4. Mitra S, Kumar M, Sharma V, Mukhopadhyay D. Squash preparation: A reliable diagnostic tool in the intraoperative diagnosis of central nervous system tumors. J Cytol. 2010;27(3):81-5.
5. Kulic L, Unschuld PG. Recent advances in cerebrospinal fluid biomarkers for the detection of preclinical Alzheimer's disease. Curr Opin Neurol. 2016;29(6):749-55.
6. Chakrabarty D, Chaudhuri S, Maity P, Chatterjee U, Ghosh S. Utility of Squash Cytology in Spinal Lesions with Special Reference to Ki67 Immunostain. Acta Cytol. 2019;63(5):424-30.

CHAPTER 7

Respiratory Tract Cytology

INTRODUCTION

Sputum is a mucous-like secretion from the lung and bronchi. It contains plasma and mucus secretions from the lining and submucosal bronchial glands. This may be mixed with secretions from salivary glands and oral cavity.

Cytologic examination of a pulmonary lesion can be approached in several ways depending on the location of the lesion/neoplasm. "Sputum cytology" is exfoliative cytology based on the spontaneous shedding of cells from the lining of the bronchial tree, trachea, larynx as well as abnormal mucosal, and submucosal lesions. Carcinoma of the lungs and bronchi sheds cells into the sputum and viewing these exfoliated cells confirms the diagnosis of carcinoma.

Submucosal tumors which behave stubbornly in not exfoliating cells (carcinoid), neoplasms in the smaller bronchi, and bronchioles can be approached by the transbronchial fine needle aspiration cytology (FNAC) and bronchial brushings. Peripherally located lesions can be assessed by the transthoracic fine needle aspiration (FNA) approach. Bronchial washings are of value in disseminated lung infections like *Pneumocystis jirovecii* and in lesions of smaller segments of the bronchial tree not amenable to FNAC or brushings.

SPUTUM CYTOLOGY[1,2]

Indications

- To determine the presence of tumor and to classify it as accurately as possible. Sputum is the most easy and accessible method of screening for lung carcinoma and yields good results for centrally located lesions.
- Examination of three consecutive early morning samples should be seen before declaring a negative result in carcinoma.
- Sputum cytology is a noninvasive method of diagnosing diseases like tuberculosis, lung infections like aspergillomas, and *Cryptococcus neoformans*.
- In the detection of chronic diseases as allergic bronchitis and tuberculosis.
- Detection of viral and fungal infections
- In the diagnosis of *P. jirovecii* infection

Sample Collection

- Spontaneously produced fresh sputum is best obtained as a deep cough sample early in the morning. The patient is instructed to take a few deep breaths before coughing out from deep down the chest. It is advisable to give plenty of water to drink the previous night.
- Where sputum production is sparse, aerosol-induced sputum (induced by inhalation of a heated mixture of sodium chloride and propylene glycol or induction by using neostigmine) yields better results.
- Best results are obtained when fresh cellular samples are smeared onto slides, fixed, and stained. Ammanagi et al.[2] (2012) have suggested the "fresh pick and smear" method, which deals with examination of sputum for blood-tinged, discolored or solid particles, and preparation of smears from these particles.
- Sputum, bronchial aspirates, and mucocele fluids can be refrigerated for 12–14 hours as the mucus forms a coating around the cells and protects them against degeneration to a certain extent. However, when immediate examination is not possible prefixation of

sputum is done in 70% ethyl alcohol or Saccomanno's fixative or CytoLyt solution. However, the results are superior when examined in a fresh state.

Gross examination: It is done before subjecting the sample to smear making:

- Yellow and viscid sputum—lung abscess, pneumonia, bronchitis, and bronchiectasis
- Green colored sputum—*Pseudomonas*, hemophilia, and pneumococcal species
- White and mucoid—bronchial asthma
- Blood stained—tuberculosis, carcinoma, and mitral stenosis
- Watery and blood stained—pulmonary edema
- Rust colored sputum—pneumococcal pneumonia
- Chocolate colored (anchovy sauce like)—amebic lung abscess as an extension from the liver
- Foul smelling—suppurative infections like lung abscess, bronchiectasis, etc.
- Dittrich's plugs[3]—named after Franz Dittrich, a German pathologist, are small to round yellow blobs of mucus 0.5–3 mm in diameter with a characteristic rancid odor seen in suppurative conditions. To be differentiated from sulfur granules of actinomycosis by crushing them as a smear, staining, and examining under microscope.

Processing of Sputum

- *Saccomanno's technique of processing (is the preferred technique):*
  - Principle:
    - Uniform spread of cells on the smear due to blending of the sputum with fixative
    - Sputum is collected in a solution composed of 50% ethyl alcohol and 2% polyethylene glycol (carbowax).
    - This is subsequently broken-up in a food blender, centrifuged and the smears are prepared from the cell button.
  - Advantages:
    - Best method of processing sputum
    - Concentration of the cells is satisfactory.
    - Morphology is good as compared to other prefixation procedures.
  - Disadvantages:
    - Cell to cell relation is disrupted due to blending.
    - Tissue fragments with fungal colonies and bacterial colonies such as actinomycotic and botryomycotic colonies are disrupted.
    - Difficult to classify the type of malignant cells
    - Increased risk of aerosol infection (especially tuberculosis)

ThinPrep Technique[4]

ThinPrep (TP) is an automated liquid-based cytopreparatory technique. ThinPrep 2000, 3000, and 5000 are some of the automated analyzers available commercially, the latter can process up to 160 samples at a stretch.

Principle: Here, sputum is collected in a special CytoLyt solution with mucolytic and hemolyzing effects, leaving of a sample against a clear background devoid of red cells and mucus. It can be used to process aspirates as well as washings after bronchoscopy.

- *Advantages*:
  - Background is clean.
  - Single slide viewing reduces fatigue factor
  - Simultaneous processing of several samples
- *Disadvantage*: High cost of instrument

OTHER METHODS OF OBTAINING DIAGNOSTIC MATERIAL FROM LUNGS

Fiber-optic bronchoscope[5] permits collection of a variety of samples for analysis:

A bronchoscopy is done for:

- Direct visualization of bronchial tree
- Evaluate lung lesions where location is unknown and in unexplained positive sputum cytology.
- Material for culture and special stains for microbiology can be easily obtained.
- *Bronchial aspirate and washing/bronchoalveolar lavage:*
  - Bronchial aspirates are obtained by introducing the bronchoscope in the lower respiratory.
  - Tract and aspirating the secretions by a suction apparatus
  - A lavage or wash is when during the procedure, a saline solution is put through the bronchoscope to wash the airways and reaspirating the same.
  - From the aspirates and washings direct smears, centrifugation with smear preparation from cell buttons, centrifugation with embedding of the cell buttons as cellblocks can be done.

  Indicated when the disease extends into alveoli, e.g., opportunistic infections in immunocompromised patients, silicosis, beryllosis, *P. jirovecii* infection, etc.
- *Bronchial brushings*: Cell samples are obtained with small brushes from the surface of suspected tumor site under the visual fiber-optic bronchoscope.

  Procedure is generally performed prior to biopsy:
  - After brushing, the brush is firmly rolled onto glass slides, which are then fixed in 95% alcohol and stained.

- Agitating the brush in 5 mL of isotonic saline, centrifuging the fluid, and preparing smears from the cell button.
- *Transbronchial needle aspiration (TBNA)*: A thin flexible needle is inserted through the bronchial wall into the suspected lesion via the bronchoscope, and the cellular material is aspirated and processed as for percutaneous biopsies. Specific modification of fine needle aspiration guidance under fluoroscopic and computed tomography (CT) guidance is also performed. TBNA is greatly dependent on the skill of the operator and on the availability of cytopathology support for performing rapid on-site evaluation (ROSE) of the cytological sample.
  Indications of TBNA:
  - External bronchial compression
  - Upper lobe lesions
  - Lung neoplasm which has not breached the mucosa.
  - Hilar lesions, e.g., mediastinal tumors, Hodgkin lymphoma, sarcoidosis, and other granulomatous diseases (under guidance)
  - Intraluminal lesions which are necrotic with submucosal (carcinoids and bronchial gland tumor) extensions.
  - In the staging of intrathoracic malignancies
- *Transthoracic fine needle aspiration cytology (TTNA):* A fine needle (length 10–20 cm) is passed through the chest wall into the pulmonary and mediastinal mass, visualized by fluoroscopy, CT, or US guidance. The patient is asked to hold his breadth during the procedure. Core needle biopsies can also be performed following FNA. The yield of TTNA is lower for central than for peripheral lesions. Imprint cytology of the biopsies can be studies for a quick impression.
  Indications of TTNA: Peripheral lung cancers; diffuse infective processes
- *Endoscopic ultrasound-guided fine needle aspiration* (EUS-FNA) has become a popular method to diagnose a variety of intrathoracic masses. EUS-FNA is used to yield material from lymph stations through a transesophageal approach for staging purposes and mediastinal staging of non-small cell lung cancer (NSCLC) patients.

All material from FNAC is processed by making direct/indirect smears as FNAC specimens of other sites.

MICROSCOPY OF SALIENT LESIONS AT CYTOLOGY[6-9]

To determine that the specimen is sputum and not superficially coughed up saliva, it is essential to see the presence of either ciliated epithelial cells or alveolar macrophages or both apart from squamous epithelial cells. Presence of epithelial cells alone indicates saliva **(compare Figs. 1 and 2)**.

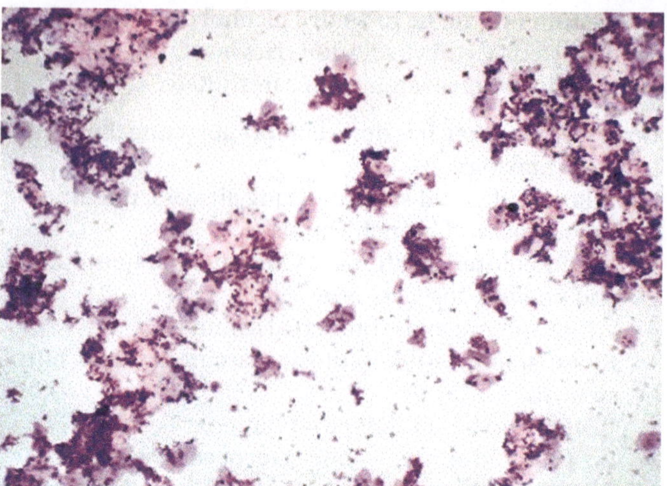

FIG. 1: Specimen composed of predominantly saliva with epithelial squames (H&E × 100).

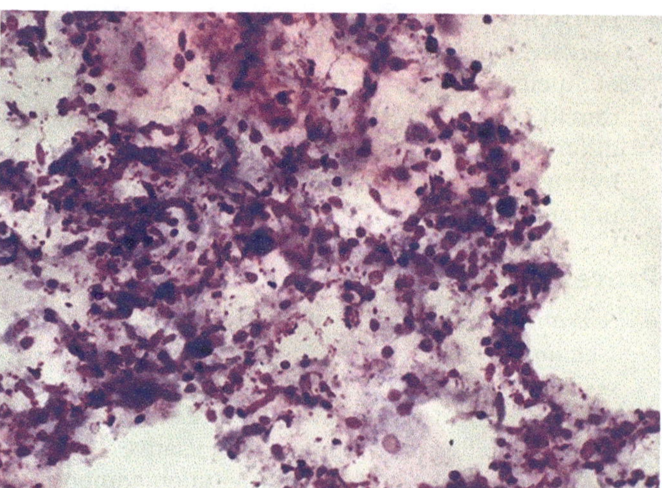

FIG. 2: Specimen composed of epithelial squames and ciliated columnar cells indicating saliva (H&E × 400).

Wet mount: The unfixed specimen may be centrifuged and then the sediment examined as a direct wet mount. If the sputum is too viscous, an equal volume of 3% sodium hydroxide may be added, then centrifuged, and the sediment examined. This helps in the detection of *Paragonimus westermani eggs, Strongyloides stercoralis larvae, Ascaris lumbricoides larvae, hookworm larvae,* and rarely *Entamoeba histolytica*. Wet mount colored with a drop of methylene blue—can be used to check out presence of cells.

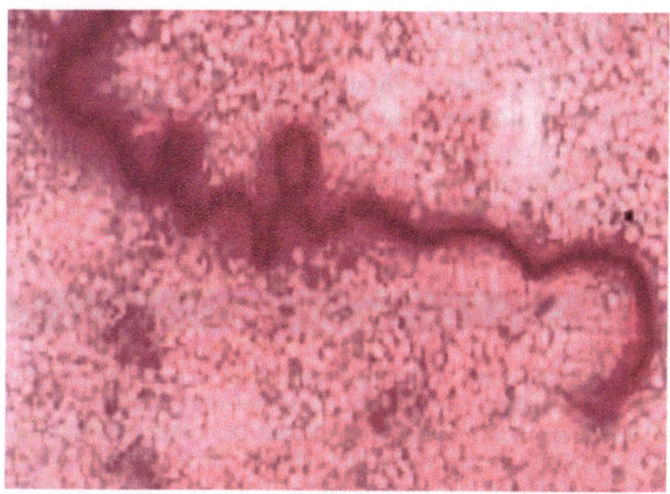

FIG. 3: Curschmann's spiral as a spiral eosinophilic structure (H&E × 400).

Stained preparation: By either H&E, Papanicolaou stain, or even Giemsa stain:

- Curschmann's spirals—coiled long thread-like and spiral-shaped stringy strands **(Fig. 3)** seen in allergic bronchitis and bronchial asthma. They appear pink and wiry by the H&E stain and cyanophilic to blue by the Pap stain. They are derived from small terminal bronchioles and submucosal bronchial gland ducts.
- Bronchial casts are elongated thread-like branching structures which are composed of fibrin and mucus and take the thickness of the bronchial tree segment from which they arise.
- Dittrich's plugs[3] composed microscopically of dense granular eosinophilic material containing necrotic cells, leukocytes, and bacteria as well as irregular clear longitudinal slits corresponding to accumulation of fat. Classically, it is associated with bacterial putrid bronchitis, lung abscesses, and bronchiectasis; in both young people and old.
- *Cells*: Neutrophils—pyogenic infections; eosinophils—parasitic infections, allergic bronchitis, and red cells.
- *Heart failure cells*: Chronic venous congestion, pulmonary infarction, and pulmonary hemorrhage.
- Actinomycosis[6,7]—radiating colonies of actinomyces surrounded by polymorphs. The disease is commonly confused clinically to be malignancy. An early diagnosis by FNAC prevents difficulties in the management of the disease.
- *Charcot-Leyden crystals:*[8] Charcot-Leyden crystals are formed from disintegration of eosinophils and composed of a protein called galectin-10, are seen in parasitic diseases and asthma. The crystals are slender and pointed and stain purplish-red in the trichrome stain.
- *Carcinoma cells:*[9] Sputum and other preparations help in picking up the spectrum of change leading to carcinoma starting from mild, moderate, and marked atypia, to carcinoma in situ and invasive carcinoma. The transition time between stages varies between patients, but on an average, the transition from mild to marked dysplasia takes 5 years and from moderate dysplasia to carcinoma in situ another 5 years. In the full-fledged forms, the cells show hyperchromatism, nuclear enlargement, high nuclear/cytoplasmic (N/C) ratio, and other features like individual cell keratinization in squamous cell carcinoma. Intracellular mucin secretion and gland formation is seen in adenocarcinoma. The latter may also show papillary and tubular structures.
- Average sensitivity of 65–75% is seen in diagnosis of carcinoma lung. The chance of detecting abnormal cells increases with (1) centrally located tumors, (2) large tumors, (3) poorly differentiated carcinomas, (4) squamous cell carcinomas rather than adenocarcinomas, and (5) increasing number of sputum samples examined.
- Small cell carcinomas show cells which resemble lymphocytes but may be larger with a round to oval cytoplasm. They also form clusters, show molding, and may be seen in "Indian file pattern".
- Gram's stain—bacteria both gram-positive and gram-negative
- Ziehl-Neelsen (ZN) stain—to detect *Mycobacterium tuberculosis*. The concentration should be at least 50,000 bacteria/mL and about 100 fields of oil immersion should be examined to declare the specimen is negative. The Revised National Tuberculosis Control Program (RNTCP) advocates a ZN staining grading system in the reporting of acid-fast bacilli (AFB) in the sputum - 3+, 2+, 1+, doubtful positive, and negative corresponding to >10 AFB per field after examining 20 fields; 1–10 AFB per field after examination of 50 fields; 10–99 AFB per 100 fields; 1–9 AFB per 100 fields; and no AFB per 100 fields.
- *Grocott methenamine silver (GMS) stain*: For fungal organisms
- *Periodic acid-Schiff (PAS) stain*: For capsule of *C. neoformans.*
- Nuclear image analysis depends on nuclear chromatin clumping, hyperchromatism and density of nucleus, semi-automated cytometry can be used to differentiate between normal and malignant changes, the sensitivity and specificity being much greater than in the use of conventional staining and screening.

- Cytology though of immense usefulness is still not a recommended tool for the screening of carcinoma lung in the high-risk group.[10,11] It is recommended that high-risk group should be screened by low-dose computed tomography (LDCT), i.e., a CT scan machine combined with sophisticated computers to produce multiple, cross-sectional images, or pictures.

CONCLUSION

Sputum is the most easily accessible sample in diagnosing respiratory diseases with the introduction of imaging and endoscopy complex lesions from smaller segments of the bronchial tree and other thoracic masses can be easily sampled by FNAC for cytology.

REFERENCES

1. Mehta AC, Marty JJ, Lee FY. Sputum cytology. Clin Chest Med. 1993;14(1):69-85.
2. Ammanagi AS, Dombale VD, Miskin AT, Dandagi GL, Sangolli SS. Sputum cytology in suspected cases of carcinoma of lung (Sputum cytology a poor man's bronchoscopy!). Lung India. 2012;29(1):19-23.
3. Martínez-Girón R, Martínez-Torre S. Dittrich's plugs in sputum: morphological observations. Cytopathology. 2012;23(4):278-9.
4. Choi YD, Han CW, Kim JH, Oh IJ, Lee JS, Nam JH, et al. Effectiveness of sputum cytology using ThinPrep method for evaluation of lung cancer. Diagn Cytopathol. 2008;36(3):167-71.
5. Cameron SE, Andrade RS, Pambuccian SE. Endobronchial ultrasound-guided transbronchial needle aspiration cytology: a state of the art review. Cytopathology. 2010;21(1):6-26.
6. Lazzari G, Vineis C, Cugini A. Cytologic diagnosis of primary pulmonary actinomycosis: report of two cases. Acta Cytol. 1981;25(3):299-301.
7. Patel KB, Gupta G, Shah M, Patel P. Pulmonary actinomycosis in fine needle aspiration cytology. J Cytol. 2009;26(2):94-6.
8. University of Delaware. (2008). Diagnostic Parasitology: Charcot-Leyden Crystal. [online] Available from https://www1.udel.edu/mls/dlehman/medt372/Ch-lyd.html [Last accessed March, 2024].
9. Thunnissen FB. Sputum examination for early detection of lung cancer. J Clin Pathol. 2003;56(11):805-10.
10. Colson YL, Shepard JO, Lennes IT. New USPSTF Guidelines for Lung Cancer Screening: Better but Not Enough. JAMA Surg. 2021;156(6):513-4.
11. Potter AL, Bajaj SS, Yang CJ. The 2021 USPSTF lung cancer screening guidelines: a new frontier. Lancet Respir Med. 2021;9(7):689-91.

CHAPTER 8

Gastrointestinal Cytology

INTRODUCTION

The scope of cytology as a means of diagnosis has not only encompassed organ aspiration and exfoliation into fluids but enabled cytology impressions into far-reaching organs within the body. This fact is well illustrated in the gastrointestinal tract (GIT) cytology. The combined use of endoscopy, endoscopy brushings, imaging (ultrasound), and fine needle aspiration (FNA) has expanded the boundaries of GIT cytology. Endoscopists can now reach to sample mural as well as extramural lesions adjacent to the GIT.

INDICATIONS FOR PERFORMING GASTROINTESTINAL TRACT CYTOLOGY EXAMINATION

- The newer techniques have made it relatively easier to collect not only cytologic but also histologic specimens from most gastrointestinal sites enabling cytology to become complementary to histology.
- Allows for screening programs to be implemented.
- To detect Barr bodies in oral mucosa
- In inflammations, viral, and fungal infections
- In the diagnosis of malignancy/carcinomas of any part of the GIT
- In the diagnosis of lymphomas, unnecessary surgery is avoided.
- Brush cytology and fine needle aspiration cytology (FNAC) of mural and extramural lesions
- Adjacent lymph node aspirations in metastatic disease help in staging
- Mucosal and submucosal lesions can be diagnosed.
- In biliary stenosis and bile cytology

ADVANTAGES OF CYTOLOGY OVER BIOPSY

- Cytology samples have larger surface areas as compared to biopsy facilitating diagnosis.
- Cytologic evaluation provides rapid interpretation, is a less invasive technique than open biopsy, and provides a cost-effective modality for the diagnosis and management of gastrointestinal lesions.
- Enables treatment without invasive procedures
- Crush artifacts of biopsy which hinder interpretation can be avoided.

SAMPLE COLLECTION[1]

Exfoliative Cytology

- *Oral mucosal scrapings*: This is done on intramucosal irregularity, ulcers and suspicious lesions as well as on surface of mucosal masses where an intraoral carcinoma is suspected. The scrape is done gently with an edge of a slide and material spread on another slide and fixed immediately and stained. Also it is done in the detection of Barr bodies.
- *Lavage or washing of the organ under suspicion*: A saline wash of the mucosal surface mainly of the stomach is done by introducing the fluid by a plastic or rubber tube and then collecting the exfoliated cells from the saline sample. The procedure may also be used in large bowel cytology.
- *Endoscopically directed brush cytology*: Brushes are introduced through the endoscope and the brushing done firmly over the surface to collect the exfoliated cells. The brush sample when obtained is pulled just back within the Teflon sheath and the whole sheath

withdrawn through the scope. Several ranges of brushes are available and multiple samples can be collected at a time. It is preferable to obtain a brush sample before the biopsy because the latter results in bleeding which obscures the lesion and affects the quality of the cytological sample.

- *Endoscopically directed jet wash* may also be used and is known to yields good results.
- *Balloon cytology:*[2] It is used to study esophageal samples (in Barrett's esophagus and to detect dysplasia and suspected carcinoma). In this method, a flexible tube with an attached balloon is swallowed to just beyond the cricopharynx (15 cm from teeth). The deflated balloon is passed into the stomach and then inflated with about 20 mL of air. As it is pulled up gently, it meets resistance at the cardioesophageal junction. It is then deflated by 5–10 mL of air. This allows it to cross the gastric junction, the balloon is reinflated and withdrawn along the entire length of the esophagus, then after deflation again, the balloon and catheter are withdrawn and the cells are transferred from it onto glass slides, immediately fixed in 95% alcohol and stained. Innovative techniques using nipple-like projections on the balloon surface for better collection of samples have been developed.
- *Salvage cytology:* All brushes, biopsy forceps, or the cytology brush channel of the endoscope are rinsed with saline solution. The sample is then centrifuged or filtered to produce smears and cellblocks.

Fine Needle Aspiration Cytology: Guided and Nonguided

- *Fine needle aspiration technique* is usually performed either directly on palpable masses or under guidance. It can be used on all abdominal masses including upper GIT, lower GIT, and mesenteric lesions. Bleeding parameters are checked before doing intra-abdominal aspiration and the standard technique using a syringe holder and a 10-cc syringe is used.
- *Transmucosal fine needle aspiration biopsy:* Fine needle aspiration can be done submucosal, mural, and extrinsic mass lesions via direct endoscopy or visualization under guidance (endoscopic ultrasonography). This is also used for preoperative staging as it permits sampling of adjacent lymph nodes and masses as well as suspected distant metastases. The material obtained is processed for smears and cellblock preparations, and can also provide material for ancillary techniques.

Imprint Cytology

Imprints are taken from endoscopic biopsy samples and serve as adjunct to biopsy reading.

Processing

- The specimen sample must be processed immediately for optimal results. Air-dried smears, alcohol-fixed smears, transport media for ThinPrep, and cellblock preparations from excess material are taken.
- The presence of a pathologist at the time of the procedure for "rapid on-site evaluation" reduces the chance of inadequate specimens.[3]
- FNA material embedded in formalin-fixed cellblocks can be reliably used in immunohistochemical studies as well as interpretation.
- Material from aspirates can be taken for molecular studies.

Interpretation

Normal Mucosa Oral Cavity

- Superficial squamous epithelial cells
- Intermediate squamous epithelial cells
- Parabasal and occasionally basal cells
- Occasional inflammatory cells

Squamous Cell Carcinoma: Oral Cavity

- Atypical squamous cells
- Pleomorphic squamous epithelial cells with hyperchromatic nuclei
- Increased nuclear/cytoplasmic (N/C) ratio
- Dense cytoplasm; cells with cytoplasmic tails

Barr Bodies[4]

- Smear shows normal squamous epithelial cells
- Nucleus shows a dot-like plano-concave densely stained structure against the inner lining of the nuclear membrane, i.e., the Barr body (sex chromatin or unextended chromosome) **(Fig. 1)**.
- The cells which contain this are called chromatin-positive and others are called chromatin-negative cells. Barr body can be found in many cell types but can be conveniently examined in the buccal mucosa.
- In females, the Barr body is seen up to or >20% of cells. It is absent in the males.
- The test is done on buccal smears where "X" chromosome is suspect.
- Barr body represents one of two X chromosomes of female cell. There is no Barr body seen in a male. In a normal female, one Barr body is seen in a cell nucleus **(Fig. 1)**.

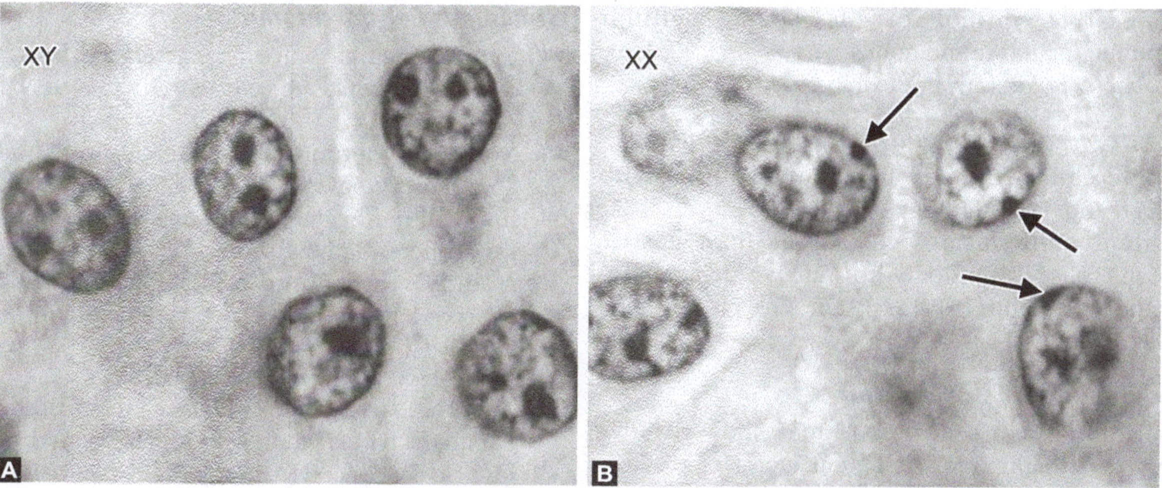

FIGS. 1A AND B: (A) Absence of Barr body in nuclei of squamous cells. (B) Buccal mucosa smear shows a Barr bodies (arrows) in squamous cells from a female.

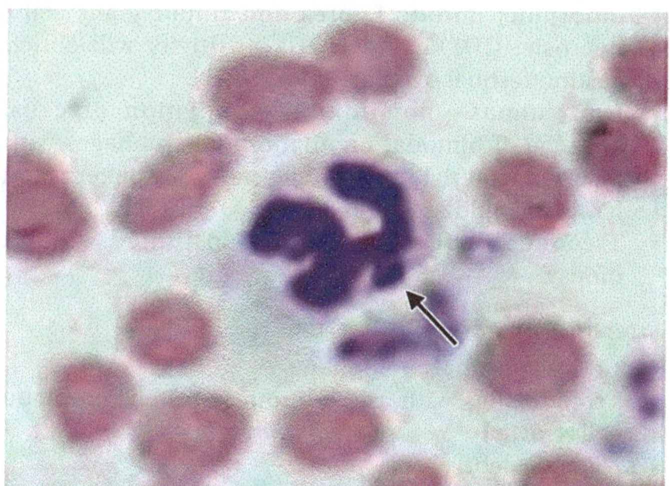

FIG. 2: Barr bodies can also be seen in the peripheral smear. They appear as a drumstick (arrow) over the lobe of a neutrophil.

- Number of Barr bodies in a cell will depend upon the number of X chromosomes in the cell, i.e., number of Barr bodies = number of X chromosomes - 1. For example, in an individual with 47,XXX complement, there are 3X chromosomes. Therefore, the number of Barr bodies is 3 - 1 = 2.
- A Turner's syndrome patient having 45, XO complement has only one X chromosome. Therefore, the number of Barr bodies is 1 - 1 = 0, i.e., no Barr body.
- The sex chromatin body of the neutrophils of females is a small mass, usually adjacent to the nuclear membrane that stains deeply with hematoxylin and is about 0.7–1.2 µm in diameter. It takes the form of a drumstick projecting from one of the nuclear lobes of about 2–3% (extreme range 1–17%) of the segmented neutrophils in the blood. They are connected to the lobe by a single fine strand **(Fig. 2)**.

Normal Esophagus

- Mature squamous cells if superficial and intermediate type.
- Occasional parabasal cells
- Occasional squamous pearls
- Occasional respiratory epithelial cells in wash preparations

Esophagitis

- *Viral*: Ground-glass nuclei, eosinophilic inclusions [cytomegalovirus (CMV)], and multinucleation
- *Fungal*: Fungal organisms (*Candida albicans*), inflammatory cells, and cytoplasmic debris

Barrett's Esophagus

- Glandular cells in sheets and clusters
- Goblet cells
- Dysplasia (if present)

Squamous cell carcinoma: Esophagus (similar to appearances as carcinoma oral cavity mucosa)

Stomach: Normal Pattern

- Minimal spontaneous exfoliation from undiseased mucosa
- Honeycomb pattern on surface view; palisade of nuclei in profile
- Nuclei are uniform, round, or oval with a distinct nuclear membrane and prominent small nucleoli.
- Cytoplasm—granular or vacuolated
- Whole crypts may be seen.

Gastritis

- Clusters of gastric epithelial cells against a background of polymorphonuclear exudate
- Nuclear changes mimicking carcinoma in both acute and chronic forms

- Regenerative epithelial cells—strong cellular basophilia; regular round nuclei
- *Helicobacter pylori* may be seen in mucus.

Chronic Atrophic Gastritis and Intestinal Metaplasia

- Atrophic cells—rounded or cuboidal forms with enlarged and dark staining nuclei
- Intestinal metaplasia—cells larger than gastric mucosal cells, distended with mucus. Alcian blue-periodic acid-Schiff (AB-PAS) stain gives purple hue to these cells.

Reactive Changes versus Carcinoma

- Cells from any part of the GIT may show reactive changes to inflammation, radiation, etc.
- Mild nuclear enlargement, prominent nucleoli, multinucleation, and cytoplasmic vacuolation
- Carcinomatous cells in comparison show not only increased nucleocytoplasmic ratio but thick nuclear membranes, prominent nucleoli, and clumped chromatin.

Dysplasia—Borderline Lesions

- Cells show enlarged nuclei with hyperchromasia and abnormal nuclear patterns (dispersed to clumped chromatin) pose a diagnostic dilemma
- Repeat cytology, multiple biopsies, and follow-up

Carcinoma—Adenocarcinoma[5]

- Carcinomas are by far the most common malignancy of the GIT. With the exception, esophagus and anal region, where squamous cell carcinomas are common, most carcinomas are adenocarcinomas.
- Adenocarcinoma cells are seen as small groups and clusters with overlapping of nuclei and loss of polarity. Loosely cohesive cells and scattered single cells may also be seen.
- The cytoplasm is finely granular to vacuolated; early intracytoplasmic lumina.
- The tumor cell nuclei are large, pleomorphic, have irregular nuclear membranes, and show prominent nucleoli.
- Papillary/tubular structures
- Findings of Barrett's intestinal metaplasia may be present.

Bile Cytology in Stenosis/Periampullary Carcinoma[6]

- Pleomorphic epithelial cells with ductular differentiation
- Exact site of origin may not be arrived at pancreatic duct, bile duct, and intestinal mucosa.

Squamous Cell Carcinoma[5]

- Cytologic smears are characterized by single and dispersed neoplastic cells with increased N/C ratio in several cells.
- Nuclear hyperchromasia, dense and moderate to abundant cytoplasm
- Intercellular bridges, evidence of pearl formation in well-differentiated tumors
- A "dirty" background indicating tumor diathesis is observed. Individual cell keratinization observed.

FNAC Smears—Guided or Nonguided

- Tuberculosis—yields clusters of epithelioid cells, Langhans type of giant cells, necrosis; may be positive for acid-fast bacilli (AFB) on Ziehl-Neelsen (ZN) stain
- Carcinoma—increased N/C ratio, hyperchromatism of nuclei, etc.
- Leiomyosarcoma—spindle-shaped cells with pleomorphic; mitotic figures and tumor giant cells; necrosis; CD117 and DOG1 positivity will clinch gastrointestinal stromal tumor (GIST).
- Lymphomas—monotonous population of cells, absence of bimodal population, macrophages with ingested material representing starry sky pattern, and lymphoglandular bodies
- Treatment can sometimes be instituted without biopsy.

Intestinal Ameboma

- Native intestinal components
- Trophozoites with and without ingested red blood cells (RBCs)
- Necrotic debris
- Cystic forms may be seen.

Anorectal Cytology[7]

The incidence of anal squamous cell carcinoma in human immunodeficiency virus (HIV)-positive MSM is twice as common as that of HIV-negative MSM (men who have sex with men: homosexual men). Meta-analysis has shown human papillomavirus (HPV) prevalence to be 71%, 91%, and 88% in anal cancer, high-grade squamous intraepithelial lesions (HSILs), and low-grade squamous intraepithelial lesions (LSILs), respectively. Screening programs have been outlined for anal cancer though controversy exists regarding such screening with the Centers for Disease Control and Prevention (CDC), United States Preventive Services Task Force (USPSTF), American Cancer Society (ACS), not support routine screening.

- Such programs use exfoliative cytology techniques to detect anal squamous intraepithelial lesions (ASILs), comparable to the cervical Pap test, and the criteria of reporting exactly similar to the Bethesda system 2001 (TBS 2001), i.e., specimen adequacy, interpretation with regard to presence of squamous intraepithelial lesion (SIL).
- Anal squamous cell carcinoma arises within the anal canal, extending from the anal verge to the rectal mucosa (3–4 cm). Histologically, the proximal margin is at the anal-rectal transformation zone. Anal-rectal cytology specimens sample the entire length of the anal canal mucosa with a moistened swab inserted about 5 cm into the anal canal and pressed firmly against the mucosa while slowly rotating and withdrawing it (Palefsky et al. 1997)[8]
- Once collected, specimens are prepared by the conventional smear or liquid-based cytology, such as ThinPrep or SurePath.
- *Specimen adequacy*: Specimen adequacy is based primarily upon specimen cellularity and morphological quality of the sample. As outlined in TBS 2001, minimum cellularity for conventional anal-rectal cytology smears is 2,000–3,000 nucleated squamous cells for conventional smears, 1–2 nucleated squamous cells per high-power field (hpf) for ThinPrep specimens, and 3–6 nucleated squamous cells per hpf for SurePath specimens.[9,10]
- Normal anal-rectal cytology tests are reported as "negative for intraepithelial lesion or malignancy" (NILM). Anal Pap tests with squamous epithelial cell abnormalities are further categorized into atypical squamous cells of undetermined significance (ASC-US), LSIL, HSIL, atypical squamous cells, cannot exclude HSIL (ASC-H), or squamous cell carcinoma.[11]
- NILM contain no abnormal squamous cells and shows exfoliated parabasal, intermediate, and superficial squamous cells. Reactive cellular changes associated with inflammation, radiation, and infectious organisms, such as *Trichomonas vaginalis*, *Candida* species, or herpes simplex virus (HSV) may be seen.
- Atypical squamous cells of undetermined significance are used to describe the presence of abnormal squamous cells that do not meet the diagnostic criteria of LSIL. Typically, ASC-US cells are superficial or intermediate-type cells with an enlarged nuclear area 2.5–3 times that of the normal intermediate cell nucleus, an increased ratio of N/C area, nuclear hyperchromasia/clumping, and nuclear membrane irregularities.
- Changes associated with LSIL are also seen within superficial and intermediate type squamous cells and are characterized by a nuclear area >3 times that of the normal intermediate cell nucleus, hyperchromasia, and chromatin clumping. Nuclear membrane irregularities, binucleation, or multinucleation may also be seen. Koilocytes, LSIL cells characterized by cytoplasmic haloes with distinct borders are pathognomonic of HPV-infected cells, are infrequently identified in anal-rectal cytology samples.
- A HSIL is identified as smaller, less mature parabasal-type, or metaplastic squamous cells. HSIL cells have a high N/C ratio seen in aggregates or as individual cells. Nuclear hyperchromasia and nuclear membrane irregularities are apparent.
- Samples with features suggestive but not qualitatively and/or quantitatively diagnostic of HSIL are interpreted as ASC-H (cannot exclude high-grade lesion). Squamous cell carcinoma is characterized by cells with marked nuclear abnormalities that have marked variation in cell size and shape, such as kite and tadpole cells.
- All patients with NILM should return to the routine screening pool. For these patients, anal-rectal cytology tests should be repeated within 1–2 years for all HIV-positive MSM.
- All patients with ASC-US or worse on anal-rectal cytology should be referred for anoscopy.
- During anoscopy, the mucosa of the anal canal is visually inspected using an anoscope. An acetic acid solution is applied to assess for areas of mucosal acetowhitening. When acetowhite lesions are detected, additional features, such as color, contour, surface, and vascular patterns to determine the nature of the lesion—HPV-related or reactive—and, if applicable, the severity of the lesion is assessed. These features are similar to those described for the cervix. Lesions are biopsied as clinically indicated to confirm presence and severity of intraepithelial neoplasia. Lesions of frankly invasive squamous cell carcinoma are also biopsied to confirm the diagnosis.
- At biopsy, anal intraepithelial neoplasia (AIN) is categorized as grade 1, 2, or 3, corresponding to mild, moderate, and severe/carcinoma in situ. Invasive squamous cell carcinoma is defined by an abnormal proliferation of squamous cells penetrating the basement membrane, invading the underlying stroma and is often associated with brisk inflammation and a desmoplastic reaction.

In conclusion, anal cytology is a good predictor of an on developing squamous cell carcinoma and adequate sampling may pick up early/low-grade lesions which may then be referred to an oncologist. Screening may become a recommendation for high-risk individuals in future.

CONCLUSION

The interpretation of GIT cytology may prove simple in certain cases or may be fraught with pitfalls, many of which are the result of contamination of the specimen by normal enteric mucosal elements. The pathologist's challenge is to differentiate lesional from nonlesional native tissue. Once the lesional tissue has been identified, reactive and reparative lesions need to be differentiated from infectious and neoplastic diseases.

Awareness of these errors can improve diagnostic accuracy and prevent false-positive diagnoses. Requisite patient information, on-site evaluation, and effective communication are important to improve diagnostic accuracy.

REFERENCES

1. Shariff S, Kaler AK. Principles and Interpretation of Laboratory Practices in Surgical Pathology. New Delhi: Jaypee Brothers Medical Publishers (P) Ltd.; 2016.
2. Patel AA, Strome M, Blitzer A. Directed balloon cytology of the esophagus: A novel device for obtaining circumferential cytologic sampling. Laryngoscope. 2017;127(5):1032-5.
3. Yadav M, Ramrakhiani D, Yadav A, Nijhawan S. Role of Rapid Onsite Evaluation (ROSE) of EUS-FNAC in Diagnostic Yield of Solid Mass Lesions. J Med Res. 2016. Int J Med Res Prof. 2016;2(3);163-8.
4. ScienceDirect. (2017). Barr Body. [online] Available from https://www.sciencedirect.com/topics/biochemistry-genetics-and-molecular-biology/barr-body [Last accessed March, 2024].
5. Conrad R, ShobhaCastelino-Prabhu, Cobb C, Raza A. Role of cytopathology in the diagnosis and management of gastrointestinal tract cancers. J Gastrointest Oncol. 2012;3(3):285-98.
6. Sugimoto S, Matsubayashi H, Kimura H, Sasaki K, Nagata K, Ohno S, et al. Diagnosis of bile duct cancer by bile cytology: usefulness of post-brushing biliary lavage fluid. Endosc Int Open. 2015;3(4):E323-8.
7. Bean SM, Chhieng DC. Anal-Rectal Cytology: The Other Pap Test. 2010. Labmedicine. 2010;41(3).
8. Palefsky JM, Holly EA, Hogeboom CJ, Berry JM, Jay N, Darragh TM. Anal cytology as a screening tool for anal squamous intraepithelial lesions. J Acquir Immune Defic Syndr Hum Retrovirol. 1997;14(5):415-22.
9. Hoots BE, Palefsky JM, Pimenta JM, Smith JS. Human papillomavirus type distribution in anal cancer and anal intraepithelial lesions. Int J Cancer. 2009;124(10):2375-83.
10. Daling JR, Weiss NS, Hislop TG, Maden C, Coates RJ, Sherman KJ, et al. Sexual practices, sexually transmitted diseases, and the incidence of anal cancer. N Engl J Med. 1987;317(16):973-7.
11. Solomon D. The Bethesda System for Reporting Cervical Cytology: Definitions, Criteria, and Explanatory Notes, 2nd edition. New York, NY: Springer; 2004. p. 191.

CHAPTER 9

Female Genital Tract

INTRODUCTION

The cytological specimens collected from the female genital tract (FGT) include cervical smears, vaginal smears, and aspiration from the posterior fornix of vagina (vaginal pool smear) as well as endometrial smears. Cervical smears and Papanicolaou stain are the essence of cervical cancer screening. Endometrial cytology though not so popular is practiced in Institutions and is a useful procedure in the diagnosis of abnormal uterine bleeding.

ENDOMETRIAL CYTOLOGY

Endometrial cytology[1-7] is usually done in women with abnormal uterine bleeding. It may be combined with other procedures to yield a high sensitivity. A combination of transvaginal ultrasonography and endometrial cytology may be an effective way to diagnose endometrial cancer and hyperplasia. This combined method in literature has resulted in 100% sensitivity, 99.1% specificity, 92.9% positive predictive value, and 100% negative predictive value in diagnosing endometrial carcinoma. In endometrial hyperplasia, the method resulted in 100% sensitivity, 89.6% specificity, 40.0% positive predictive value, and 100% negative predictive value.

Endometrial Specimen Collection

- Smears from the posterior fornix show exfoliated endometrial cells
- Endocervical smears show endometrial cells
- Endometrial brush cytology
- Intrauterine aspirations

Vaginal pool smear: The technique allows collection of cells under direct vision from the posterior fornix pool using an unlubricated speculum. It is a collection of exfoliations of cells of the vaginal wall, cervix, cervical canal, endometrium, using a Pasteur pipette. When a speculum is not employed, the pipette is gently introduced into the vagina until resistance is encountered.

The advantages are that the smears can be obtained in the presence of an intact hymen. Vaginal smears are used for hormonal studies. The vaginal smear is efficient in the detection and diagnosis of endometrial cancers but fails to detect nearly 50% of all precancerous lesions. Yet it complements the cervical smear and offers several major advantages, particularly in women past the age of 40 years. Cells from endometrium, the fallopian tube, the ovary, and occasionally from other distant sites are found in the vaginal pool smear and usually not in the direct smear of the uterine cervix.

Endometrial aspiration and brushings:[6,7] The best yield occurs by the aspiration through the cannula and brush techniques **(Fig. 1)**. Various cannulas and brushes are available for obtaining the sample from the uterine cavity—rigid metal cannulas, thin, flexible laryngeal cannulas with beveled ends, Ayre's endometrial rotating brushes, etc. Cannulas are fixed to syringes and aspirations performed at various levels as the cannulas are pulled out slowly. If the aspiration is unproductive, the uterine cavity can be lavaged with 2 cc of a sterile, normal saline solution which is introduced through the tubing and sprayed inside; the contents are withdrawn; mixed with alcohol ether mixture, centrifuged, and the sediment spread onto glass slides and stained.

In the same manner, the tube with the brush within is inserted high up into the cavity. The outer casing or tube is pulled down 3–4 cm; the brush is turned to collect the cells; pulled back into the tube which is then removed.

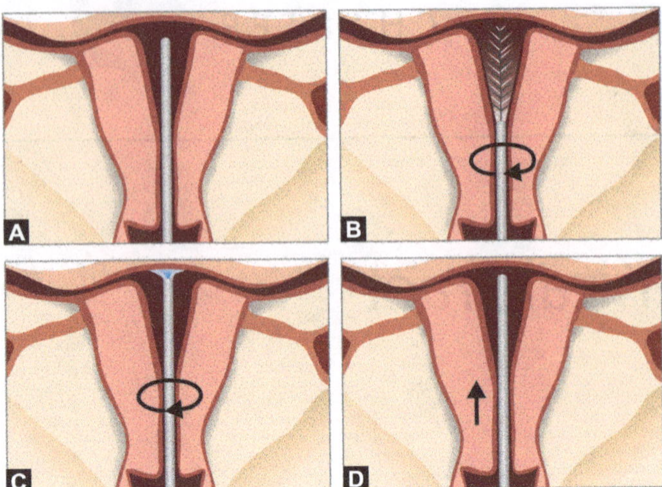

FIGS. 1A TO D: Method of collecting endometrial sample by brush (Li brush). (A) Cannula with brush within; (B) Brush ejected from cannula and rotating to collect sample; (C) Rotation to collect sample from fundus; and (D) Cannula moves forward to close on brush and is withdrawn.

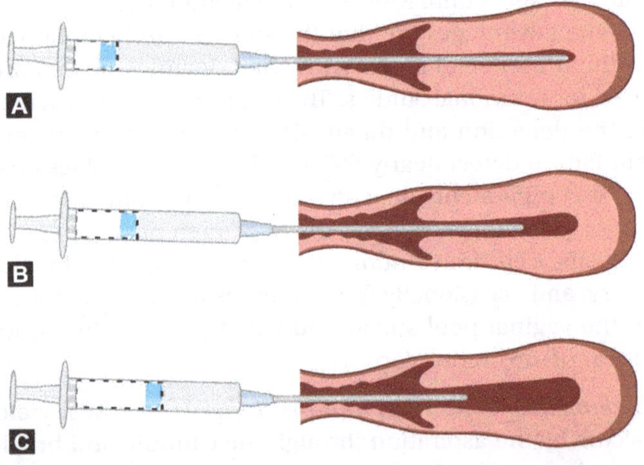

FIGS. 2A TO C: Aspiration through endometrial cavity through a syringe.

Endometrial aspiration procedure **(*Fig. 2*)**: After preliminary visualization and cleaning of the cervix, a sterile endometrial cannula is introduced into the endometrial cavity without preliminary dilatation of the endocervical canal. A 20-mL syringe attached to this provides the negative pressure necessary for aspiration of material.

The material is aspirated and subsequently expressed on a slide, smeared, and fixed in the usual cytological fixative. Alternatively, the material is placed in a fixative, spun, and embedded in paraffin and examined as microbiopsies.

The advantages are that the method provides a reliable means for the diagnosis of early endometrial carcinoma and information about the status of the endocervical canal.

Cytological sample brushings using the above devices are collected in vials and processed using a ThinPrep® 2000 automated slide processor.[2,4,5] The slides are stained using the Pap stain.

Interpretation

Benign: In all benign conditions, the cellular material is characteristically uniform, i.e., the nuclei are round to oval, equal in size, and have a uniform granular chromatin structure and the nuclear membranes well delineated and smooth.

Malignant endometrial cells:[1,2,7] The malignant endometrial cells are characteristically irregular, and have irregular nuclear membranes except in well-differentiated tumors show increased chromatin irregularly arranged (hyperchromasia). In differentiated forms, the cells are often found typically arranged back to back. Rosette-like patterns indicate papillary growth. Undifferentiated cells which have no clear cytoplasmic details reveal their glandular origin by the characteristic group formation, overlapping of the nuclei, eccentric positioning of the nuclei, and vacuolization of the cytoplasm. When adenoacanthoma is present, metaplastic as well as adenocarcinomatous cells are found which are similar to cells originating from squamous carcinoma.

CERVICAL CYTOLOGY

Cervical/Pap Smear[8,9]

It is the universally accepted screening procedure for carcinoma of the cervix and entails examination of a smear from the lower part of the endocervical canal.

The Pap smear is usually done in combination with a pelvic examination. As a screening test, it is a recommended procedure after age of 20 years. In women older than age of 25 years, the Pap test may be combined with a test for human papillomavirus (HPV), a sexually transmitted infection that can cause cervical cancer, every 5 years. In some cases, the HPV test alone may be done instead of a Pap smear.

- The focus on HPV has gained importance in the last decade as compared to even Pap smear.
- According to the International Agency for Research on Cancer (IARC) classification, high-risk human papillomavirus (hrHPV) is of 14 types: HPV16, HPV18, HPV31, HPV33, HPV35, HPV39, HPV45, HPV51, HPV52, HPV56, HPV58, HPV59, HPV66, and HPV68. High-risk papillomavirus is an etiological agent for cancer of the cervix, vulva, and vagina. HPV16 and HPV18 represent approximately 60% for adenocarcinoma of the endocervix (ADC-CX).[10]

- Screening of cervical cancer includes three procedures: Cytology evaluations of a sample acquired from the cervix, detection of hrHPV deoxyribonucleic acid (DNA) or ribonucleic acid (RNA), and cotesting (combination of microscopy and HPV nucleic acid testing).

Advantages of Pap Smear

- It is simple office procedure, is painless, and is performed without anesthesia.
- It is an easy screening procedure for cervical carcinoma and precursor lesions.
- Detection done either manually or on automated device is sensitive to detecting premalignant changes of the cervix in a high percentage of cases.
- It has brought down incidence of cervical carcinoma in most countries.
- It detects presence of microorganisms

Patient Preparation and Procedure[8]

- No intravaginal douching of any type as preparation is needed.
- Installation of drugs should be avoided for at least 1 week, and the patient should abstain from coitus for 1–2 days before the examination.
- A smear should not be taken during menstrual bleeding as it would show only blood and debris.
- Lubricants should not be used while examining, as it can mask cells during smear examination.
- Mucus is wiped out with a cotton swab before taking the smear.
- *Spatulas*: A variety of wooden and plastic spatulas are available. The *Ayre spatula* was developed in 1947 and has been widely used. It is especially designed with a bifid end; one end of the scraper slightly longer than the other so that the spatula fits snugly against the external os. The scraper is rotated 360°, the longer end used as a pivot at the external os **(Fig. 3)**. Smears obtained with the Ayre's spatula result in adequate yield and are easy to screen.
- *Preparation of smear:* After taking the smear, the spatula is rotated evenly on a glass slide in multiple clockwise swirls as shown in the **Figure 3** and fixed immediately. If the smear does not appear satisfactory, a repeat smear can be done during the same examination.
- Most gynecologist smear one slide with endocervical material and a second slide with ectocervical material.
- *Other spatulas*:
  - *Wooden spatulas* are the least expensive and serve as good sampling devices, but have the disadvantage of "trapping cells". This leads to false-negative results. Therefore, modifications generally include variably sized hooks and extension of tips which easily reach into the endocervical canal.
  - The pointed *Ayres bury spatula* is a wooden spatula with an extended tip designed to sample cells from both endocervix and the transformation zone (TZ) of the cervix. The disadvantage is that this method is traumatic to the patient and the edge of the scraper may not fit well into the external os and sometimes fail to sample the squamocolumnar junction.
  - *Multispatula:* It consists of two parts—a body and a long central portion which slides with the body. The main advantage of multispatula is to increase the endocervical cell content. At the cervical end, the body has two wing-like protuberances which surround the central portion. The sliding into the endocervical canal is controlled by a button and allows an endocervical penetration of 8 mm when fully extended.

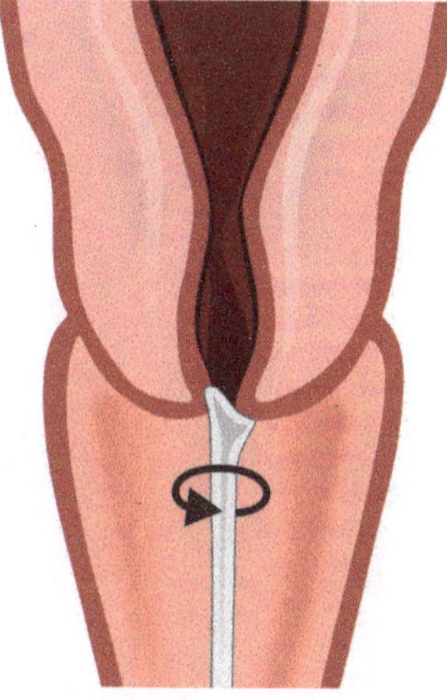

FIG. 3: Smear being taken by Ayre's spatula.

- *Brushes in use include* ***(Fig. 4)****:*[11]
  - *Cytobrush:* A cervical brush for the sampling of endocervical cells **(Fig. 4)** is superior to the Ayre spatula and yields better results. It consists of a metal wire core with perpendicular plastic bristles attached to it at one end in a wedge-shaped manner. The bristles bend easily; the narrow tip of the wedge can easily be inserted into a small cervical os. The instrument is highly effective in obtaining adequate endocervical material. Transfer of cells is accomplished by *rolling the brush* across the slide.

The disadvantage with the Cytobrush is the trauma that occurs to the cervix as a result of the stiff bristles on the instrument which may obscure the transformation zone and thus create a bloody smear which hampers morphology.

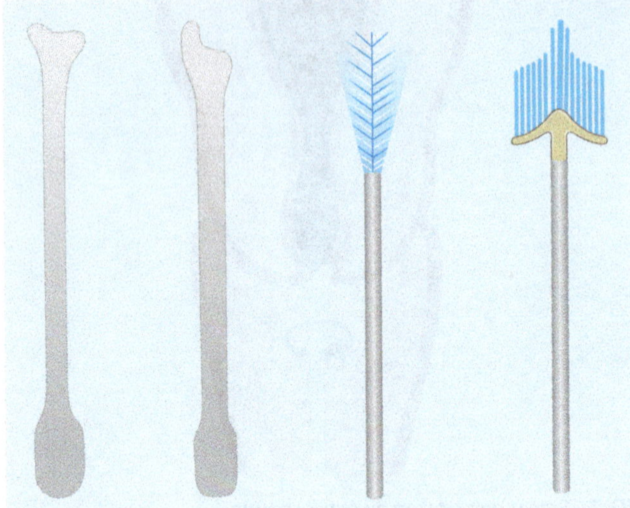

FIG. 4: Sampling devices (from left to right—Ayre's spatula; modified Ayre's spatula; Cytobrush; and Cervex Brush).

- The *Cervex Brush* combines features of both the spatula and the Cytobrush. The plastic bristles extend parallel to the plastic handle and are attached to one end in an inverted "V"-shape manner. This samples an adequate amount of cytologic material from both the ecto- and endocervix onto a slide, with far less trauma to the patient, resulting in thinner better-preserved smears with monolayers and less blood. The bristles are softer and thicker than those of the Cytobrush, the longer strands extend into the canal, while the shorter strands spread over the portio and lateral ectocervix.

  Both endo- and ectocervical components are well represented by this technique.

  It is to advantage in patients with cervical stenosis and in postmenopausal women with high indrawn transformation zones. The disadvantage is that it is the most expensive of all the sampling devices.
- *Combined spatula and Cytobrush technique* is a very effective sampling combination for both the endocervix and the ectocervix. Smears are taken with the brush initially, followed by the spatula **(Fig. 5)**. Smears are prepared after both collections using the entire length of the slide; rolling the brush on one side and then smearing with the spatula in a monolayer, on the unused side of the slide.

Rehydration of Unfixed Dried Smears before Staining

Unfixed, air-dried gynecological smears received from peripheral areas should be rehydrated before staining. The simplest rehydration technique is to place air-dried cytological specimens in 50% aqueous solution of glycerin for 3 minutes followed by two rinses in 95% ethyl alcohol, and then stain by the Papanicolaou method.

Liquid-based cytology (LBC): It is an ideal method for preparation of a monolayer of cells for viewing against a clean background from liquid-based gynecologic cytology samples. The idea was developed in 1970. The main disadvantage is the cost of the instrument.

Two systems of LBC are available:
- *ThinPrep*: Several models are available and workloads of up to 20,000 samples per annum can be carried out.

  The cells are collected in the ThinPrep vial of the preservative solution using a broom type device or endocervical brush/spatula as a collection device. The vial is processed by both—the semiautomated T2000 processor and fully automated T3000 processor.

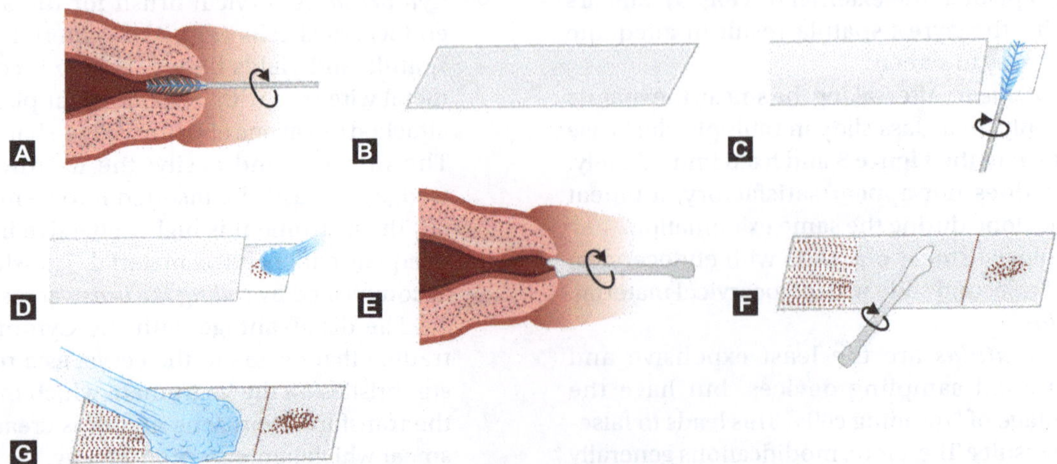

FIGS. 5A TO G: The combined spatula and Cytobrush method. (A to D) Material being smeared after brush collection; and (E to G) Ayre's spatula and smearing.

TP-2000 is a bench top model which is loaded manually with individual pots and consumables. The T3000 and T5000 are fully automated and convert vials into slides ready for staining without any intervention and allow up to 80–160 vials respectively in a batch.

In either case, the method of sample collection remains the same (as shown in **Fig. 5**). The fluid in the vial is agitated to break up cell clusters, mucus, and cell debris. A series of negative pressures draw the fluid through the ThinPrep membrane. Red blood cells, mucous cells, and neutrophils pass through the filter, while epithelial cells block the pores of the filter, leading to a pressure differential across the filter. This pressure gradient determines when sufficient cells have become stuck on the filter. The filter is then removed and dabbed onto an electrically charged slide, causing the cells to transfer onto the glass slide and get stained.

- *SurePath*: Layering of cell sample on to a liquid density gradient by vortexing and centrifugation the vortex breaks up large cell aggregates, mucus, and blood. Density gradient centrifugation separates the cellular elements which form a pellet, from inflammatory cells and debris. The pellet remixed and placed in a settling chamber and applied to a glass slide by gravity sedimentation. Even layered circle of cells on slide (13 mm) are monolayered, automatically stained by SurePath processer.

All laboratories using LBC should ensure that their staff undergoes adequate training in handling the instrument and is capable of trouble shooting and participate in external quality assurance (EQA) programs. Cytopathologists should be familiar with appearances of LBC smears.

American Cancer Society Recommendations for Cervical Cancer Screening

Cervical cancer screening is effective in reducing incidence of cervical carcinoma and deaths leading from it. The recent American Cancer Society (ACS) recommendations for cervical cancer screening are given in **Table 1**.[12]

Screening with an HPV test (for *hrHPV testing)* alone is more sensitive than a Pap smear. The 2018 USPSTF guideline included HPV testing alone, cotesting, and Pap testing as equal options. The new ACS guidelines prefer HPV testing alone over the other two tests.

These new screening recommendations of ACS differ with respect to the 2012 recommendations by the following:[12,13] (1) The preferred screening test is HPV testing every 5 years; (2) Cotesting (doing both HPV and Pap) and cytology alone is acceptable where access to United States Food and Drug Administration (US-FDA) approved primary HPV testing is not available; (3) The recommended age to start screening is 25 years rather than 21 years; (4) Primary HPV testing and cotesting are recommended starting at the age of 25 years rather than age of 30 years; and (5) Cytology alone is acceptable every 3 years in the absence of the other two.

Reporting of cervical smear: The Bethesda system[14,15] is presently the accepted system for reporting cervical cytology in most centers across the globe. Introduced in the year 1988 at the National Cancer Institute, Bethesda, Maryland, USA, it was later modified in 1991 and 2001 and

TABLE 1: American Cancer Society (ACS) recommendations for cervical cancer screening in the years 2020, 2012 in comparison to the USPSTF (United States Preventive Services Task Force) screening programme.

	2020 ACS	2012 ACS	2018 USPSTF
Age 21–24 years	No screening	Pap test every 3 years	Pap test every 3 years
Age 25–29 years	• HPV test every 5 years (preferred) • HPV/Pap cotest every 5 years (acceptable) • Pap test every 3 years (acceptable)	Pap test every 3 years	Pap test every 3 years
Age 30–65 years	• HPV test every 5 years (preferred) • HPV/Pap cotest every 5 years (acceptable) • Pap test every 3 years (acceptable)	• HPV/Pap cotest every 3 years (preferred) • Pap test every 3 years (acceptable)	• Pap test every 3 years • HPV test every 5 years • HPV/Pap cotest every 5 years
Age 65 and older	No screening if a series of prior tests were normal	No screening if a series of prior tests were normal	No screening if a series of prior tests were normal and not at high risk for cervical cancer

(HPV: human papillomavirus; USPSTF: United States Preventive Services Task Force)

2014, after critical feed backs on the validity of the report as well as development of advances in techniques such as LBC and detection of high-risk HPV infection implications.

The system provides a uniform format for cervical/vaginal cytology reporting specifically commenting on specimen adequacy as well as emphasizing communication of clinically relevant information.

The following are the salient features of the format of reporting based on the revised Bethesda System 2014 (The Pap test and Bethesda 2014)[9,14] as given by the authors.[16]

Specimen Type

Indicate conventional smear (Pap smear) versus liquid-based versus other

Specimen Adequacy

- *Satisfactory for evaluation*: Mention presence or absence of endocervical/transformation zone component and any other quality indicators, e.g., partially obscuring blood, inflammation, etc.
- *Unsatisfactory for evaluation (specify reason)*:
  - Specimen rejected/not processed *(specify reason)*
  - Specimen processed and examined, but unsatisfactory for evaluation of epithelial abnormality because of (*specify reason*)

GENERAL CATEGORIZATION (OPTIONAL)

- Negative for intraepithelial lesion or malignancy
- *Other*: See "interpretation/result"(e.g., endometrial cells in a women ≥45 years of age)
- *Epithelial cell abnormality*: See "interpretation/result"(specify "squamous" or "glandular" as appropriate)

Interpretation/Result

Negative for Intraepithelial Lesion or Malignancy

When there is no cellular evidence of neoplasia, state this in the general categorization above and/or in the interpretation/result section of the report, whether or not there are organisms or other non-neoplastic findings.

- *Nonneoplastic findings (optional to report)*:
  - *Nonneoplastic cellular variations*:
    - Squamous metaplasia
    - Keratotic changes
    - Tubal metaplasia
    - Atrophy
    - Pregnancy-associated changes
  - *Reactive cellular changes associated with*:
    - Inflammation (includes typical repair)
    - Lymphocytic (follicular) cervicitis
    - Radiation
    - Intrauterine contraceptive device (IUCD)
  - Glandular cells status posthysterectomy
- *Organisms*:
  - *Trichomonas vaginalis*
  - Fungal organisms morphologically consistent with *Candida* species
  - Shift in flora suggestive of bacterial vaginosis
  - Bacteria morphologically consistent with *Actinomyces* species
  - Cellular changes consistent with herpes simplex virus (HSV)

Other

Endometrial cells *(in a woman ≥45 years of age)[specify if negative for squamous intraepithelial lesion (SIL)]*.

Epithelial Cell Abnormalities

Squamous Cell

- *Atypical squamous cells (ASCs)*:
  - Of undetermined significance (ASC-US)
  - Cannot exclude high-grade squamous intraepithelial lesion (HSIL) (ASC-H)
- *Low-grade squamous intraepithelial lesion (LSIL)*: (Encompassing: HPV/mild dysplasia/CIN1)
- *High-grade squamous intraepithelial lesion*:
  - Encompassing moderate and severe dysplasia, CIS/CIN2 and 3
  - With features suspicious for invasion (if invasion is suspected)
- Squamous cell carcinoma

Glandular Cell

- *Atypical*:
  - Endocervical cells [not otherwise specified (NOS) or specify in comments]
  - Endometrial cells (NOS or specify in comments)
  - Glandular cells (NOS or specify in comments)
- *Atypical*:
  - Endocervical cells, favor neoplastic
  - Glandular cells, favor neoplastic
- Endocervical adenocarcinoma in situ
- *Adenocarcinoma*:
  - Endocervical
  - Endometrial
  - Extrauterine
  - Not otherwise specified

OTHER MALIGNANT NEOPLASMS (SPECIFY)

Adjunctive Testing

Provide a brief description of the test method(s) and report the result so that it is easily understood by the clinician.

Computer-assisted Interpretation of Cervical Cytology

In case examined by automated device, specify device and result.

Educational Notes and Comments Appended to Cytology Reports (Optional)

Suggestion should be concise and consistent with clinical follow-up guidelines published by professional organizations (references to relevant publications may be included).

Changes/evolution of Bethesda System from 1988 to date: The Bethesda system of reporting is an elaborate system of reporting with classification of the smear into normal, reactive changes, and epithelial cell abnormalities and was designed to standardize reporting of cervical cytology and categorize squamous epithelial malignancies on a two-tier system, low-grade, and high-grade. The epithelial cell abnormality if present needs to be described separately into squamous cell and glandular cell in origin.

Adequacy of specimen (2001 specimen adequacy criteria)—is satisfactory:
- It has appropriate labeling and identifying information
- Relevant clinical information
- Adequate number of well-preserved and well-visualized squamous cells (spread over >10% of slide surface)
- An adequate endocervical/transformation zone component is not a must but mention should be made whether seen or not (a minimum of two well-preserved endocervical cell clusters and/or metaplastic squamous cells with each having at least 5 cells).
- An estimated 8,000–12,000 well-visualized squamous cells for conventional smears and 5,000 well-preserved and visualized squamous cells for liquid-based preparation are required to designate a specimen as adequate (this is a rough estimate made on comparison with standardized visual photographs provided and does not entail actual counting of cells).

2014 criteria—added: In postmenopausal patients, postradiation therapy, posthysterectomy this criterion cannot be strictly adhered to as transformation is much higher.

Satisfactory (2001 criteria) but limited by, if any of the following apply:
- Lack of pertinent clinical information
- Partially obscuring blood, inflammation, thick areas, poor fixation, air dry artifact, contaminant, etc., that cover <50–75% of the epithelial cells
- Lack of transformation zone component

A specimen is unsatisfactory (2001 criteria) for evaluation when:
- Lack of patient identification on the specimen or request form
- A technically unacceptable slide defined as one that is broken and as having cellular material that is inadequately preserved.
- Scant squamous well-preserved epithelial cells spread over <10% of the slide surface
- Obscuring blood, inflammation, thick areas, drying artifact, etc., which precludes interpretation of approximately 75% or more of the epithelial cell component
- However, if abnormal or neoplastic cells are present the specimen is never categorized as unsatisfactory, as the smear has served its purpose. In postmenopausal patients, absence of transformation zone component does not affect the adequacy.

2014 criteria:
- Only two categories should exist either satisfactory or unsatisfactory; as the category of "satisfactory but limited by..." creates confusion in follow up of these patients.
- Guidance for postradiation and posthysterectomy patients
- HPV testing and adequacy

Nonneoplastic changes (2001):
Organisms: The common infections recognized in cytology are:
- *Trichomonas vaginalis* infection is a very common infection with approximately 29% of females harboring the organism. It is characterized by gray-colored pear-shaped organism ranging in size from 8 to 30 µm commonly seen at the edge of the squamous cells. A faint blue colored nucleus and axostyle can be appreciated in some cases. Associated findings are lilac coloration of the smear, perinuclear halos, exfoliation of parabasal cells, and presence of leptothrix organism and clusters of neutrophils seen as "balls" (buckshot appearance).
- *Candida albicans* infection is another common infection seen in about 20% of the pregnant women, women taking oral contraceptives, diabetics, and immunocompromised patients. Some show budding yeast forms and pseudohyphae which stain lightly with eosin. Epithelial changes show degenerative changes.

- *Herpes simplex infection:* Majority of genital herpes infections are caused by HSV type-II which is venereally transmitted. Cytological features include multinucleated giant cells 50–100 μm in size containing about 50 nuclei which appear structureless or ground glass. Amphophilic intranuclear inclusions and nuclear molding are also seen.
- *Actinomyces:* It is seen in about 1% of IUCD users. These appear as cotton wool colonies surrounded by inflammatory cells predominantly polymorphs.

Reactive cellular changes are associated with:

- *Inflammation (includes typical repair)* shows an abundance of polymorphs and microorganism in the background often masking epithelial cells. The epithelial cells show frayed cell borders, loss of staining characteristics, and cytoplasmic vacuolation. The nuclei show mild hyperchromatism, swelling, loss of structure, and other degenerative changes such as pyknosis and karyorrhexis. Also seen are sheets of metaplastic squamous cells of immature type indicating repair.
- *Radiation-associated changes* in epithelial cells are frequently encountered in cancer patients and they can persist for many years. Radiation-induced atypia closely mimics malignancy. The changes include (1) enlarged and bizarre nuclei with wrinkling and smudged chromatin; (2) enlargement of cells with coarse vacuolation of cytoplasm, multinucleation, and phagocytosis; and (3) giant squames with multiple swollen structureless nuclei are common. It is often difficult to distinguish radiation atypia from malignant cells. The presence of mitosis is a reliable guide to recurrence or presence of malignant cells.
- *Intrauterine contraceptive device-associated changes* show discrete or clusters of endometrial cells often showing enlarged nuclei with mild atypia, the so-called IUCD cells. Associated *Actinomyces* may be seen.
- *Posthysterectomy* shows mainly parabasal cells mimicking malignancy at times.
- *Atrophy smears* show sheets of parabasal cells showing cellular pleomorphism and degenerative change with swollen irregular cells and large pale nuclei. Cell death is manifested by nuclear pyknosis, karyolysis, and karyorrhexis. Nuclear threads may also be seen. As the cells are highly fragile, many bare nuclei are seen, multinucleate giant cells may be found. This picture is easily mistaken for atypical epithelial cells.

2014 criteria: In addition to above, mimics of epithelial abnormalities were expanded to include many more changes, e.g., stromal decidual change.

GENERAL CATEGORIZATION (OPTIONAL) (2001/2014)

Negative for intraepithelial lesion or malignancy or other... (age criteria of endometrial cells in a woman was changed from ≥40 to ≥45 years in 2014 criteria as predictive value for endometrial carcinoma decreased significantly. Endometrial evaluation to be done only in postmenopausal women).

EPITHELIAL CELL ABNORMALITY

Epithelial Cell Abnormalities 2001

Squamous Cell

The term atypical squamous cells of undetermined significance (ASC-US) of the 1988 and 1991 categories of classifications had been modified in the 2001 Bethesda. This category included cells for which a reliable interpretation of SIL could not be made through the cells contained features that were more marked than reactive changes. It was suggested that qualifiers, such as ASC-US, favor reactive or ASC-US, and favor neoplastic should be used. In 2001, it was considered that ASC-US though having poor interobserver reproducibility could not be eliminated as a certain percentage of it led to HSIL/carcinoma. In the Bethesda system 2001 (TBS 2001), the new category of "atypical squamous cells" emphasized the importance of predicting risk status of ASC-US by dividing it into two subcategories—atypical squamous cells "of undetermined significance" (ASC-US) and atypical squamous cells "cannot exclude HSIL" (ASC-H).

The Bethesda system (TBS) 2001 eliminated ASC-US, favor reactive with the intent that most of the specimens in this category will be downgraded to negative (e.g., if ASC-US was associated with severe inflammation, smears should be repeated after appropriate treatment. If ASC-US was associated with marked atrophy a repeat smear should follow a course of intravaginal estrogen application and repeat Pap test after 1 week).

In the TBS 2001, ASC-US was the more numerically prominent qualifier and should account for 90–95% of all ASC results. The use of the qualifier "undetermined significance" emphasized that a specific diagnosis could not be made. ASC-US would include most cytology results previously categorized as ASC-US-NOS and ASC-US favor SIL. ASC-US excluded cytology suggestive of HSIL. As per 2001 criteria, pathologists should remember that the ASC-US category was not a license for equivocal diagnosis and its use should be minimized. The rate of ASC-US should not exceed >5% of PAP smears reported in any laboratory and it should not exceed 2–3 times the rate of LSIL reported.

Atypical squamous cells, cannot rule out a high-grade lesion (ASC-H): ASC-H was interpreted as cytologic changes that are suggestive of HSIL but lacked criteria for definitive interpretation; it was created to include an intermediate category between ASC-US and HSIL.

ASC-H was the less common qualifier accounting for 5–10% of all ASC cases and the risk of an underlying high-grade lesion is higher in this category than in the ASC-US. The positive predictive value for HSIL (CIN 2 and 3) in ASC-H is higher than in ASC-US. ASC-H is more likely than ASC-US to be caused by a precancerous change and the risk of a high-grade precancerous lesion in women with ASC-US is 15% and for those with ASC-H is probably 38%. Immediate colposcopy is recommended due to knowledge that CIN 2 and 3 is identified in up to 94% of women with this initial Pap test interpretation.

2014 guidelines for ASC: ASC continues to be defined as the general category with subcategories as ASC-US and ASC-H. Guidance is provided to enable laboratories to use these categories along with HPV results.

2006 and 2012 consensus guidelines for management of abnormal cervical screening:[17,18] As per the American Society for Colposcopy and Cervical Pathology (ASCCP), the following are recommended for ASC-US:

- For ASC-US cytology, immediate colposcopy is not an option. The *serial cytology option* for ASC-US incorporates cytology at 12 months, not 6 months and 12 months, and then if negative, cytology at every 3 years.
- DNA testing for high-risk (oncogenic) type of HPV is recommended as cotesting.
- HPV-negative and ASC-US results should be followed with cotesting at 3 years rather than 5 years.
- Women whose HPV test results are positive and cytology results are negative should repeat cotesting in 12 months (first option) or undergo immediate HPV genotype-specific testing for types 16 or 16/18 (second option).
- Colposcopy is indicated for all women with HPV-DNA +ve and ASC-US, regardless of genotyping result.
- Those found to have CIN on biopsy should be managed according to the ASCCP guidelines.
- Endocervical sampling is preferred for women who are HPV positive but in whom no lesions are identified at colposcopy.
- Postcolposcopic management option for women with ASC who are HPV positive but in whom CIN is not identified at colposcopy (and in whom endocervical sampling is not done) can be subjected to repeat HPV-DNA testing at 12 months or repeat cytological testing at 6 and 12 months.
- HPV-DNA testing is not recommended at intervals <12 months.
- A loop electrosurgical excision procedure (LEEP) should not be used to treat women who have ASC in the absence of biopsy confirmed CIN.

Management of cases reported as ASC-H is colposcopy and biopsy.

Low-grade Squamous Intraepithelial Lesion

The lesion LSIL encompasses HPV/mild dysplasia/CIN 1 (2001).

Low-grade squamous intraepithelial lesion (CIN 1) appears as flat polygonal cells of superficial or intermediate cells with nuclear size 2–4 times that of intermediate cell nuclei with mild irregularity, hyperchromasia, and minimal chromatic clumping.

Koilocytes must satisfy the following criteria: (1) nuclear abnormality, (2) thick cellular margins, and (3) cytoplasmic clearing.

These two lesions (HPV and CIN 1) are clubbed together because (1) the HPV spectrum is same both in koilocytic atypia and CIN 1; (2) the progression rate to high-grade lesion is almost the same, i.e., about 15%; (3) the rate of biopsy confirmation is also similar; and (4) morphological features are quite similar and overlap in both areas.

LSIL 2014 criteria continue as above

Management options for LSIL: Colposcopy is recommended as the sole management option in those with LSIL. Between 15 and 30% of women with LSIL on Pap testing will have CIN 2 and 3 diagnosed on colposcopy and subsequent cervical biopsy. High-risk HPV-DNA is usually tested to be positive for such LSIL patients.

Those with no CIN identified at colposcopy can either have repeat cytological testing at 6–12 months or HPV-DNA testing at 12 months.

Postmenopausal women with LSIL can be followed with repeat cytology in 4–6 months or HPV-DNA testing at 12 months after a course of intravaginal estrogen for a period of 1 week.

High-grade Squamous Intraepithelial Lesion

It encompasses moderate and severe dysplasia, CIS/CIN 2 and CIN 3 with features suspicious for invasion (if invasion is suspected).

High-grade squamous intraepithelial lesion is characterized by smaller cells of basal or parabasal cells with rounded borders, showing dense cytoplasm and pronounced nuclear abnormalities like markedly increased nuclear/cytoplasmic (N/C) ratio, hyperchromasia, nuclear abnormalities, nuclear irregularity, and coarse chromatin. Large numbers of abnormal cells are found in clumps or sheets so-called "microbiopsies". Larger cells showing pronounced nuclear abnormalities are also included in HSIL.

2014 Bethesda criteria for HSIL remain the same.

Management options for HSIL: A diagnosis of HSIL accounts for only about 0.5% of Pap test results. Three quarters of these usually result in CIN 2, 3, or greater.

- HSIL patients must undergo colposcopy and endocervical (TZ zone) histological confirmation.
- If the high-grade lesion is identified at colposcopy, immediate LEEP of the transformation zone may be done in patients at risk of being lost to follow up or those for whom fertility is not an issue.

Squamous cell carcinoma: As used in TBS, squamous cell carcinoma indicates a probable invasive carcinoma which shows malignant cells in the background of blood, pus and necrotic material called tumor diathesis. Cytologically it is possible to distinguish large cell keratinizing, large cell non keratinizing and small cell carcinomas though not necessarily in the per view of TBS lesion.

Management: Refer to oncology center.

Glandular Cells

The Pap test was not introduced to screen for glandular lesions but the increase in incidence of adenocarcinoma and challenging appearances the abnormal glandular cells has made it incumbent that their morphology be familiar. In 1988 TBS used the term "atypical glandular cells of undetermined significance (AGUS)" to describe cells showing glandular differentiation with nuclear atypia that exceeds obvious reactive or reparative changes but lack unequivocal features of adenocarcinoma. It was suggested that qualifier such as "favor reactive" and "favor neoplastic" should be used. The spectrum of AGUS ranged from benign appearing reparative findings to adenocarcinoma in situ.

The TBS Bethesda 2001 recommended that the term AGUS be replaced with the term "atypical glandular cell" (AGC) and the "favor reactive" be eliminated. As far as possible an attempt should be made to indicate the origin of AGC as being either endocervical, endometrial or unqualified. The finding of AGC needs to be addressed as this is associated with a high percentage of high-grade disease (10-39% either glandular or squamous)

In addition, "adenocarcinoma in situ" (a new term in TBS 2001) and AGC "favor neoplastic" are treated as separate entities.

Atypical endocervical/endometrial/glandular cells NOS: This designation encompasses inflammatory changes or reparative changes in glandular cells or atypia which may be onset of neoplasia but insufficient for a diagnosis of neoplasia. They are less commonly encountered than ASC-US cells (forming 0.5% of cases). These lesions include a morphologic spectrum of cells and whenever possible endocervical cells must be differentiated from endometrial cells.

Atypical endocervical cells favor neoplastic show mild nuclear abnormalities, those favoring neoplastic process show hyperchromatic crowded groups, loss of honeycomb pattern with overlapping, loss of polarity, rosettes and feathering, nuclear size 3–5 times that of benign endocervical cells, nuclear irregularity, and coarse chromatin.

Atypical endometrial cells: Normal appearing endometrial cells in a postmenopausal woman who is not receiving hormonal therapy is always abnormal. Endometrial atypical cells are seen in small groups with slightly enlarged nuclei, scanty cytoplasm with ill-defined borders, and small nucleoli. Presence of these cells indicates either endometrial polyps, hyperplasia, or neoplasia and sampling of the lower uterine segment is advised as AGUS endometrial cells are associated with squamous or glandular neoplasia in many instances.

Management of atypical glandular cells: Presence of atypical glandular cells warrants further investigations such as colposcopy and endocervical curettage as well as HPV testing. Cervical cytology alone has a sensitivity of 50–72% in identifying glandular dysplasia. Women aged >35 years with unexplained vaginal bleeding should also undergo endometrial sampling along with colposcopy and endocervical sampling.

Cold knife conization is the recommended next step for women with an initial cytology of AGC—favor neoplasia or adenocarcinoma in situ.

Adenocarcinoma: Diagnosis of adenocarcinoma indicates a probably invasive carcinoma. The origin of the tumor may be specified if possible.

NHS RECOMMENDATIONS FOR REPORTING CERVICAL CYTOLOGY

The last decade incorporated major changes to the National Health Service Cervical Screening Programme (NHSCSP).[19] These included the introduction and implementation of LBC sampling, and the implementation of hrHPV testing for triage of borderline and low-grade abnormalities. That revision of the program includes:

- *The NHSCSP[19] adopted the revised British Society for Clinical Cytology (BSCC) terminology for reporting cervical cytology*:
  - Division of the category "borderline change" into "squamous" and "endocervical" categories
  - Division of dyskaryosis into "low-grade" and "high-grade" categories (the latter encompassing moderate and severe dyskaryosis)
  - Division of glandular neoplasia into "endocervical" and "noncervical" categories
- *Guidance on the management of abnormal cytology results has been linked to this terminology*: Management guidance has been updated in the light of hrHPV testing for triage of low-grade cytological abnormality.

CONCLUSION

Persistent HPV infection with high-risk subtypes causes high-grade dysplasia in the cervix. High-grade changes that persist for 1 or 2 years are more likely to lead to malignancy, and therefore, HPV testing/screening every 5 years is mandatory after 25 years of age. It takes approximately 3–10 years for high-grade changes in cervical cells to lead to carcinoma. Cervical cancer screening by Pap smear detects these changes. Those with high-grade changes can get treated (conization) to have these dysplastic changes removed. Women with low-grade changes can be tested more frequently to see the progress of these.

Standardization in the reporting of these abnormal findings has to be strictly adhered to for universal acceptance and communication and therefore the Bethesda System of reporting cervical cytology.

REFERENCES

1. Remondi C, Sesti F, Bonanno E, Pietropolli A, Piccione E. Diagnostic accuracy of liquid-based endometrial cytology in the evaluation of endometrial pathology in postmenopausal women. Cytopathology. 2013;24(6):365-71.
2. Ma K, Yang X, Chen R, Zhao J, Dong Y, Zhang NY, et al. Liquid-based endometrial cytology associated with curettage in the investigation of endometrial carcinoma in postmenopausal women. Taiwan J Obstet Gynecol. 2016;55(6):777-81.
3. Minagawa Y, Sato S, Ito M, Onohara Y, Nakamoto S, Kigawa J. Transvaginal ultrasonography and endometrial cytology as a diagnostic schema for endometrial cancer. Gynecol Obstet Invest. 2005;59(3):149-54.
4. Akahane T, Kitazono I, Yanazume S, Kamio M, Togami S, Sakamoto I, et al. Next-generation sequencing analysis of endometrial screening liquid-based cytology specimens: a comparative study to tissue specimens. BMC Med Genomics. 2020;13(1):101.
5. Wang Q, Wang Q, Zhao L, Han L, Sun C, Ma S, et al. Endometrial Cytology as a Method to Improve the Accuracy of Diagnosis of Endometrial Cancer: Case Report and Meta-Analysis. Front Oncol. 2019;9:256.
6. Ayre JE. Rotating endometrial brush: new technic for the diagnosis of fundal carcinoma. Obstet Gynecol. 1955;5(2):137-41.
7. Han L, Ma S, Zhao L, Liu Y, Wang Y, Feng X, et al. Clinical Evaluation of Li Brush Endometrial Samplers for Diagnosing Endometrial Lesions in Women With Intrauterine Devices. Front Med (Lausanne). 2020;7:598689.
8. Directorate General of Health Services, Ministry of Health and Family Welfare. Manual for Cytology. Directorate General of Health Services, Ministry of Health and Family Welfare, Government of India; 2005.
9. Nayar R, Wilbur DC. The Pap test and Bethesda 2014. Cancer Cytopathol. 2015;123(5):271-81.
10. Saxena SK, Kumar S, Goel MM, Kaur A, Bhatt MLB. Recent advances in Human Papillomavirus infection and management. InTechOpen; 2018.
11. Shariff S, Kaler AK. Principles and Interpretation of Laboratory Practices in Surgical Pathology. New Delhi: Jaypee Brothers Medical Publishers (P) Ltd.; 2016.
12. National Cancer Institute. (2020) ACS's Updated Cervical Cancer Screening Guidelines Explained. Subscribe. [online] Available from https://www.cancer.gov/news-events/cancer-currents-blog/2020/cervical-cancer-screening-hpv-test-guideline [Last accessed March, 2024].
13. World Health Organization. WHO Guidelines for Screening and Treatment of Precancerous Lesions for Cervical Cancer Prevention. Geneva: World Health Organization; 2013.
14. Nayar R, Wilbur DC. The Bethesda System for Reporting Cervical Cytology, Definitions, Criteria, and Explanatory Notes. Cham, Switzerland: Springer; 2015.
15. Solomon D, Davey D, Kurman R, Moriarty A, O'Connor D, Prey M, et al. The 2001 Bethesda System: terminology for reporting results of cervical cytology. JAMA. 2002 Apr 24;287(16):2114-9.
16. Koss LG, Melamed MR. Koss' Diagnostic Cytology and Its Histopathologic Bases. Philadelphia: Lippincott Williams and Wilkins; 2006.
17. Massad LS, Einstein MH, Huh WK, Katki HA, Kinney WK, Schiffman M, et al. 2012 updated consensus guidelines for the management of abnormal cervical cancer screening tests and cancer precursors. J Low Genit Tract Dis. 2013;17(5 Suppl 1):S1-S27. Erratum in: J Low Genit Tract Dis. 2013;17(3):367.
18. Wright TC Jr, Massad LS, Dunton CJ, Spitzer M, Wilkinson EJ, Solomon D, et al. 2006 consensus guidelines for the management of women with abnormal cervical cancer screening tests. Am J Obstet Gynecol. 2007;197(4):346-55.
19. NHS Cancer Screening Programmes. (2013). Reporting and classification of cervical cytology. [online] Available from https://assets.publishing.service.gov.uk/government/uploads/system/uploads/attachment_data/file/436753/nhscsp01.pdf [Last accessed March, 2024].

CHAPTER 10

Fine-needle Aspiration Cytology

INTRODUCTION

Fine-needle aspiration cytology (FNAC) or fine-needle aspiration biopsy (FNAB) is a minimally invasive and cost-effective technique with a high diagnostic accuracy. The diagnostic accuracy depends on the experience of the reporting cytologist, the site and the type of lesion sampled, the adequacy of material, and the quality of specimen preparation. It is a diagnostic procedure which is immensely popular in diagnosing not only superficial swellings in various organ systems but has also earned a reputation in the last two to three decades in diagnosing deep-seated lesions due to the accessibility of the lesion by an image-guided needle. The ability to remove cellular material for diagnostic purposes as well as ancillary techniques like flow cytometry, and molecular studies in neoplasia have made FNAC an essential tool in the field of diagnosis.

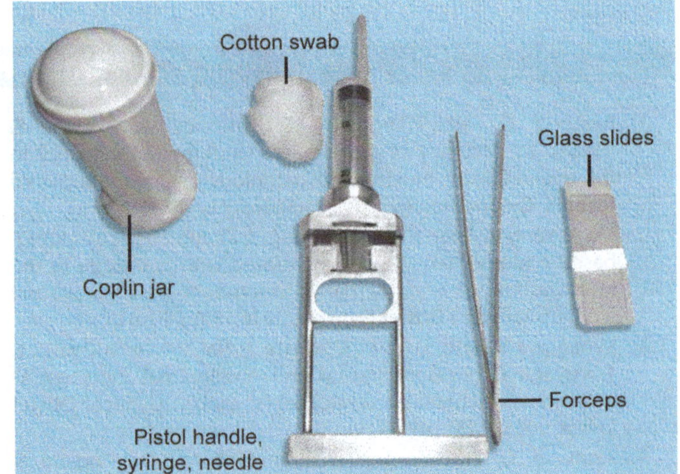

FIG. 1: Requirements for fine-needle aspiration cytology (FNAC): Coplin jar contains absolute alcohol for insertion of smears once they are made.

PROCEDURE

Fine-needle aspiration cytology can be performed as an office procedure in a matter of a few minutes and the report available on the same day thereby alleviating patient anxiety and fear. In experienced hands, it is a useful tool in guiding patient management and avoiding unnecessary surgery.

- The patient is explained about the procedure, and his willingness is taken. All attempts are made to relieve anxiety. An informed consent form and patient/guardian signature should be obtained on having filled it up. Written consent is an institutional policy.
- The procedure is streamlined in most institutions and requires a metal syringe holder and a 10–20 cc sterile disposable syringe **(Fig. 1)**. The needle with the syringe holder popularly the Cameco syringe holder is inserted into the swelling and once within it material withdrawn under negative pressure **(Fig. 2)** with 2–3 brisk strokes along the same tract.
- For larger lesions, a single-entry multidirectional technique is used as shown in the **Figure 3**. The direction of the aspiration **(Figs. 2 and 3)** is changed as the syringe is drawn up without completely coming out of the nodule, not when it is deep down in the lesion thus avoiding tears in tissue; resulting in a single puncture multidirectional technique. The force of the cutting motion needed to obtain an adequate sample must be adjusted for the body site and characteristics of the lesion. The entire procedure should be finished in a few seconds and practice makes perfection!
- Soon after aspiration, material appears in the hub of the needle, the suction is then released and needle

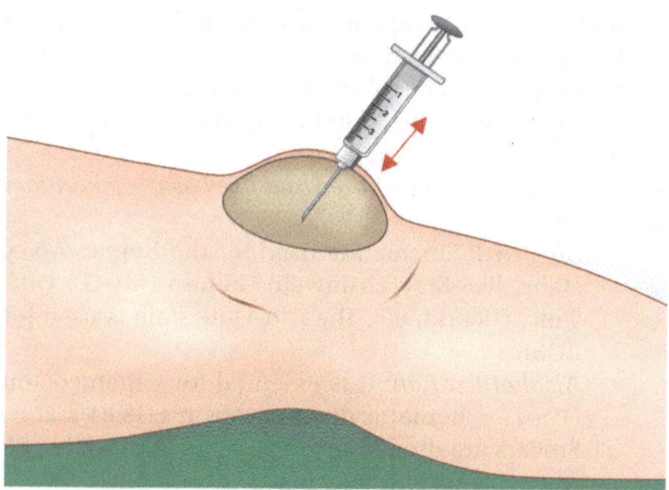

FIG. 2: Single entry point of needle into swelling.

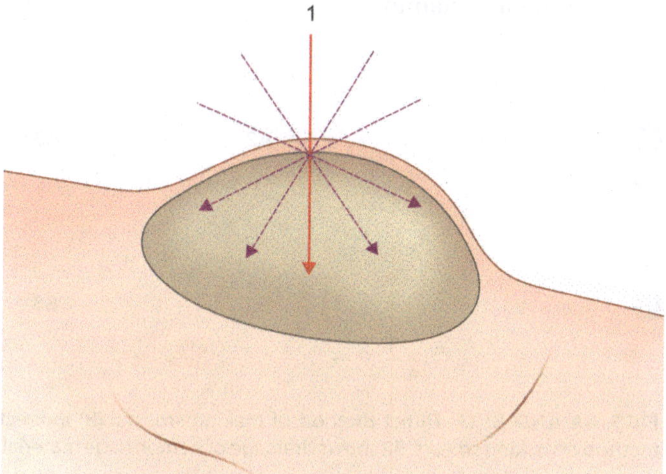

FIG. 3: To show single entry, multidirectional technique.

withdrawn smoothly. Failure to release negative pressure within the lesion causes the aspirated material to enter the syringe instead of remaining in the hub of the needle. The needle is detached from the syringe, air drawn in the syringe, which is refixed and the aspirate expelled onto a glass slide and smears made.

- All subcutaneous nodules, breast swellings as well as thyroid lesions are aspirated with a regular 22 or 23 gauge needle whereas sharp lumbar puncture needles are used for deep-seated abdominal organs and liver. Various needle lengths to match location of the lesion can be obtained. An ultrasound or computed tomography (CT) guidance should be used. Bleeding parameters are checked out for all intra-abdominal aspirates.
- A technique popular with thyroid aspirations (to avoid bloody material) is needling, i.e., aspiration without attaching the syringe or applying negative pressure; as the intention is to collect the material in the hub of the needle and then expel it from the needle, while making smears.
- Rarely intraoperative FNAB may be performed for a quick on table diagnosis and whenever required material is to be obtained for ancillary tests such as cell block preparations, molecular studies, flow cytometry, or microbiological studies like culture, etc.
- In cystic lesions, as much fluid as possible is removed and the cyst fluid is taken for analysis. In cystic lesions, particularly of the thyroid, breast and salivary gland, residual nodules/solid areas in cystic walls have to be aspirated to exclude cystic change in a neoplasm as the cyst may obscure a small malignant tumor.
- Needles should be discarded using a sharps disposal container.
- Local pressure is usually adequate to control post-procedural bleeding at superficial sites. Patients who have undergone deep FNAB should be followed for complications. They may be kept under observations for a period of 6–8 hours.
- Specimen adequacy is assessed during FNAC by using a rapid stain such as Diff-Quik or toluidine blue stain. Although no universal criterion for adequacy exists, a multiparameter assessment is usually performed which includes cellularity, organ-specific architectural features, and cellular elements. Rapid on-site evaluation (ROSE) reduces several false-negative reports due to inadequacy.
- Slides should be marked with the patient's name or specific identifier.
- A written report should follow the procedure and should contain information with regard to site of biopsy, age of the patient, medical record number, and collection data. A brief microscopic description and impression should be included. Comments/suggestions may be given at the end of the report. The report should include data that are legible and accurate and must be sent to persons that are authorized to receive and use the information.
- All reporting personnel should attempt to correlate cytological findings with histological material if available or on a follow-up biopsy if performed.
- Special anatomical areas require special precautions and positioning.

Figure 4 shows a thyroid aspirate with the neck being extended for easy accessibility.

Figures 5A and B show a specially designed instrument with a needle guide, used in prostatic aspiration while doing a per rectal examination. The needle guide protects the tip of the needle till it reaches the lesion.

Smear Making and Staining

The needle tip is brought into light contact with the slide and the material expelled gently onto a slide.

- There are two fundamental methods of making smears obtained by fine-needle aspiration (FNA)—direct and indirect. Direct smear is for a cellular aspirate. An ideal aspirate is white and creamy with numerous cells suspended in a small amount of tissue fluid without admixture with blood. The smear is made using another slide which is placed at an incline to the one with the aspirate so that the edge of the inclined slide is on the cellular material. Using gentle uniform pressure, the second slide is pulled across resulting in uniform thickness of the smear. The indirect method is for bloody aspirates and deals with tilting the slide with the expressed material so as to drain out the blood and then making smears as in the direct method **(Figs. 6A and B)**.
- *Smears should be prepared and fixed as per laboratory protocols*:
  - *Air-dried*: Smears are used for the Romanowsky stains like May-Grünwald Giemsa (MGG), Diff-Quik, Giemsa, etc. The Diff-Quik stain is used for ROSE.
  - *Alcohol fixation*: It is essential for Papanicolaou (Pap) or hematoxylin and eosin (H&E) stains. Smears are dipped in absolute alcohol while still wet as soon as they are made.
  - In FNAC smears of bloody material, the smear is given one dip in 1% acetic acid before bringing it to water and staining.

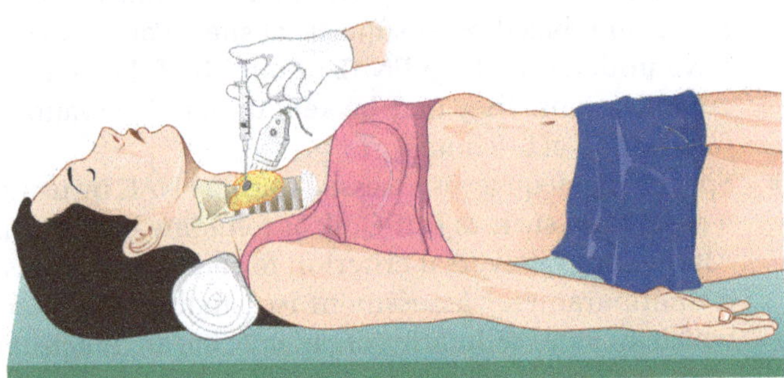

FIG. 4: Procedure for thyroid aspiration with extended neck position using support beneath.

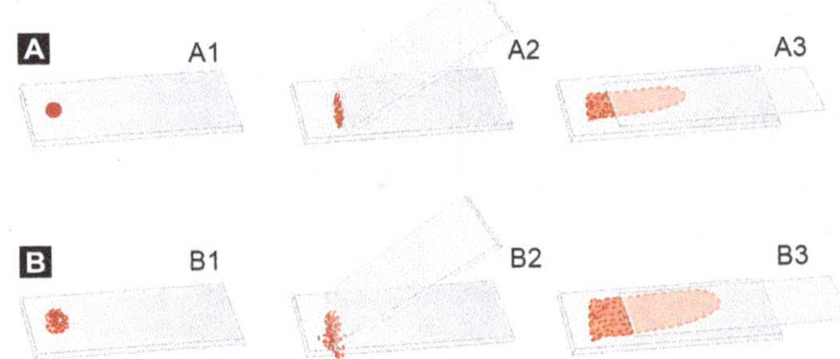

FIGS. 6A AND B: (A) Direct method of making smears; (B) Indirect method of making smears. B2 shows drainage of hemorrhage material.

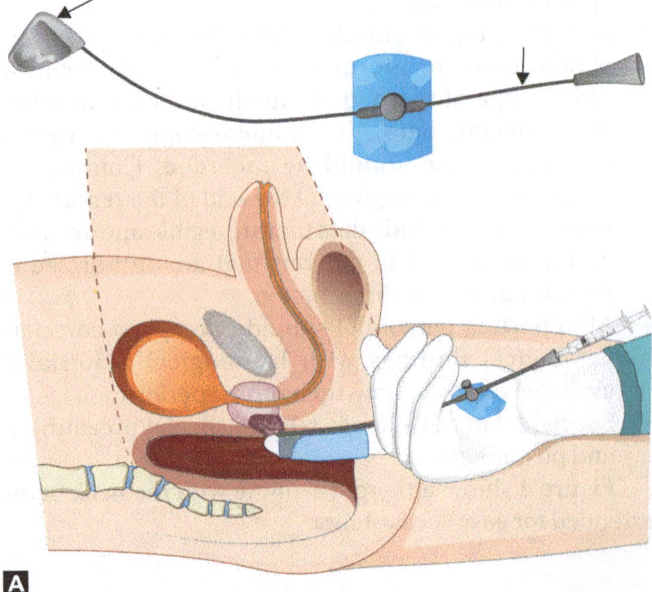
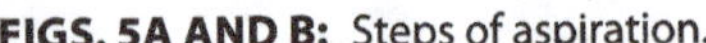

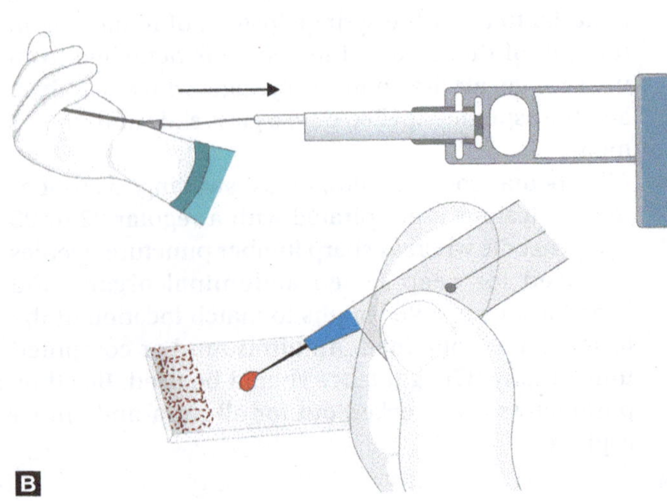

FIGS. 5A AND B: Steps of aspiration.

Cell Block Technique for FNAC Material and Immunohistochemistry

Tissue fragments/blood clots are picked up with a forceps and wrapped in a small piece of filter paper as above. This is placed in a tissue cassette with a label; fixed in 10% neutral buffered formalin and then processed as a paraffin block. The procedure is used for sediments also. In case of paucity of the later, the sediment can be embedded in the egg albumin/agar gel.

Fixing in 10% neutral buffered formalin preserves antigens for IHC apart from showing excellent morphology.

FINE-NEEDLE ASPIRATION CYTOLOGY REPORTING CRITERIA

Standard criteria are available in literature for reporting FNA samples. Given below are some standard protocols required to be followed in certain organ systems. Outlining all cytological in various lesions is out of scope of this book. A few important guidelines are provided.

The Bethesda System of Reporting Thyroid Pathology[1-3]

Palpable thyroid nodules are common and seen in about 5% of the population. The first line of diagnosis is to do an FNAC and FNAC of the thyroid is widely accepted as a simple, quick, outpatient, and safe procedure in order to select which type of nodules should be subjected to surgery. FNA saves countless unnecessary thyroid surgeries while appropriately triaging patients with malignant nodules for the same.

- The Bethesda System of Reporting Thyroid Cytopathology comprises distinct categories which provide room for a standard reporting system where thyroid FNA is considered, avoids dubious and multiplicity of category names, narrative reports, and borrowed terminology from surgical pathology. Besides this, it also provides risk of malignancy (ROM) in each category and management modalities as a guide to the treating clinician. These figures and percentages of risk of malignancies are authenticated and supported by meta-analyses and confirmation.
- The system was introduced after much deliberation which occurred at a conference held in Bethesda, Maryland in the year 2007, where 154 participants from various specialties including cytologists, pathologists, clinicians, and endocrinologists met and came to a consensus opinion. The categories put forward then and continued even after the 2017 revision which are as follows:
    - *Category 1 [Nondiagnostic (ND) or unsatisfactory (UNS)]*: 1–3%
    - *Category 2*: Benign
    - *Category 3*: Atypia of undetermined significance (AUS) or follicular lesion of undetermined significance (FLUS)
    - *Category 4*: Follicular neoplasm or suspicious for a follicular neoplasm (specify if Hürthle cell in type)
    - *Category 5*: Suspicious for malignancy
    - *Category 6*: Malignant
- Risk of malignancy and clinical management in each category are given in **Table 1**.

TABLE 1: Diagnostic category, risk of malignancy (ROM), and clinical management.

Diagnostic category	ROM	Management
Nondiagnostic/UNS	5–10%	Repeat aspiration
Benign	0–3%	Clinical and US follow-up
AUS/FLUS	10–30%	Repeat FNA, molecular testing or lobectomy
Follicular neoplasm or suspected for FN/Hürthle cell neoplasm	25–40%	Molecular testing and lobectomy
Suspicious for malignancy	50–75%	Near total thyroidectomy or lobectomy
Malignant	97–99%	Near total thyroidectomy or lobectomy

(AUS: atypia of undetermined significance; FLUS: follicular lesion of undetermined significance; FN: follicular neoplasm; FNA: fine-needle aspiration; UNS: unsatisfactory)

Category 1: Insufficient for Diagnosis (Unsatisfactory/Nondiagnostic)

- Limited cellularity
- Cyst fluid only
- Poor fixation and preservation of cells

About 2–20% of FNAs constitute the category "insufficient for diagnosis".

Inadequate sample and unsatisfactory for diagnosis are used synonymously in this category.

To know what is a limited sample at cytology, it is important to be aware of an adequate specimen at aspiration. The Bethesda system (TBS) states that a sample is considered satisfactory for evaluation if *at least six groups* of benign follicular cells are seen; each group composed of *at least 10 cells*.

Exceptions to this would be:

- *Solid nodules with cytologic atypia*:
    - *Colloid nodules*: Any specimen that contains abundant colloid is considered adequate (and benign).
    - *Solid nodules with inflammation*: Inflammatory cells seen and can be reported benign cyst fluid with macrophages alone is considered inadequate.

Macrophages do not contribute to cellularity. If considered adequate then such a specimen may contribute to a false-negative in presence of a cystic papillary carcinoma.

Poor morphology due to inadequate preservation of cells, drying artifacts, all hinder assessment of morphology and contribute to an unsatisfactory sample.

Nonrepresentative aspirates showing respiratory epithelial cells from trachea, skeletal muscle, etc., are considered inadequate.

Management of Category 1

- Nodules with initial ND/UNS are reaspirated after an interval period of 3 months. Immediate aspiration is not done to prevent false-positive interpretations due to reactive or reparative changes.
- If immediate reaspiration is carried out, it should be done under ultrasound guidance.
- Repeat aspiration gives results in approximately 60% of cases. Most of the ND/UNS prove to be benign.
- After two successive ND/UNS specimens, a close clinical follow-up with US or surgery may be done if clinical features are suspicious.

Category 2: Benign (Negative for Malignant Cells)

- This includes all lesions which are unequivocally benign—consistent with benign follicular nodule (includes adenomatoid nodule and colloid nodule), follicular adenoma. Graves' disease, Hashimoto's (lymphocytic) thyroiditis in the proper clinical context, etc. Difference between macrofollicular adenoma and hyperplastic nodule (HN) is not possible at cytology or even on histologic examination.
- Also includes granulomatous thyroiditis

Nodular Goiter

- Abundant thick or thin colloid
- Follicular cells in monolayered sheets, poorly cohesive clusters, and single cells
- Involutional cells with minimal cytoplasm and oxyphilic follicular cells
- Hyperplastic cells with feathery and fragile cytoplasm, many bare nuclei
- Pigment-laden histiocytes (foam cells)
- Degenerative features such as cell debris and macrophages
- Retrogressive changes in goiter FNA yields brownish colloid-like fluid with altered blood
- Smears show macrophages that may contain hemosiderin and sparse degenerating follicular cells.

Chronic Thyroiditis

- *Hashimoto's (autoimmune) thyroiditis*: Sheets of lymphocytes with bimodal population.
  - Follicular cell epithelium with infiltrating lymphocytes
  - Hürthle cell change
  - Plasma cells

Subacute (De Quervain's) thyroiditis **(Fig. 7)**: Sheets of inflammatory cells including lymphocytes, macrophages, and epithelioid-like cells.

- Numerous giant cells in clusters
- Necrotic background with neutrophils and debris

Acute Suppurative Thyroiditis

- Tender thyroid enlargement, fever, and high erythrocyte sedimentation rate (ESR)
- Smears show neutrophils, necrotic cells, and debris
- Intracellular bacteria, (usually gram-positive cocci), may be present.

Macrofollicular Adenoma

- Monolayered sheets of follicular cells with maintained polarity and spacing
- Benign appearing nucleus
- Rare macrophages; minimal hemosiderin

Graves' Disease/Nodule in Graves' Disease

- Colloid-free bloody background
- Increased cellularity with monolayered sheets with rounded borders

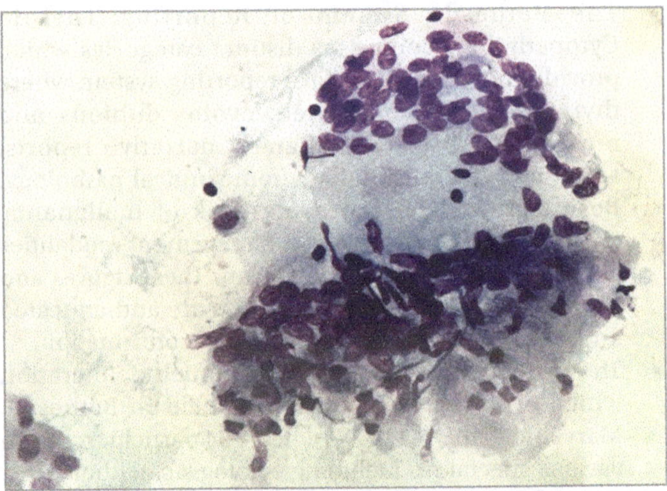

FIG. 7: De Quervain's thyroiditis showing a cluster of multinucleate giant cells (Pap, ×400).

- Increased granularity of cells better appreciated in Giemsa stain
- Fire flares at the periphery also well seen in Giemsa stained smears
- Marked anisonucleosis
- Atypical nuclear changes on patients with therapy
- Hürthle cell changes

Management of Category 2

- The false-negative rate of a benign interpretation is low (0–3%), nevertheless patients *are followed with repeated assessment by palpation or ultrasound at 6–18 months intervals.*
- If the nodule shows significant growth or "suspicious" sonographic changes, repeated FNA is considered.
- As per the American Thyroid Association, 2015, a nodule with a high suspicion of ultrasound pattern should be subject to repeat aspiration within 12 months.
  - Nodules with a low to intermediate US pattern, repeat US should to done after 12–24 months and a guided FNA performed if necessary
  - Nodules with very low US suspicious pattern, FNA repeated only after 24 months.

Category 3: Atypia of Undetermined Significance or Follicular Lesion of Undetermined Significance

- Some thyroid FNAs are not easily classified into either the benign, suspicious for malignancy, or malignant categories.
- Such cases represent a minority of thyroid FNAs and are reported as AUS or FLUS in cases of atypical follicular cells or any other cell type or atypia.
- Cells (follicular, lymphoid, or other) are with *architectural or nuclear atypia.*
- It may also be a compromised specimen with presence of focal atypia.

  Examples of this category may be reported in the following instances:
  - Prominent population of microfollicles in an aspirate that does not otherwise fulfill the criteria for "follicular neoplasm" or predominance of Hürthle cells in a sparsely cellular aspirate with scant colloid.
  - Intranuclear inclusions in occasional cells but no other features of a papillary thyroid carcinoma (PTC)
  - A minor population of follicular cells show nuclear enlargement, often accompanied by prominent nucleoli
  - An inadvertent air-drying of alcohol fixed smears leads to suboptimal nuclear detail.
  - Occasional cells show intranuclear cytoplasmic inclusion (INCI)/grooves

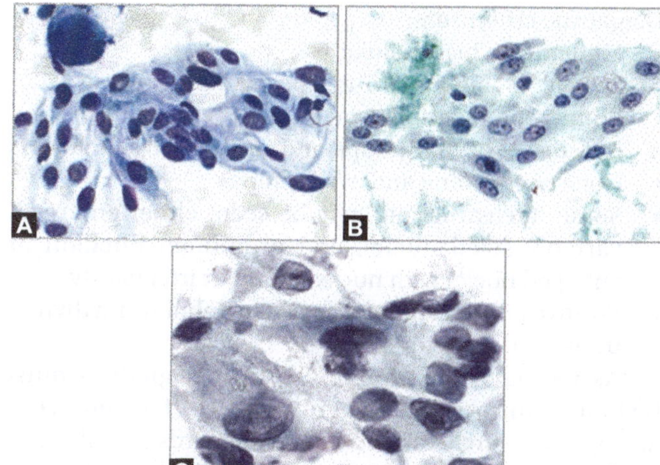

FIGS. 8A TO C: Cyst lining cells showing atypia (Bethesda atlas 2017).

  - Carbimazole/methimazole therapy and ionizing radiation may give rise to atypical nuclear changes and enlargement.
  - An atypical lymphoid infiltrates (in which repeated aspirate for flow cytometry is desirable), but the degree of atypia is insufficient for the general category "suspicious for malignancy."
  - Cyst lining cells in multinodular goiter (MNG) with elongated cell appearances, squamoid appearances with pavementing, and nucleus may show prominent nucleoli **(Fig. 8)**.
  - The ROM for an AUS nodule is difficult to ascertain because only a minority of cases in this category have surgical follow-up.
  - Those that are resected represent a selected population of patients with repeated AUS results or patients with worrisome clinical or sonographic findings.

Management of Category 3: Atypia of Undetermined Significance

- Repeat FNA
- Molecular testing
- Lobectomy

Microarray-based studies: To differentiate suspicious PTC from benign tissue, atypia in follicular lesions, etc.

Gene classifier system for further characterization of nodules with an indeterminate thyroid cytology is available.

Category 4: Suspicious for Follicular Neoplasm or Lesion/Specify if Hürthle Cell Type

All follicular lesions suspected as being follicular or Hürthle cell lesions are placed in this category.

Diagnostic criteria are:

- Moderate to high cellularity
- Bloody, usually colloid-free background
- Prominent microfollicular pattern
- Rosettes, syncytial groups, and equal-sized cell clusters
- Nuclear crowding and overlapping
- Some nuclear atypia may be seen, either enlarged, variably sized nuclei, and prominent nucleoli or enlarged nuclei with nuclear contour irregularity
- Positive immunostaining for thyroglobulin and thyroid transcription factor-1 (TTF-1)

As per TBS, the "microfollicle" designation must be limited to crowded, flat groups of <15 follicular cells arranged in a circle that is at least two-thirds complete.

Figure 9 shows how to assess follicular patterned lesions and the rationale for diagnosing follicular neoplasm.

Hürthle cell neoplasm: Criteria are—

- Moderately to markedly cellular aspirate
- Exclusively (or almost exclusively) of Hürthle cells
- Enlarged, central, or eccentrically located round nucleus
- Prominent eosinophilic nucleolus
- Small cells with high nuclear/cytoplasmic (N/C) ratio (small cell dysplasia).
- Large cells with at least twice the nuclear size (large cell dysplasia).

Management of category 4 is surgical excision and diagnosis, usually lobectomy or hemithyroidectomy.

Category 5: Suspicious for Malignant Cells

It includes suspicious for papillary carcinoma, medullary carcinoma, metastatic carcinoma, lymphoma, or others.

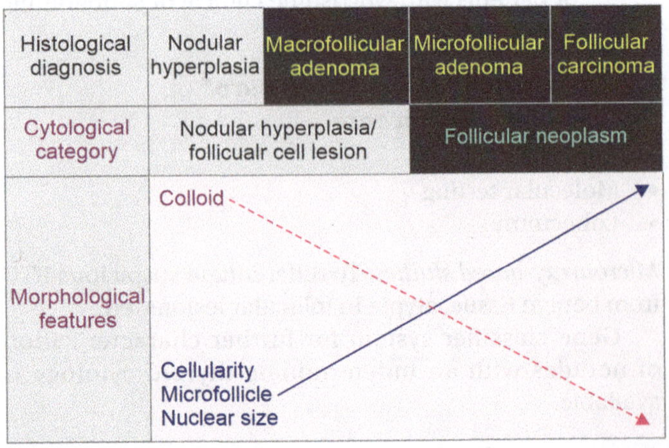

Histological diagnosis	Nodular hyperplasia	Macrofollicular adenoma	Microfollicular adenoma	Follicular carcinoma
Cytological category	Nodular hyperplasia/ follicualr cell lesion		Follicular neoplasm	
Morphological features	Colloid Cellularity Microfollicle Nuclear size			

FIG. 9: Assessment of follicular patterned lesions and the rationale for diagnosing follicular neoplasm.

- This category is like the one used in other organs, where a strong suspicion of carcinoma occurs but still some hesitancy occurs due to lack of an adequate sample size. It invariably turns out to be malignant on excision.
- Many thyroid cancers, most especially PTC, can be diagnosed with certainty by FNA.
- But, the nuclear and architectural changes of some PTCs are subtle and focal. This is particularly true of the follicular variant of PTC, which can be difficult to distinguish from a benign follicular nodule
- Other PTCs may be incompletely sampled and yield only a small number of abnormal cells. Such cases occur with some regularity, and they are best classified as "suspicious for malignancy," or qualify as "suspicious for papillary carcinoma."

Suspicious for Lymphoma

- Cellular sample composed of numerous monomorphic small to intermediate-sized lymphoid cells with mild nuclear irregularity or the smear is sparsely cellular and contains atypical lymphoid cells.
- Absence of bimodal population

Suspicious for Medullary Carcinoma

- Sample sparsely or moderately cellular
- Monomorphic population of noncohesive small or medium-sized cells with high N/C ratio (? lymphoid lesion/? medullary carcinoma)
- Absence of amyloid

Management of Category 5

- Surgery—total thyroidectomy
- In large tumors >4 cm, total thyroidectomy is considered because they have a high risk to undergo malignant transformation.
- Lymphomas/medullary carcinomas—flow cytometry, immunoreactivity for calcitonin, synaptophysin, and chromogranin

Category 6: Positive for Malignant Cells

It includes positive for papillary carcinoma, medullary carcinoma, anaplastic carcinoma, lymphoma, metastatic, and others (other than follicular carcinoma).

Papillary Carcinoma

- Cellular smears
- Cells forming syncytial aggregates and sheets focally with a distinct "anatomical border" and nuclear crowding and over lapping, and thick nuclear membranes.

- Flat sheets, three-dimensional tissue fragments, and papillary tissue fragments with or without a fibrovascular core
- Enlarged, ovoid, strikingly pale nuclei, finely granular, and powdery chromatin (PAP)
- Intranuclear cytoplasmic inclusions and nuclear grooves
- Dense cytoplasm and distinct cell borders
- Squamoid or histiocyte-like and "metaplastic" epithelial cells
- Scanty, viscous, stringy (chewing gum) colloid—variable
- Psammoma bodies—variable
- Macrophages and debris (evidence of cystic degeneration), multinucleate giant cells, and lymphocytes—variable
- Dual immunostaining for keratin and vimentin; positive immunostaining for CK19, CD44, and Hector Battifora mesothelial-1 (HBME).

Variants of papillary carcinoma
- May not show all classic features of papillary carcinoma listed above.
- *Nuclear features are subtle. Therefore, these are invariably categorized as suspicious for carcinoma (category 5). The variants are*:
    - *Follicular (and macrofollicular encapsulated)*:
        - Oncocytic variant
        - Warthin tumor-like variant
        - Cribriform-morular variant
        - Adenoid cystic variant
        - Variant with fasciitis-like stroma
        - *High-grade variants*: Tall cell, columnar, and diffuse
        - Sclerosing and solid/trabecular variants

Medullary Carcinoma

- Cellular specimen with dispersed cells, some clustering; round, ovoid, plasmacytoid or spindle cells singly or in small cluster; cells have moderate to abundant cytoplasm and eccentric nuclei; and chromatin has salt and pepper appearance
- Moderate anisonucleosis, scattered very large nuclei, and binucleate and multinucleate form.
- Uniform, stippled ("neuroendocrine") nuclear chromatin
- May have pink azurophilic granules and intranuclear pseudoinclusions
- Amyloid is present occasionally.

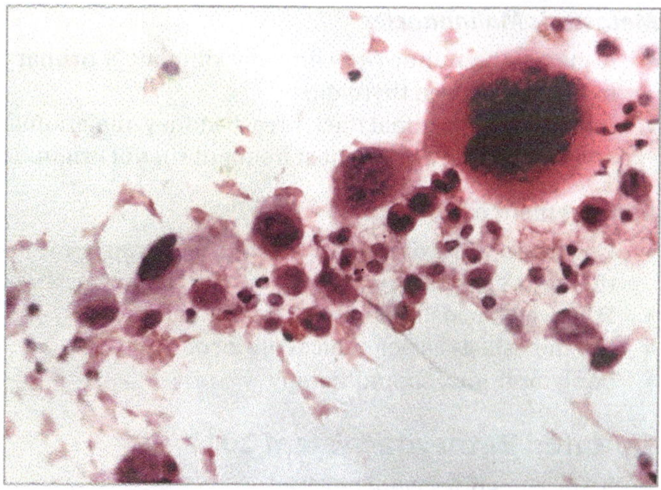

FIG. 10: Smear shows anaplastic epithelial cells with nuclear pleomorphism, hyperchromatism, and tumor giant cells (H&E, ×400).

Anaplastic Carcinoma (Undifferentiated Carcinoma) (Fig. 10)

- Necrotic background with pleomorphic malignant cells
- Multinucleate, bizarre giant cells and/or spindle/squamoid cells showing marked atypia, some with moderate to abundant cytoplasm
- Frequent, abnormal mitoses

Poorly Differentiated Carcinoma (Insular Carcinoma)

- Small follicular cells arranged in crowded insulae and morulae
- Some necrotic debris may be seen.

Lymphoma

- Lymphoma may involve the thyroid secondarily. Primary thyroid lymphoma is rare (1–5% of thyroid malignancies).
- Most are of B-cell lineage and mucosa-associated lymphoid tissue (MALT) type and occur in a background of Hashimoto's thyroiditis.
- High-grade lymphomas show large abnormal lymphoid cells of blastic type
- In elderly females with rapid thyroid enlargement and pressure symptoms, clinically mimicking anaplastic carcinoma
- A mixed cell population including plasma cells, suggestive of a florid reactive process in low-grade lymphoma.

Metastatic Malignancies

- A metastatic tumor can clinically simulate a primary neoplasm or even thyroiditis.
- Lung, gastrointestinal tract, breast, kidney, melanoma, and lymphoma are the most frequent sites of origin.

Management of Category 6

- Complete surgical resection with preoperative radiotherapy or chemotherapy.
- Followed by postoperative chemotherapy
- For metastasis as per clinical protocol
- For lymphoma, chemotherapy

Updated Bethesda System 2017

- Same categories were retained.
- Each category has an implied cancer ROM that ranges from 0 to 3% for the "benign" category to virtually 100% for the "malignant" category, and, in the 2017 revision, the malignancy risks were updated based on recent (post 2010) data and clinical management
- Reclassification of some thyroid neoplasms was done, e.g., *noninvasive follicular thyroid neoplasm with papillary-like nuclear features (NIFTP)*. Diagnostic criteria for this were outlined and it had implications with reduced ROM. Therefore, clinical management was different with a better prognosis.
- Follicular variant of papillary thyroid carcinoma (FVPTC) is of two types: Infiltrative or nonencapsulated and diffuse variant.
- It occurs in young females and is aggressive.
- FVPTC with an infiltrative growth pattern is associated with frequent lymph node metastases, a risk of recurrence, and BRAFV600E mutations, *similar to conventional PTC ("BRAF-like PTCs")*.
- *FVPTC*: The encapsulated FVPTC is characterized by a follicular growth pattern with no papillae formation and total tumor encapsulation and the diagnosis rests on finding characteristic nuclear features of PTC.
- 50–75% of the encapsulated FVPTC show RAS mutations: Closer to follicular adenoma and carcinoma; PAX8 and PPARγ translocation; and THADA fusion. BRAF and RET are absent.
- *Two types*: (1) Encapsulated FVPTC with invasion (30%) tends to spread in a fashion similar to follicular thyroid carcinoma, with distant lung and bone metastases and infrequent lymph node metastases **(Fig. 11)** and (2) NIFTP—most encapsulated FVPTCs show no invasive growth—NIFTP a very low-risk tumor that *likely represents a preinvasive stage of invasive encapsulated FVPTC*. Cytology—hypercellular, syncytial sheets, and microfollicles/rosettes; nuclear features subtle, minimal colloid; absent—papillae, multinucleate giant cells, INCI, and psammoma bodies **(Fig. 12)**.

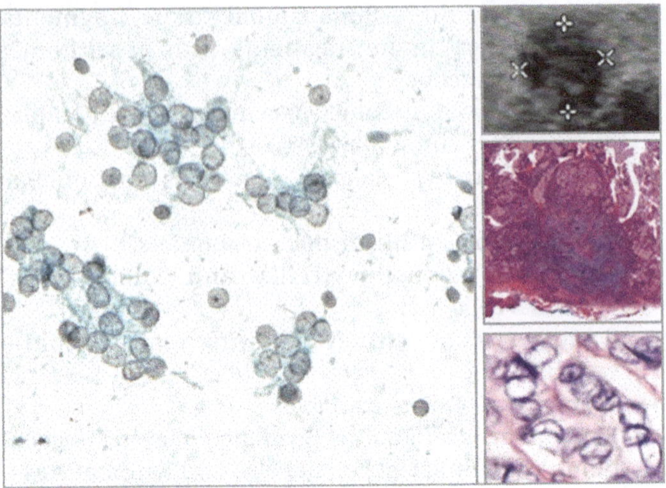

FIG. 11: At cytology, may be interpreted as suspicious for PTC (25–35%), FN/SFN (25–30%), or AUS/FLUS (10–20%) (Bethesda atlas 2017).

(AUS/FLUS: atypia of undetermined significance/follicular lesion of undetermined significance; FN/SFN: follicular neoplasm/suspicious for a follicular neoplasm; PTC: papillary thyroid carcinoma)

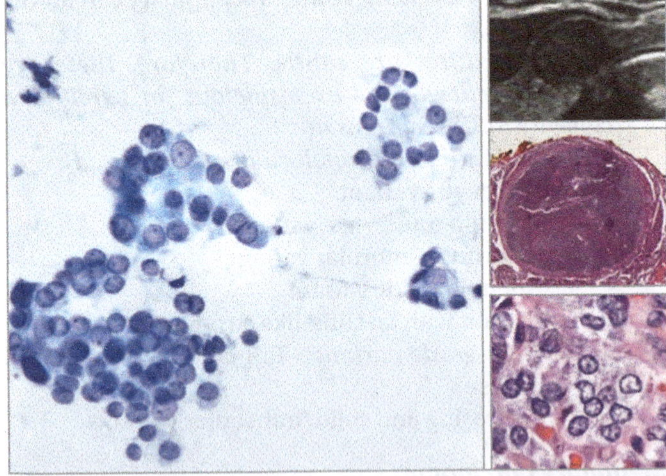

FIG. 12: At cytology: Follicular pattern; slightly enlarged and pale nuclei; may be interpreted as FN/SFN; AUS/FLUS; NIFTP (Bethesda atlas 2017).

(AUS/FLUS: atypia of undetermined significance/follicular lesion of undetermined significance; FN/SFN: follicular neoplasm/suspicious for a follicular neoplasm; NIFTP: noninvasive follicular thyroid neoplasm with papillary-like nuclear features)

The Bethesda System for Reporting Thyroid Cytopathology (TBSRTC) is a simple method of reducing interobserver variability in reporting thyroid FNAs. It improves dialog between the pathologists and clinicians by way of communicating cancer risk in each category and providing guidelines in the surgical management of patients. It helps in comparison of data across institutions for statistical purposes.

It is hoped that this terminology if applied universally, will be a valuable step toward uniformity and consensus in the reporting of thyroid FNA interpretations.

The Milan System for Reporting Salivary Gland Neoplasms[4-10]

The American Society of Cytopathology and International Academy of Cytology (IAC) recently put forth at a conference at Milan in 2018, a six-tiered international classification scheme called the "Milan System for Reporting Salivary Gland Cytopathology" (MSRSGC). The Milan System for Reporting Salivary Gland Cytopathology referred to as "MSRSGC" was introduced to provide guidelines toward diagnosis of salivary gland pathology for treatment and management according to the ROM in the various categories. This categorization was attempted to limit and restrain the number of false-negative and false-positive cases. Akin to the Bethesda System of Thyroid Cytology, it aims at a uniform system of reporting for easy comparison between institutions, categorization of lesions, statistical analysis, and communication to clinicians with regard to standardization in management.

The various categories in this system are:
- *Category 1*: Nondiagnostic (ND)
- *Category 2*: Nonneoplastic (NN)
- *Category 3*: Atypia of undetermined significance
- *Category 4*:
  a. *Neoplasm*: Benign (NB)
  b. *Neoplasm*: Salivary gland neoplasm of undetermined malignant potential (SUMP)
- *Category 5*: Suspicious for malignancy (SM)
- *Category 6*: Malignant (M)

Category 1: Nondiagnostic

- Category created just as in TBSRTC.
- Constitutes about 10–20% of salivary gland FNA
- *Diagnostic criteria*: Insufficient cellular material <60 lesional cells for a cytologic diagnosis (without atypia)
- Nonneoplastic acinar cells only in the setting of a clinically defined nodule
- Nonmucinous cyst fluid only
- Poorly prepared slides with artifacts (e.g., air-drying, obscuring blood, and poor staining)
- Estimated ROM is 25%. This somewhat high ROM most likely reflects sampling limitations at the preanalytic level.
- Similar to other cytology reporting systems, an attempt should be made to limit the rate of nondiagnostic FNAs to 10% or lower.
- For repeat aspirates from a previous nondiagnostic salivary gland FNA, radiographically guided FNA is highly recommended to reduce sampling errors.

Exceptions to these nondiagnostic cytologic criteria include mucinous cyst contents as this may represent mucoepidermoid carcinoma where cellular elements have not been aspirated, aspirates with atypia (which would in fact represent AUS category), and specimens that contain abundant acellular matrix material (representing pleomorphic adenoma (PA) thereby coming into benign neoplasm) or abundant inflammatory cells without an epithelial component (falling actually into AUS category—either inflammation or lymphoma).

Category 2: Nonneoplastic

- Nonneoplastic lesions of the salivary gland are common and constitute 15–25% of salivary gland aspirates; and, clinically, they can be misinterpreted as neoplasms because of the presence of a mass.
- A pitfall of salivary gland aspirates diagnosed as nonneoplastic is the possibility of a false-negative diagnosis because of inadequate sampling.
- In the MSRSGC, the nonneoplastic category includes benign conditions such as reactive, metaplastic, sialadenitis, sialolithiasis, and inflammatory processes including acute, chronic, and granulomatous sialadenitis.
- Common false-negative conditions are lymphoid rich tumors, low-grade lymphoma, Hodgkin lymphoma, lymphoepithelial carcinoma, etc. and cystic tumors such as mucoepidermoid carcinoma.
- Benign or bland lymphocytes (interpreted as in the reactive lymph node), necessitates flow cytometry or some other method of immunophenotyping to avoid a false-negative diagnosis.
- The suggested ROM for the nonneoplastic category is expected to be lower than 10% if strict criteria of inclusion are applied.
- The ROM for aspirates of nonneoplastic salivary gland tumors ranges in various studies from 0 to 20%, which seems to be an overestimate as a follow-up surgical excision in the nonneoplastic aspirates is rare.

Category 3: Atypia of Undetermined Significance

- The MSRSGC introduced a diagnostic category designated as "AUS" for a limited subset of salivary gland FNAs which should be ≤10%.
- *Diagnostic criteria*: Limited cellular atypia; lacks qualitative or quantitative features for diagnosing a neoplasm
- The aim of this diagnostic category is to reduce the number of false-negative results in the nonneoplastic category and the number of false-positive results in the neoplasm category.
- The AUS category is heterogeneous, exhibiting morphologic overlap between nonneoplastic and neoplastic processes.

- Different scenarios in the AUS category include (1) reactive and reparative atypia; (2) low cellularity samples that are suggestive, but not diagnostic, of a neoplasm; (3) cystic lesions with abundant mucin and/or a scant epithelial component, and (4) parotid gland aspirates indefinite for a lymphoproliferative disorder; (5) metaplastic changes indefinite for a neoplasm, e.g., squamous and oncocytic.
- The ROM is approximately 20%. FNAs classified as AUS often will have preanalytic issues (e.g., preparation artifact or sampling limitations). A majority of salivary gland FNA samples classified as AUS will represent reactive atypia or, in some cases, poorly sampled neoplasms.

Category 4: Benign Neoplasm

- The *neoplasm-benign* subcategory is used for those aspirates in which a definitive diagnosis of a particular benign neoplasm can be made unequivocally based on certain cytomorphologic features specific for the neoplasm.
- Constitutes about 30% of salivary gland aspirates
- The most common entities included in the benign neoplasm category are PA **(Fig. 13)**, Warthin tumor (adenoma lymphomatosum papilliferum), schwannoma, lipoma, and hemangioma.
- The ROM for the neoplasm-benign category is expected to be low (<5%), and the majority of these lesions can be managed by conservative surgical resection or, in selected cases, patients may be followed clinically to avoid potential surgical complications, patient hesitancy, or contraindications to surgical procedures.
- To maintain the low ROM associated with this category, stringent cytomorphologic criteria need to be used.

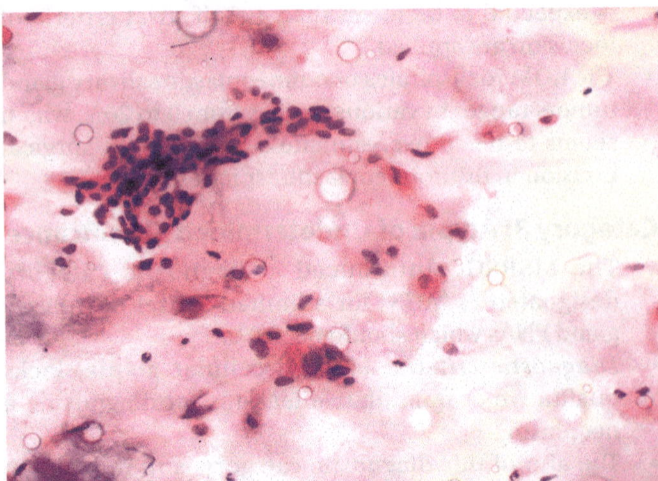

FIG. 13: Aspirate from a case of pleomorphic adenoma showing bland ductal cells of the neoplasm against a background of myxoid material (H&E, ×100).

Neoplastic Category: Salivary Gland Neoplasm of Undetermined Malignant Potential

- The SUMP category is used for salivary gland FNAs in which the morphologic features are compatible with a neoplastic process, but a specific diagnosis cannot be assigned to unequivocally.
- Of much concern would be where a malignant neoplasm (usually low-grade) cannot be entirely ruled out at FNA.
- FNAs diagnosed as SUMP proves to be neoplasms both benign and malignant entities. The SUMP category can be further divided based on the presence of basaloid, oncocytic, or clear cell features. Basaloid cells reflect presence of a basal cell neoplasm ranging from an adenoma to a basal cell carcinoma. Matrix-producing carcinomas with basaloid cells can be falsely interpreted as pleomorphic or basal cell adenoma. These should be reported as SUMP with basaloid features.
- Oncocytic cells may reflect either a benign oncocytoma or malignant oncocytoma or even an Warthin-like variant of mucoepidermoid carcinoma and should be diagnosed as SUMP with oncocytic features.
- Clear cells may show lesions which range from PA (myoepithelial component); mucoepidermoid carcinoma or adenocarcinoma. These should be reported as SUMP with clear cells
- If the aspirates contain many lymphocytes besides neoplastic cells, the differentials would be mucoepidermoid carcinoma with lymphoid cuffing, acinic cell carcinoma with lymphoid infiltrates; this would then be SUMP.
- The presence of a cystic component may reflect mucoepidermoid carcinoma in which case it may be accompanied by some extracellular mucus or cystic change in any other neoplasm. This further expands the differential.
- The important thing is that the features suggest a neoplasm but the type cannot be specified at cytology.
- Clinical management in most cases of SUMP is conservative surgical resection.

Category 5: Suspicious for Malignancy

- This category is similar to the corresponding conventional diagnostic category used in other reporting systems such as the Bethesda category or even Breast reporting.

- The cytomorphologic features of suspicious for malignancy are characterized by an aspirate that is highly suggestive of a malignant neoplasm, but the definitive diagnosis not made either due to very few cells in the aspirate; clinically definitely points toward being malignant but cells show morphological artifacts; instances where a limited sample containing few markedly atypical lymphoid cells suggestive of lymphoma.
- Limited cytologic features of a specific malignancy, e.g., adenoid cystic carcinoma with limited cellular atypia or hyaline globules, mucoepidermoid carcinoma with limited mucus cells or extracellular mucin, and secretory carcinoma with limited cytoplasmic vacuolization or papillary formations
- Suspicious cytologic features in a subset of cells but admixed with predominant features of a benign lesion, e.g., carcinoma and PA
- Many specimens diagnosed as suspicious for malignancy potentially could benefit from the application of ancillary studies or are subjected to frozen section before resection/radical surgery.
- The estimated ROM is 60%.

Category 6: Malignant

- Most neoplasms in this category are carcinomas; primary and metastatic carcinomas to the salivary gland/salivary gland lymph nodes; lymphomas and sarcomas.
- Once the FNA is diagnosed as malignant **(Fig. 14)**, an attempt to make a specific diagnosis. Based on the 2017 edition of the *World Health Organization Classification of Head and Neck Tumors*, it should be done.

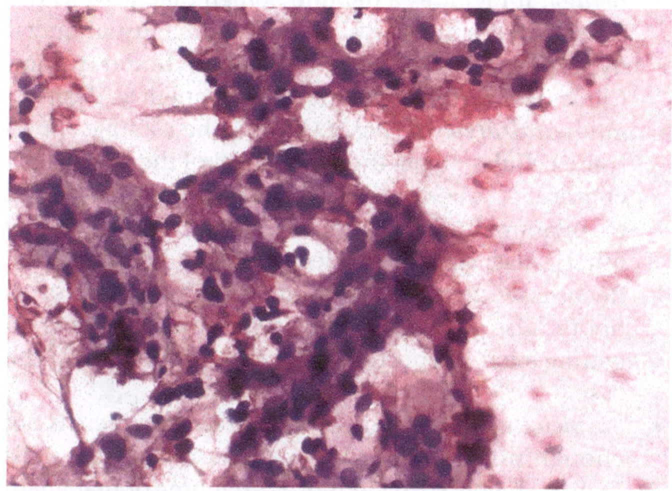

FIG. 14: Aspirate from a mucoepidermoid carcinoma (high grade) showing the epidermoid component (H&E, ×400).

TABLE 2: Various categories in the Milan system and the associated risk of malignancy (ROM) and their management.

Category	ROM	Clinical management
Nondiagnostic	25%	Clinical and radiology correlation repeat FNA
Nonneoplastic	10%	Clinical follow-up and radiology correlation
Atypia of undetermined	20%	Repeat FNA significance
Benign neoplasm	05%	Conservative surgery
Salivary gland neoplasm of uncertain malignant potential (SUMP)	35%	Conservative surgery
Suspicious for malignancy	60%	Surgery
Malignant	≥90%	extensive surgery

(FNA: fine-needle aspiration)

- Even more important is that the tumor should be graded, when possible, as low-grade versus high-grade for purposes of clinical management.

The various categories in the Milan system and the associated risk of malignancy are given in **Table 2.**

Breast Aspiration Cytology[3,11-17]

Introduction

- Breast cancer is a heterogeneous disease with varied morphological and biologic behavioral characteristics. The host response to tumor varies from individual to individual.
- For many decades, invasive breast carcinomas were classified according to histological type, grade, and expression of hormone receptors.
- This has been now overtaken to a more meaningful molecular classification based on advances in technology such as molecular and gene prolific studies.
- The primary objective in treating breast cancer is to establish an accurate diagnosis and to achieve the ultimate optimal result in therapy.

Diagnosis: Triple Assessment

- The accepted management for diagnosis of a lesion discovered in the breast by any means is the "triple-approach technique"
- Several studies have shown that a combination of clinical examination, imaging (mammography or ultrasound), and FNAC or core biopsy will give an accurate diagnosis on the breast lesion.
- The triple approach is considered positive if any one of these investigative modalities is positive.
- In 99.6% of cancers, it is positive; in <1% of cancers it is negative

Fine-needle Aspiration Cytology as a Tool in Triple Approach

- Triple assessments of breast lesions consist of clinical, radiological, and pathological evaluation. Hence, one of the current clinical approaches to palpable breast masses is to get cytopathologic evaluation before going to a definitive surgery.
- The results can be made available rapidly, enabling a one-stop diagnostic result in clinics.
- Excellent results with FNA and triple assessment are reported in the literature.
- In general, FNAC is more suitable as compared to tissue biopsy for patients on anticoagulants and for lesions close to the skin, chest wall, vessels, and implants or for very small lesions and those that are deep-seated and difficult to reach.
- This approach has an accuracy of over 90% for palpable breast lesions when all three components are concordant for benign or malignant disease.
- *Routine practice uses the following major diagnostic categories when reporting a FNAC of a breast lesion*:
  - *Nondiagnostic*: C1
  - *Benign*: C2
  - *Atypical/equivocal*: C3
  - *Suspicious*: C4
  - *Malignant*: C5
- National Health Service Breast Screening Programme (NHSBSP) guidelines for cytology practice have employed the above categories for more than two decades in the reporting of screening results. The NHSBSP began in 1988. It aimed at inviting all women aged 50–70 years for mammographic screening once every 3 years. The program now screens 1.3 million women each year, about 75% of those invited, and diagnoses about 10,000 breast cancers annually.
- *Breast aspirates*: Cytological diagnosis and treatment decisions should be audited against outcome, which may be clinical rather than histological. The NHSBSP reporting guidelines for FNA specimens of the breast (C1—inadequate; C2—benign; C3—atypia, probably benign; C4—suspicious for malignancy; and C5—malignant) are now acceptable. The use of C4 category avoids poor quality samples being overcalled while C3 provides a mechanism for follow-up, clinical discussion, and repeat biopsy in equivocal cases. Such cases should be reviewed in a multidisciplinary setting in order to minimize the chances of a false-positive result. The C3 and C4 categories should be used as sparingly and their outcome monitored. It must be emphasized here that the text report rather than C1–C5 reporting may be used for making management decisions as the reporting categories are a convenient way of recording data for audit purposes but not sufficient grounds for deciding clinical management.

International Academy of Cytology Yokohama System for Reporting Breast Fine-needle Aspiration Biopsy Cytology: Five Category Stratification[15]

- Recently in 2016, however, an IAC Yokohama system for classification of breast lesions was established that provided a comprehensive approach of FNAC practice and reporting of breast lesions across the globe. Experts from various specialties, such as cytopathology, radiology, surgery, and medical oncology met at this international congress. According to the IAC classification system, there are five categories of cytological diagnoses for breast lesions: (1) insufficient material, (2) benign lesions, (3) atypical lesions, (4) suspicious for malignancy, and (5) malignant lesions.
- This IAC Yokohama system defines the same above five categories as the NHSBSP for reporting breast cytology, each with a clear descriptive term for the category, a definition, a ROM and a suggested management algorithm.
- The system emphasizes that a high standard for the performance of the FNAB; the making of direct smears from a cellular aspirate, and well-trained experienced cytopathologists to interpret the material are crucial factors for an accurate result.
- *Nondiagnostic*: It refers to aspirates that are inadequate for a diagnosis to be arrived at nonrepresentative samples; artifacts like broken slide, poor staining, crush artifact, covered by blood, etc. The management is a guided repeat aspiration.
- *Benign*: It includes a definite benign diagnosis as per criteria in literature, e.g., fibroadenoma, usual ductal hyperplasia; papilloma; benign phyllodes tumor. Clinical follow-up or excision if the patient so desires.
- *Equivocal/atypical* ***(Fig. 15)***: Here, the aspirate shows some cellular atypia though the rest of the smear may conform to a benign lesion. The changes may be due to inflammation, radiation effect, reactive due to any other cause; such that a clean chit could not be given. Recommendation is to do an excision biopsy so as not to miss any suspicious lesion. Most clinicians on getting such a report do not excise but follow up the case.
- *Suspicious*: For a diagnosis it is given when there is not enough material showing malignancy but the cells seen are highly suspicious of a carcinoma or malignant neoplasm. On excision, it invariably turns out to be malignant. Generally, such a report is supplemented by a frozen section.

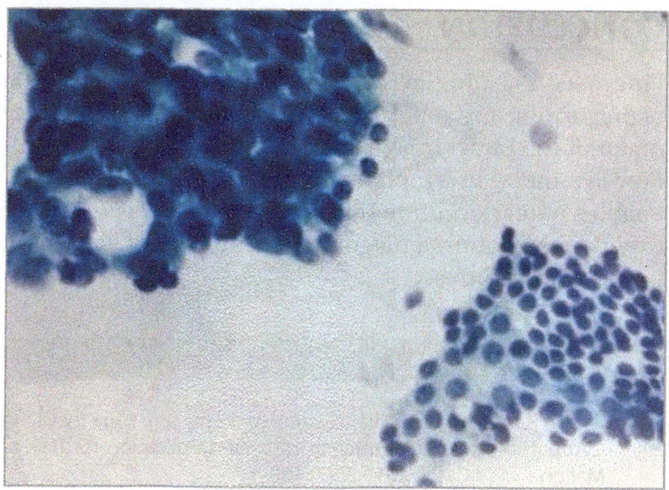

FIG. 15: Stained by the Pap stain shows two sheets of ductal cells; the ones in the right lower corner show unequivocal benign cells with fine nuclear chromatin. The group of cells in the left upper corner show overlapping with mild nuclear enlargement. It is neither definitely malignant nor benign. Also, it is reported as C3 category.

- *Malignant*: When the aspirate shows unequivocal malignant cells, a diagnosis is made. The excision shows malignancy in almost 100% of cases.
- Two recent publications have shown a range of "ROM" for the insufficient/inadequate category of 2.6–4.8%, benign 1.4–2.3%, atypical 13–15.7%, suspicious of malignancy 84.6–97.1%, and malignant 99.0–100%.
- The current practice of breast FNAB has resulted in the increasing use of ultrasound guidance and ROSE.
- With ROSE, the performance data showed a positive predictive value of 96.4%, negative predictive value of 97.6%, and a ROM of a FNAB categorized as "insufficient" to be 2.6%, "benign" 1.7%, "atypical" 15.7%, "suspicious of malignancy" 84.6%, and "malignant" 99.5%.
- Reporting cytology by these categories helps in uniformity and standardization of FNA reports, better communication between cytologists and clinicians; reduces interobserver variability and helps in statistical and epidemiological data share.

Core Biopsy over Fine-needle Aspiration Cytology

- Core biopsy is presently rapidly replacing FNAC as a procedure of choice for the triple assessment of the breast problems.
- Core biopsy is considered a more reliable predictor of the pathology and can distinguish between benign and malignant tumors and between in situ and invasive cancers.
- In the majority (83%) of core biopsies, the findings reflect histology at excision
- It gives a good guide to the grade and histological type of the cancer and can be used instead of excision biopsy.
- Also used to assess the receptor [estrogen (ER) and progesterone (PR)] status

Be it so, FNAC is still being used as one of the prongs of triple assessment and the debate between using core over FNA is an ongoing one, with hard core cytologists defending the procedure as a simple, cost-effective, noninvasive, and easily performable office procedure which can be repeated any number of times and is quick to reassure patient anxiety as compared to a core.

Sensitivity, Specificity, and Predictive Value of a Positive Result in FNAC

Many times it becomes necessary to ratify results obtained at cytology with histopathology, which is generally used by all cytologists as gold standard. The various indices calculated using histopathology as gold standard can be:

Sensitivity: Sensitivity means positive in disease. As per Frable 1984, it can be calculated as follows:

$$\text{Sensitivity} = \text{Positive in disease} = \frac{\text{True positive} \times 100}{\text{True negative} + \text{False positive}}$$

(In a nutshell, it means if 100 FNAC smears are compared to the histological paraffin sections; what percentage of these smears gives the correct diagnosis. In different centers, it varies from in-between 85–100%, i.e., in approximately 85–100% of cases, a correct diagnosis is given at cytology).

Specificity: Means negative in disease (Frable, 1984)

$$\text{Specificity} = \text{Negative in disease} = \frac{\text{True negative} \times 100}{\text{True negative} + \text{False positive}}$$

(If 100 FNAC smears with a negative diagnosis are compared to the corresponding paraffin sections; what percentage of these smears could definitely be told that there was no disease at cytology. Varies at center from 95 to 100%)

Predictive value of the positive result: Means when histology is taken into consideration, what percentage of cases are predicted at cytology.

$$\text{Predictive value of a positive result} = \frac{\text{True positive} \times 100}{\text{True negative + False positive}}$$

Example: In 200 histologically proven breast lesions, it was seen that at FNAC, 165 cases were reported as being carcinomas (true positive at FNAC); 27 cases were reported as being negative at FNAC.

CONCLUSION

Fine-needle-aspiration cytology is a very easy technique of diagnosing any superficial or deep-seated lesion in any organ of the body. Imaging and ancillary techniques like flow cytometry in lymphoma aspirates, etc. supporting it, enables a near accurate diagnosis in many cases. Under experienced hands, a diagnosis can be arrived at without invasive procedures.

REFERENCES

1. Ali SZ, Cibas ES (Eds). The Bethesda System for Reporting Thyroid Cytopathology Definitions, Criteria, and Explanatory Notes. 2nd edition. Cham, Switzerland: Springer; 2018.
2. Renuka IV, Saila Bala G, Aparna C, Kumari R, Sumalatha K. The bethesda system for reporting thyroid cytopathology: interpretation and guidelines in surgical treatment. Indian J Otolaryngol Head Neck Surg. 2012;64(4):305-11.
3. Shariff S. Fundamentals of Surgical Pathology, 2nd edition. New Delhi: Jaypee Brothers Medical Publishers (P) Ltd.; 2010.
4. Wei S, Layfield LJ, LiVolsi VA, Montone KT, Baloch ZW. Reporting of fine needle aspiration (FNA) specimens of salivary gland lesions: A comprehensive review. Diagn Cytopathol. 2017;45(9):820-7.
5. Faquin WC, Rossi ED, Baloch Z, Barkan GA, Foschini MP, Kurtycz DFI (Eds). The Milan System for Reporting Salivary Gland Cytopathology. Cham, Switzerland: Springer; 2018.
6. Rossi ED, Wong LQ, Bizzarro T, Petrone G, Mule A, Fadda G, et al. The impact of FNAC in the management of salivary gland lesions: Institutional experiences leading to a risk-based classification scheme. Cancer Cytopathol. 2016;124(6):388-96.
7. Lee JJL, Tan HM, Chua DYS, Chung JGK, Nga ME. The Milan system for reporting salivary gland cytology: A retrospective analysis of 1384 cases in a tertiary Southeast Asian institution. Cancer Cytopathol. 2020;128(5):348-58.
8. Rossi ED, Faquin WC, Baloch Z, Barkan GA, Foschini MP, Pusztaszeri M, et al. The Milan System for Reporting Salivary Gland Cytopathology: Analysis and suggestions of initial survey. Cancer Cytopathol. 2017;125(10):757-66.
9. Mairembam P, Jay A, Beale T, Morley S, Vaz F, Kalavrezos N, et al. Salivary gland FNA cytology: role as a triage tool and an approach to pitfalls in cytomorphology. Cytopathology. 2016;27(2):91-6.
10. Kala C, Kala S, Khan L. Milan System for Reporting Salivary Gland Cytopathology: An Experience with the Implication for Risk of Malignancy. J Cytol. 2019;36(3):160-4.
11. Layfield LJ, Baloch Z. Categorical systems for reporting of cytology specimens: Following the footsteps of Bethesda-like reporting systems. Diagn Cytopathol. 2020;48(10):859-61.
12. The uniform approach to breast fine-needle aspiration biopsy. National Cancer Institute Fine-Needle Aspiration of Breast Workshop Subcommittees. Diagn Cytopathol. 1997;16(4):295-311.
13. Field AS, Schmitt F, Vielh P. IAC Standardized Reporting of Breast Fine-Needle Aspiration Biopsy Cytology. Acta Cytol. 2017;61(1):3-6.
14. Wang HH, Ducatman BS. Fine needle aspiration of the breast. A probabilistic approach to diagnosis of carcinoma. Acta Cytol. 1998;42(2):285-9.
15. Field AS, Raymond WA, Rickard M, Arnold L, Brachtel EF, Chaiwun B, et al. The International Academy of Cytology Yokohama System for Reporting Breast Fine-Needle Aspiration Biopsy Cytopathology. Acta Cytol. 2019;63(4):257-73.
16. Embaye KS, Raja SM, Gebreyesus MH, Ghebrehiwet MA. Distribution of breast lesions diagnosed by cytology examination in symptomatic patients at Eritrean National Health Laboratory, Asmara, Eritrea: a retrospective study. BMC Womens Health. 2020;20(1):250.
17. Wong S, Rickard M, Earls P, Arnold L, Bako B, Field AS. The International Academy of Cytology Yokohama System for Reporting Breast Fine Needle Aspiration Biopsy Cytopathology: A Single Institutional Retrospective Study of the Application of the System Categories and the Impact of Rapid Onsite Evaluation. Acta Cytol. 2019;63(4):280-91.

CHAPTER 11

Conjunctival Impression Cytology

INTRODUCTION

The technique of impression cytology of the conjunctiva was established by Egbert et al. in 1977 for the study of goblet cells. It is a noninvasive office procedure which is a window to the study of exfoliated conjunctival surface epithelial cells by a simple technique.[1]

APPLICATIONS OF THE PROCEDURE[1-7]

- Eye disorders, such as keratoconjunctivitis sicca (KCS), and vitamin A deficiency reflect changes in the conjunctiva which can be assessed by conjunctival impression cytology (CIC). It is of immense help in identifying subclinical vitamin A deficiency cases in a population where the prevalence rate of this deficiency is manifest.
- In patients with various other ocular surface disorders before they become symptomatic.
- It is also useful in contact lens users and dry eyes.
- CIC can also be studied in several disorders: Epithelial cell storage diseases such as mucopolysaccharidosis, ocular cicatricial pemphigoid, changes of viral and chlamydial infection, and in patients with open-angle glaucoma who are on antiglaucoma therapy.

PRINCIPLE OF THE TEST

- The conjunctiva is a thin translucent mucous membrane that covers the anterior surface of the eyeball turning onto the inner aspect of the eyelids and continuous with the corneal epithelium.
- Conjunctival goblet cells are present amidst the epithelial cells throughout the conjunctival surface and arise from the basal layer of the epithelium and mature gradually to enlarge as they reach the surface.
- These mucin secreting goblet cells are more concentrated on the medial side.
- Chronic inflammation and severe conditions leading to dry eyes cause destruction of goblet cells and this can be assessed by the imprint cytology.
- On the other hand in cases of "limbal stem cell deficiency", the conjunctival epithelium extends over the cornea where goblet cells are present on the corneal surface and their presence ascertained.
- CIC is based purely on squamous and goblet cell abnormalities of the exfoliated cells of the conjunctival epithelium.

PROCEDURE OF OBTAINING SMEARS

- Smears are obtained by impression on a cellulose acetate membrane millipore filter paper of 0.025–0.22 µm thickness.[1]
- The paper is cut into 5 mm parallel strips, which again are trimmed into triangular shapes.
- They are marked with various anatomical regions, like bulbar, fornical, palpebral conjunctiva, etc., to identify the location of the surface cells.
- The eyes should be dry, or if teary, then wiped dry before the application.
- The paper strips (which are gas sterilized using ethylene oxide) are applied on the conjunctiva with the dull surface down with or without topical anesthesia.
- They are held in contact with the conjunctiva for 5–10 seconds.
- A blunt end forceps holds the pointed tip of the paper to peel it off.

- They are then peeled off from the conjunctiva (the cells coming off with it), are laid onto a glass slide with cells down, gentle pressure is applied to the paper making the cells adhere to the slide.

FIXATION AND STAINING

- Fixation is done by dipping the slide into a Coplin jar containing 95% ethyl alcohol and stained; or the filter paper with the specimen is fixed for approximately 10 minutes in alcohol and then stained and later mounted onto the slide with the cell surface up.
- Fixation can also be done in a solution containing glacial acetic acid, formaldehyde, and ethyl alcohol in a 1:1:20 volume ratio. In either method, xylene dips make the filter paper transparent. A Hematoxylin and eosin (H&E) stain, Papanicolaou, and periodic acid-Schiff (PAS) stain is done.

INTERPRETATION

- The greatest density of goblet cells is in the nasal palpebral conjunctiva, with decreasing densities in the temporal and palpebral conjunctiva, bulbar conjunctiva near the fornices, and the bulbar conjunctiva near the limbus.
- Normal cells are flat with a prominent nucleus with a low nuclear-cytoplasmic ratio. Limbal epithelial cells are smaller, more densely packed, and have a higher nuclear-cytoplasmic ratio.
- For classification of the morphological changes of the conjunctiva, several grading systems have been developed. The first grading system *published by Nelson et al. (1983, 1988)*[1,5] is based on the morphological appearance of the conjunctival epithelial and goblet cells. This grading system was scaled from 0 to 3, based on the morphology of the epithelial cells, their staining behavior, the nuclear-cytoplasmic ratio as well as the density and the PAS staining of the goblet cells. This classification system is still widely used.

Grading System for the Changes on Cytology: Three Grade System

- *Grade 0*: Epithelial cells are small and round with eosinophilic cytoplasm. Nuclei are large and basophilic with a nuclear-cytoplasmic ratio of 1:2. Goblet cells are abundant, plump, and oval and have intensely PAS-positive cytoplasm.
- *Grade I*: Epithelial cells are slightly larger and are more polygonal and have eosinophilic stained cytoplasm. Nuclei are smaller with nuclear-cytoplasmic ratio of 1:3. Goblet cells are decreased in number but still are plump and oval and have intensely PAS-positive cytoplasm.
- *Grade II*: Epithelial cells are large and polygonal, occasionally multinucleated with variably staining cytoplasm. Nuclei are small with a nuclear-cytoplasmic ratio of 1:4 or 1:5. Goblet cells are markedly decreased in number, are smaller, less intensely PAS positive and have faintly defined cellular borders.
- *Grade III*: Epithelial cells are large and polygonal with basophilic staining cytoplasm. Nuclei are small, pyknotic and in many cells are completely absent. Nuclear-cytoplasmic ratio is 1:6 or greater. Goblet cells are completely absent.
- Other grading systems are those of *Tseng*[4] *(1985—six grades) and Adams*[6] *(1979).*

CONCLUSION

By doing CIC, not only goblet cell study is possible but material can be taken for sophisticated investigations, like DNA analysis, etc. There are numerous clinical and research applications on conjunctival cytology; it has however not yet become a routine diagnostic tool. The ability to obtain multiple samples of the ocular surface at one sitting with minimal discomfort to the patient makes this an ideal investigation for ocular surface disorders.

The cytologist and ophthalmologist need to develop a standardized approach and universal acceptance is the key to its validity as a diagnostic tool.

REFERENCES

1. Nelson JD, Havener VR, Cameron JD. Cellulose acetate impressions of the ocular surface. Dry eye states. Arch Ophthalmol. 1983;101(12):1869-72.
2. Egbert PR, Lauber S, Maurice DM. A simple conjunctival biopsy. Am J Ophthalmol. 1977;84(6):798-801.
3. Chen M. (2022). Impression Cytology. [online] Available from https://eyewiki.aao.org/Impression_Cytology [Last accessed March, 2024].
4. Tseng SC. Staging of conjunctival squamous metaplasia by impression cytology. Ophthalmology. 1985;92(6):728-33.
5. Nelson JD. Impression cytology. Cornea. 1988;7(1):71-81.
6. Adams AD. The morphology of human conjunctival mucus. Arch Ophthalmol. 1979;97(4):730-4.
7. Singh R, Joseph A, Umapathy T, Tint NL, Dua HS. Impression cytology of the ocular surface. Br J Ophthalmol. 2005;89(12):1655-9.

CHAPTER 12

Role of Cytology in Autopsy

INTRODUCTION

Clinical autopsy is an essential exercise meant to give an answer to the cause of death. As a norm, a full autopsy is performed, other times a limited autopsy may be done. Whether a full or limited autopsy is done, a cytology examination of samples from the body are of immense importance toward contributing to diagnosis.

A limited autopsy focuses on an organ-specific problem. Cytology if performed gives an overview of the body condition, e.g., urine collected from a jaundiced person would be yellow and indicate hepatitis. Presence of ascites would indicate either cirrhosis and portal hypertension or malignant effusion.

The advantages and utility of postmortem cytology in its various forms—fluid examination, fine needle aspiration (FNA), touch preparations, scrapings, etc., in both neoplastic and nonneoplastic conditions have been established as contributing to the final diagnosis.

DECLINING CLINICAL AUTOPSIES

Declining autopsy rates are an indisputable fact, in places due to religious sentiments or possibly that performing the autopsy may prove a health hazard to the pathologist [acquired immunodeficiency syndrome (AIDS)-related era]. Other reasons for a decrease in autopsy rates include the widespread use of antemortem imaging, blood tests, biopsies, and cytology, which lead to the sometimes incorrect assumption that the cause of death is already known and that an autopsy is thus redundant and unnecessary. A pathologists' distaste for the autopsy procedure unfortunately aids and abets the death of the autopsy. The role of cytology in contributing to diagnosis where such factors hinder a regular clinical autopsy is of paramount importance.

VARIOUS APPLICATIONS OF CYTOLOGY AT AUTOPSY[1-6]

- Fluid sampling for cytologic study is a quick and inexpensive technique that can provide a rapid diagnosis. Body cavity effusions may be aspirated before incision and the specimen centrifuged and smears made. This can yield answers with regard to the etiology of the effusion—malignancy or absence of the same or otherwise.
- Cerebrospinal fluid (CSF) may be obtained through lumbar puncture or direct cisternal puncture (posterior fossa). It helps to confirm or rule out central nervous system (CNS) disorders.
- Urine samples can be obtained by suprapubic aspirate or from bladder washings; examination of the same will confirm or exclude neoplasms of the urinary tract and infections.
- Bone marrow samples showing well-preserved cytomorphology can be obtained soon after death through a sternal or iliac crest aspiration or can be squeezed from a resected rib after it has been sectioned across.
- In forensic autopsies spermatozoa can be recovered and identified by the Papanicolaou stain from vaginal and anal swabs up to 72 and 24 hours postsexual assault, respectively.
- Needle-core/FNA biopsy may be employed in the autopsy setting, permitting the harvest of fluids and/or fresh tissue for autolysis-free histology, cellblock preparations, and additional ancillary studies (microbiology, molecular, immunohistochemical, or genetic testing).
- Postmortem cytology may be of particular use in diagnosis in those parts of the world where more sophisticated laboratory facilities are not readily available.

- A positive fluid cytology in effusions suggests an advanced stage, though the categorization of tumor may still be difficult for the cytopathologist.
- Scrape cytology is a simple, rapid, accurate, and inexpensive adjunctive cytodiagnostic technique and its routine utilization in malignant neoplasms could aid in expanding the cytological appearances and knowledge of these malignant neoplasms.
- Postmortem cytology provides for rapid confirmation of macroscopic findings, allowing for more comprehensive provisional reporting to clinicians, legal investigators, and decedents' families.
- Various cytodiagnostic methods can be used in autopsy and forensic pathology investigations and represent a viable alternative for obtaining diagnostic information when conventional autopsy is not feasible.

ADVANTAGES OF POSTMORTEM CYTOLOGY

- Postmortem cytology has the potential to cut autopsy costs either by providing a rapid, relatively inexpensive cytodiagnosis, or by offering a screening tool with which pathologists can select cases that require histology and ancillary studies such as immunohistochemistry or a full autopsy.
- A potential for minimal disruption of the corpus in an era when next-of-kin full-autopsy consent has become more difficult to obtain, and decedent "public relation" officers, trained to communicate with family members, are rare to find.
- Cytodiagnostic techniques have the potential to choose cases for contribution to a full autopsy, especially in an academic institution, where complete autopsies are needed to train residents and multidisciplinary conferences.

DISADVANTAGES

- Autolytic changes may have set in if collection is delayed.
- A reliance on cytology alone may not be enough for diagnosis.
- A laid-back approach to an alert and quick collection of cytological material may defer the performance of this.

CONCLUSION

Undoubtedly cytodiagnostic autopsy techniques contribute to pathology education, quality assurance, and provide a means of immediate feedback and more specific answers, and preclude the need for removing organs in cases where religious or ethnic beliefs forbid violation of the body.

REFERENCES

1. Gillan WDH. Conjunctival impression cytology: a review. S Afr Optom. 2008;67(3):136-41.
2. Padmini C, Kumari PA, Rao, DR. Role of conjunctival imprint cytology in detecting vitamin A deficiency in cancer patients: A case-control study. J Med Nutr Nutraceut. 2014;3(2):89-93.
3. Uram-Tuculescu CG, Fuller CE. Postmortem cytology: Alive and well in the practice of autopsy and forensic pathology. Cancer Cytopathol. 2015;123(8):447-8.
4. Andrade L, Massarente VL, Tormin SC, Ribeiro KB, Pozzan G, Saieg MA. Use of cytology as an auxiliary diagnostic tool in autopsies. Cancer Cytopathol. 2016;124(11):785-90.
5. Schnadig VJ. Cytology as a diagnostic tool in the autopsy suite. Cancer Cytopathol. 2016;124(11):773-5.
6. Rao S, Sadiya N, Joseph LD, Rajendiran S. Role of scrape cytology in ovarian neoplasms. J Cytol. 2009;26(1):26-9.

CHAPTER 13

Automation in Cytology

INTRODUCTION

Automation in laboratory is performance of a test or procedure without or by minimal assistance by technical staff. Analytical machines fed by the test sample perform the required test with least interference by the analyst. Automation is well established in both hematology and biochemistry. With the advent of automation in cytology laboratories have explored the usage of these to not only process samples but also for cell viewing and detection of abnormalities.[1-3]

AUTOMATED INSTRUMENTS[4,5]

A *cytocentrifuge*, sometimes referred to as a cytospin, is a semiautomated special type of centrifuge used to concentrate cells in small quantities of fluid specimens onto a microscope slide due to centrifugal forces; best application in cerebrospinal fluid (CSF). Two such instruments in use are the Shandon Cytospin-Cytocentrifuge and the Sakura Auto smear.

Figure 1 shows the funnel shaped cuvette assembly which collects the cells onto the glass slide, the fluid being absorbed into the filter paper. A monolayer of well-preserved cells collects over just a 6 mm of slide space.

Automated Pap processing: Its inroads into cytology started with the introduction of the concept of nuclear size and nuclear optical density being used to analyze cell morphology.

Though the Pap smear with manual screening has been responsible for a very significant reduction in mortality of cervical cancer over the past 40 years, concern had arisen over false-negative cases, with subsequent repercussions,

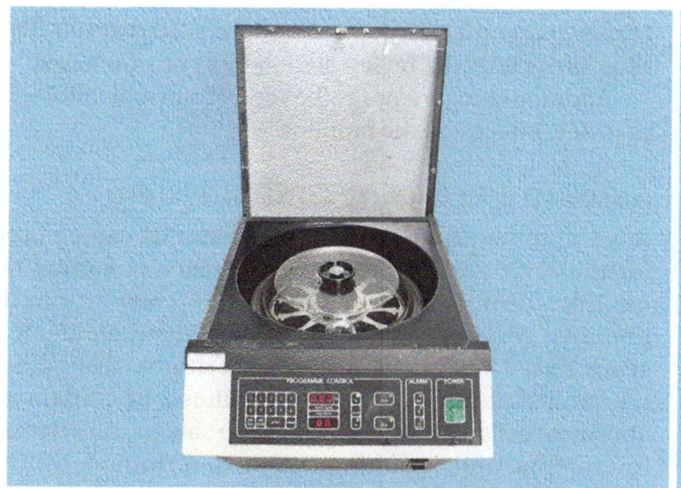

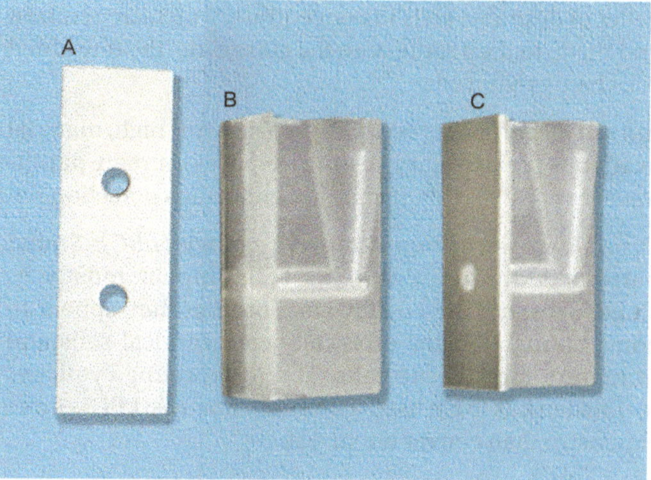

FIG. 1: Shandon Cytospin. On the right (A) Shandon cards; (B) Reusable cuvette; and (C) Shandon premade cuvettes with attached filter card.

their effects on patients, and the associated medicolegal implications. In addition, shortages of cytotechnologists, being exacerbated by new regulations limiting the number of slides that may be examined per day, had caused deep concern about the workload. Automated screening machines allowed detection of numerous samples at the same time without the fatigue factor setting in. The most challenging cases in screening are the ones which occur in the nondetection of abnormalities due to conventional preparation artifacts—thick smears, overlapping of cells and background blood or mucus obscuring detail.

The introduction of the *ThinPrep 2000 system* in the 1990s for use in screening for the presence of atypical cells, cervical carcinoma cells, or precursor lesions [low-grade squamous intraepithelial lesion (LSIL) and high-grade squamous intraepithelial lesion (HSIL)] (as defined by the Bethesda System for Reporting Cervical Cytology) revolutionized cancer screening amazingly and was intended as a replacement for the conventional method of Pap smears. It was the only Food and Drug Administration (FDA) approved slide processor. ThinPrep 2000 was introduced as a manually operated processor; subsequent to this the introduction of ThinPrep 3000 and ThinPrep 5000 processed up to 60–160 slides per batch, being fully automated and easy to use. The increased cost of the Pap test by this procedure is nullified by avoiding repetition on samples, less of call back of the patients, and procedure cost of colposcopy due to better interpretation with superior processing and increased sensitivity of the test compared to conventional smears. ThinPrep 5000 can be used on gynecology, nongynecology, and urolyte samples.

The *Surepath* is a semiautomated machine and works on the principle of density gradient. The cells are treated through a density gradient centrifugation and allow a pellet of desirable cells to concentrate, which are remixed and made to then settle onto the glass slide, the unwanted cells being removed.

Advantages of both procedures: Sensitivity is high; material available for ancillary testing, such as human papillomavirus (HPV), chlamydia, and gonorrhea detection.

Disadvantages of liquid-based cytology (LBC): Smear pattern is altered. Epithelial cells appear mostly as single cells and are slightly smaller than they appear in conventional smears, especially endocervical cells and immature metaplastic cells. The interpreting cytology/technician has to get used to the appearances. LBC is more expensive than conventional test.

Pap screening AutoAnalyzers: Besides processors AutoAnalyzers of smears are available.

An ideal analyzer system should:

- Be able to comment on smear adequacy.
- Scanning should be rapid, reliable, and reproducible.
- The system should select suspicious cells (or slides) as programmed and present them to the cytologist for a final check.
- Sensitivity of the automated device should be more than the sensitivity of the conventional method.

Automated screening systems in use for Pap smear analysis and thereby quality control purposes are described here.

PAPNET System[4,5]

The PAPNET system is a system from Neuromedical Systems uses conventionally prepared systems. It is composed of two components:

1. *Scanning function*: It is an electronic camera mounted over a microscope which scans the slides. It uses neural networks and algorithmic methodology to detect abnormal cells. The camera is programmed, slides are scanned, and about 128 digital images of potential abnormal cells or cluster of cells containing abnormal features are stored on a digital tape or on CD-ROM. The cases are triaged as negative and review. All the negative cases are filed and review cases are thoroughly examined.
2. *Review function*: The images are displayed on a video screen and are inspected and evaluated by the cytologist. The abnormal location of suspected field seen on the monitor can be assisted in location with the manual microscope.

Advantages: It is a totally interactive system. All cases are presented for review on the monitor. Less consumption of time due to automation in search.

Disadvantages: It is a costly procedure, priced at 400–500/slide as the PAPNET review station must be purchased.

Additional cost requires the time of a cytotechnologist to review images on the monitor.

AutoPap 300 Quality Control System

It is a noninteractive automatic system that can be used for the review of negatives and primary screening for quality control purpose; examines conventionally prepared cervical smears and assigns them an atypical score based on mathematical algorithms. The slides are ranked according to their likelihood of containing abnormal cells. The level at which the smears are selected for microscopic examination is determined by the operator. Thus the operator may decide what percentage of slides to analyze.

The Becton Dickinson FocalPoint GS Imaging System

Location-guided screening in cervical cytology presently offers a potentially significant advance over routine manual screening. Becton Dickinson (BD) FocalPoint GS imaging system uses SurePath Pap test slides for a computer-assisted field-of-view (FOV) screening and is intended to assist cervical cancer screening to detect evidence of squamous carcinoma, HSIL, LSIL, adeno-carcinoma and their precursor conditions.

The capacity of this system is 288 slides-performance per 24 hours. The system has a high speed video microscope with three cameras operating on different focal planes leading to dynamic focusing. A strobe light is used to acquire 25 images/s; a 4× magnification map of the entire slide is taken and 1,000 fields captured at 20× magnification. A score system is used by a score being assigned to each slide (range: 0–1); these slides being ranked according to the likelihood of abnormality. Subsequently a relocation to them for visual review of up to 10 FOVs most likely to contain abnormal cells exists. The image analysis is performed using pre-set algorithms.

Computer Vision Techniques

Computer vision techniques are automated systems for cytology static image analysis; comprising a cell scanner (digital camera) which "visualizes" images by measuring the light intensity and color properties being received by their electronic sensor elements. With a stained cytology sample, the camera is trained due to its sensor elements to react to chromatin clumping and other features, like nuclear size, form, etc. and the optical images caught by the camera are converted into digital images inside the camera and stored on a magnetic disk. The computer is programmed to analyze and classify these images. The computer selects images/smears which are most likely to contain abnormal cells and presents them to the cytotechnologist for further triage under the microscope.

The computer version techniques used are (1) pattern recognition, (2) segmentation, (3) image preprocessing, (4) feature extraction (5) feature preprocessing, (6) feature selection and discrimination measures, (7) classification, etc.

GOALS OF AUTOMATION

- Improving the accuracy and high sensitivity of test results.
- Time management, i.e., large number of specimens in the shortest possible time.
- Obtaining a slide that represents the lesion to be scanned as an original sample from the patient.

RECENT ADVANCES IN AUTOMATION

Automation in Lung Lesions

- The lung cell evaluation device (LuCED) for the early detection of lung cancer in sputum based on a three-dimensional (3D) morphology. This produces 3D volumetric cell representations in isometric, submicron resolution based on CT images.
- VisionGate Inc., in collaboration with the University of Washington, is developing LuCED test to score sputum samples processed by the cell CT for evidence of cell dysplasia or cancer.
- The LuCED analyses comprise a series of steps starting with cell preparation including fixation and staining with the routine hematoxylin and eosin stain. Based on cellular prevalence counts, it is estimated that LuCED sensitivity exceeds 90% and specificity approaches 100% for patients with cancer cells in sputum.
- Cell analysis in 3D provides an unobstructed and unambiguous representation of normal and cancer cell morphology.

Automation in Urine Cytology[6]

Automated Urine Microscopy Analyzer

- Automated instruments have greatly reduced the need for manual microscopy.
- There are three systems currently available to automate manual microscopy:
  i. First is an image-based analysis system that uses a video camera and strobe lamp (stops fluid motion) to detect and sort particles based on predetermined particle dimensions.
  ii. The second type is based on principle of flow cytometry, it classifies particles based on fluorescent intensity, electrical impedance, and forward angle light scatter.
  iii. Third is a next-generation automated image-based urinalysis system, the Iris iQ200 Elite recently received the United States Food and Drug Administration (US-FDA) clearance. Images are stored and can be viewed on the workstation screen, thereby eliminating the need for manual microscopy in most cases. Only urine samples containing crystals and/or yeast require review images for confirmation.

CONCLUSION

Automation in cytology has taken a long time to materialize, but is now a reality.

It started and was stabilized in the area of Pap screening; now has found applications in the cytology of other anatomical areas; though still a long way to go.

The technology is challenging and, if given time to develop in tandem with standard good laboratory practices, and laboratory procedures, then the most effective components of these systems will prevail.

Cooperation among pathologists, clinicians, and manufacturers will ensure that the technology performs as expected and contributes to affordable and reliable patient care.

REFERENCES

1. Wojcik EM, Booth CN. Automation in Cervical Cytology. Pathol Case Rev. 2005;10(3):138-43.
2. Desai M. Role of automation in cervical cytology. Diagnost Hepatol. 2009;15(7):323-9.
3. Shah M. (2018). Automation in cytology. [online] Available from https://www.slideshare.net/MananShah133/automation-in-cytology-126348661 [Last accessed March, 2024].
4. Becton Dickinson. (2023). BD FocalPoint™ GS Imaging System: [online] Available from https://www.bd.com/en-ca/products-and-solutions/products/product-families/bd-focalpoint-gs-imaging-system [Last accessed March, 2024].
5. Becton Dickinson. (2023). Cervical Cancer Screening. [online] Available from https://www.bd.com/en-za/our-products/cervical-cancer-screening [Last accessed March, 2024].
6. Manju M. (2017). Automated Urine Analysis. [online] Available from https://www.slideshare.net/manjunathatm/automated-urine-analysis-71543720– [Last accessed March, 2024].

CHAPTER 14

Quality Systems in Cytology

INTRODUCTION

The functioning of any cytology laboratory rests not only on the managerial ability of the laboratory director but on a host of factors such as the standardization of the procedures, best performance by personnel and proficiency in the overall outcome.

In order to achieve this, all laboratories should have clear *objectives of* functioning:

- Priority on services and accuracy in reporting
- Adherence to the standard turnaround time specified by accreditation bodies
- Adherence to all standard operating procedures
- Qualified staff on technical and interpretation level
- Maintenance of quality reagents and equipment in the laboratory

QUALITY CONTROL[1-5]

In cytopathology, it involves excellence in the execution of all steps and procedures involved in a laboratory set-up, resulting in good quality reporting. An ideal laboratory set-up should adhere to quality management in the following areas:

- Infrastructure and equipment
- Proper collection and receipt of specimens
- Processing of specimens
- Staining procedures and labeling of slides
- Timely dispatch of reports
- Qualified reporting personnel
- Documentation and archives
- Managerial support
- Educational training programs for the staff—intralaboratory and interlaboratory
- External quality assessments (EQAs) and accreditation schemes

On the other hand, *laboratory quality assurance (QA)*[1-5] includes a system which enables laboratories to achieve and maintain high levels of accuracy and proficiency in all areas of quality control despite changes occurring from time-to-time in methodology, execution, and workload. The terms "quality assurance" and "quality control" are often used interchangeably in medical practice.

The term quality control refers to quality check at every step and quality assurance is a systemic monitoring of quality control practices to assure that all systems are functioning smoothly in a manner appropriate to the health needs of the society. Quality assurance comprises administrative activities implemented in a quality system so that requirements and goals toward an objective, product, service, or activity toward clients will be fulfilled (ISO 9001:2015).

Quality control and assurance are maintained by guidelines laid down for laboratory services by professional bodies. These may be both national level or international level bodies. The process of creating guidelines is a consensus for "best practices" within a specialty.

Quality Control

Infrastructure and Equipment in Laboratory

- The laboratory should be clean, well-lighted, adequately ventilated, and spacious for proper functioning. This minimizes problems in specimen handling, evaluation, and reporting.
- The area for specimen preparation and handling should be separate from the area where specimens are evaluated and reported.
- Alcohol, formaldehyde, and xylene should be carefully monitored due to misuse and possible presence of hazardous vapor concentrations.

- An adequate number of binocular microscopes of good quality and proper working order must be available.
- Laboratory instruments and equipment should be calibrated under periodic maintenance and monitoring so as to ensure accurate analytical results.
- Quality control samples within expiry period should be fed routinely every day in automated analyzers to check for accurate results in instruments.
- Cleanliness of equipment and regular maintenance are of paramount importance.

Collection of Specimens

- Cytologic specimens should be accepted and examined only if requested by a licensed medical practitioner and collected in accordance with standard procedures which conform to the laboratory.
- Standard laboratory procedures (SOPs)[6] with clear instructions for collection in black and white, as hard copies should be available in all laboratories and issued to the hospitals (both within institution and outside) as well as clinicians who feed-in specimens to the laboratory.
- The request form should include details, such as patient's name, medical/hospital record number, age and sex, date and time of specimen collection, with or without fixative, type of fixative, source or site of specimen, clinical history including pertinent physical findings, X-ray findings, and previous histological and cytological reference numbers if reported by the same laboratory or findings if reported by outside laboratories; clinician's full name with telephone number for contact and signature of the clinician requesting the examination.
- A responsible person should be entrusted to receive specimens and entry made in the relevant log system after ensuring that each specimen is given a proper accession number as it is the norm in a particular laboratory.
- The laboratory should have written criteria for rejecting specimens.
- Fixation, while the specimen is still wet, is recommended for conventional cell samples. The cytopathology laboratory should inform the particular clinician if the specimen sample is "unsatisfactory".
- All material from infectious sources [acquired immunodeficiency syndrome (AIDS) patient and hepatitis B and C patients] should have a "biohazard label" tagged on the container indicating that the contents should be handled with care.
- Proper disinfection of areas handling biohazard samples should be carried out.

Preparation, Fixation, and Staining Procedures

- Processing of fluids should be immediate and not later than 2 hours for optimal results. All laboratories should standardize these methods for optimal results and the laboratory supervisor should routinely check both methodology in processing and staining performed.
- All staining protocols should be as per SOPs and hard copies available at the staining racks.
- The reagents should be changed from time-to-time as per the workload. Maintenance of good staining requires that the stains are replaced on a regular schedule determined by either the number of slides stained or the time elapsed since stains were last replaced.
- Staining solutions and chemicals used in the cytopathology laboratory should be labeled with the time of preparation, purchase, or both. Standard methods should be followed for the in-house preparation of stains.
- *Papanicolaou stain:* It is a crucial stain for cervical cancer screening. Several automatic programmable stainers are available. Each laboratory must develop a written staining protocol for manual, automated, or for both methods which results in optimal staining of the specimen.
- *Romanowsky stain:* It is recommended for air-dried smears and highlights cytoplasmic features. Unlike the Papanicolaou stain, these stains are metachromatic. The Giemsa stain should be checked regularly for optimal staining effect.
- Giemsa and May–Grünwald Giemsa (MGG) stains should be discarded when precipitates form. Phosphate buffer solution to be discarded when turbidity develops.
- Staining solutions should be filtered regularly to avoid contamination and should be covered/closed tightly when not in use. Effective measures to prevent cross-contamination between specimens during the staining process must be used.
- A daily record is kept of the need for topping up fixatives and stains and the replacement of stains. All chemicals should be adequately stocked in the stores.
- Daily check of the quality of staining, i.e., the intensity of nuclear staining, contrast between eosinophilic and cyanophilic staining of cytoplasm, definition of nuclear chromatin, quality of dehydration of slide, and clarity of mountant should be done by the technical supervisor before slides are presented to the consultant.
- A random selection of smears should be checked at yearly intervals to determine the extent of fading of the stain due to inadequate dehydration. Well-stained slides should maintain their color for at least 3–5 years.

- *Archives*: Slide files should be maintained in such a way as they can be easily retrieved, if necessary.

Qualified Personnel

- Job descriptions at every level with clarity of hierarchical relationships is essential.
- Cytologic diagnoses are subjective, and greatly dependent on the skill and experience of the reporting person. They require examination of the individual cells, their morphology and pattern analysis in order to make a diagnosis. Proper training is essential for both professional and technical personnel. A cytotechnologist is a *person with special training in cytopathology who is responsible for screening Papanicolaou smears and determining which are test negative and which require further review* by a *pathologist.*[7-9]
- Turnover time as per international standards, workload per person (e.g., number of specimens processed per annum, number examined per day by individual cytoscreener, productivity over the years and progress charts should be maintained). *It is generally recommended that a trained cytotechnologist screens about 100 conventional Pap-stained smears in a day and about 200 monolayered cell preparations per day*. Beyond this, it is said that the fatigue factor sets in.
- Reports should be issued as per standard norms for that particular anatomical site, e.g., Bethesda system of cervical cancer reporting. These should be agreed upon by the reporting team and concerned clinician.
- *Review of abnormal gynecological cases:* A cervical cytology specimen initially evaluated by a cytotechnologist as reactive, atypical, premalignant, or malignant must be referred to a pathologist for final interpretation and report. Discordance between cytotechnologist's and a pathologist's report is a reason for continuing education. Peer review may be taken for difficult cases and an outside consultation for cases with a discrepancy and significant clinical implications. The latter constitute part of quality assurance program and documentation of all reviews is essential.
- *Rescreening of negative cases:* Most regulatory bodies governing cytology quality programs specify that at least 10% of samples interpreted as negative should be rescreened. Similarly, random 10% slides reported by a cytotechnologist should be rescreened by a pathologist. Rapid review may be done before the reports are issued or later as may be the practice of the laboratory.
- *Randomized recall:* of 10% of women who had negative reporting should be called for repeat smear at the end of 10 months.
- *Cytohistological correlation and clinical follow-up*: Exfoliative cytology screening may give rise to false-negative results. This may depend on sample collection or the capability of the reporting person. Regular cytohistological correlation is essential and rescreening of smears should be resorted to if discrepancy is found between cytology and histology.
- Causes of any discrepancy should be determined. The comparison of the histology sample on the same sample in turn depends on the reporting ability of the histopathologist. Cytohistological correlation can be a helpful educational tool used to refine methods of evaluation for both cytology and biopsy specimens. The correlation process should be documented in the laboratory quality assurance program. Negative biopsy specimens in the context of recognized squamous intraepithelial lesion (SIL) or cancer by biopsy may be the result of a surgical sampling discrepancy.
- Comments regarding such cytological discordance in the surgical pathology report may be helpful in directing further patient management. The laboratory must have a clearly defined policy regarding the methods used for cytohistological correlation. If histological material is not available, the laboratory may attempt to obtain follow-up material or information on patients by sending letters.
- Regular EQA programs will help in minimizing this error.

Dispatch of Reports

- Procedures outlined for dispatch of reports on a daily basis should be standardized. The same norms should be followed, so that any discrepancy in reports not reaching the other end can be easily picked up. Time of dispatch, acknowledgments taken and location of end point should be streamlined. A responsible person should be in charge of the procedures.
- Cause of delay in reporting should be informed to the clinician with reasons.
- Turnaround times should be adhered to.

Maintenance of Records

- *Archiving and retention of data*: Each laboratory is responsible for a good archiving of request forms, slides, and reports. Procedures should comply with standard regulatory norms.
- A record of microscope and instrument maintenance as well as instrument calibration records should be maintained as these activities are a requirement by laboratory accreditation agencies.
- *Slide storage and retrieval: Nongynecological—*
  - Cytology laboratories must retain all nongynecological slide preparations regardless of diagnosis

for a minimum period of 5 years from the date of microscopic examinations.
  - Fine needle aspiration glass slides must be retained for a minimum of 10 years.
  - Test reports must be retained for 10 years from the date of report.
  - Logs and accession records for cytology specimens must be retained for 2 years from the date of receipt.
  - Quality control records for cytology specimens must be retained for 2 years from the data that they were created and generated.
- *Gynecological specimens:*
  - All gynecological slides must be stored for a minimum period of 10 years in good condition.
  - The request forms must be stored for a minimum period of 3 years.
  - All reports must be stored for a minimum period of 10 years.

Management

- Managerial support for all categories of services is essential. The laboratory should be directed by a qualified physician with a specialist qualification in pathology including special training and expertise in cytopathology. The director or designated medical professional is responsible for proper performance and reporting of all tests done in the cytopathology laboratory.
- Subcommittees with coordinators should be set up for quality in service. Ensure participation of all staff categories, under the chairmanship of the laboratory director or second in charge so that everyone feels responsible.

Educational Schemes

- Intralaboratory educational teaching programs help staff to update their knowledge.
- The staff should be encouraged to attend continuing medical education (CME) program annually and credit points allotted for these should be recorded.
- Interlaboratory teaching programs give the staff members an indication of their proficiency levels.

QUALITY ASSURANCE: LABORATORY STANDARDIZATION

Laboratory standardization[10] is to have a uniformity in test results with the same analytical accuracy; there should be precision across measurement systems across various laboratories.

Some of the methods of quality assurance checks are:

- *The external quality assurance assessment scheme (EQAAS)* is available from various organizations/regulatory bodies both internationally and nationally, which are qualified to audit a laboratory in its various performances: *Centers for Disease Control and Prevention (CDC), World Health Organization*, and National Level Bodies such as *Academic Professional Bodies, like the Indian Academy of Cytology (IAC), American Association of Cytology, European Association of Cytology*, etc. These organizations put forth reference systems with material wherein the participating laboratories use the material provided to verify the analytical accuracy and precision of their testing methodology. The areas covered may include: proficiency testing scheme in cytotechniques, examine the quality of cytoscreener and cytopathologist's reporting, laboratory organization and performance, etc.
- *Accreditation bodies*: The accreditation boards in India are *Indian Academy of Cytology (IAC), National Accreditation Board of Laboratories (NABL), and ISO certification.*
  - Accreditation and certification of cytotechnologists and cytopathologists.
  - Liquid-based cervical cytology specimens should be included in the proficiency testing programs for laboratories that use this methodology. Laboratories using automated screening devices must follow the manufacturer's directions that have been approved by the Food and Drug Administration (FDA).
- *Internal quality assessment programs:* Review by multiple individuals in case of cervical cytology. Review without knowledge of clinical outcome.
- *Proficiency testing* is mandatory for individuals examining gynecological and nongynecological specimens. A number of state and national programs are available toward this and can be applied to. Ongoing education is a requirement for proficiency in cytology. This requirement can be fulfilled by participating in proficiency testing, intradepartmental slide review sessions, attending workshops and symposia, teaching cytotechnology students, pathology students and fellow, and independent study.
- A cytopathologist is responsible for the management of the cytopathology laboratory. Final responsibility for all activities performed in the laboratory is with the registered cytopathologist managing the laboratory.

- The position of each employee in the pathology laboratory should be recorded in an organization flowchart.
- *Reporting personnel and workload*: Medical regulations require that individual examining a gynecological cytology specimen be a qualified cytopathologist or pathologist in a certified laboratory. In the primary screening of cervical smears, it is required to examine and evaluate every cell in the smear, to detect relatively low number of abnormal cells, <50 cells, scattered among large number of normal cells (300,000-500,000).

  These individuals may examine up to a maximum of 100 slides per 24 hours (average 12.5 slides per hour) and in not <8 hours. It is advised to screen smears for not >2 hours without break. It is advised that screeners should screen not >6 h/day. This is the case for primary screening and each laboratory should establish individual workload limits for each cytotechnologist and the limits reviewed 6 monthly using laboratory defined performance standards. All specimens must be reported using descriptive nomenclature easily understood by clinicians.
- *Referral laboratories:* The laboratory in charge is responsible for selecting referral laboratories. The referring laboratories must report all test results from the referral laboratory without alterations. All opinions given should be recorded and conveyed to the treating clinician.
- *Indexing in cytology:* It should be done for comparison of statistics and research purposes.

CONCLUSION

Quality control and quality assurance lead to quality management. This is overseeing all activities and tasks in the laboratory needed to maintain a desired level of excellence.

Quality assurance and management result in the determination of a quality policy which in turn creates and implements quality assurance, thereby constantly resulting in improvement.

REFERENCES

1. American Society of Cytopathology. (2000). Quality control and quality assurance practices. [online] Available from https://www.academia.edu/66584040/Quality_assurance_in_reporting_Cervical_Cytology [Last accessed March, 2024]
2. Donabedian A. The quality of care. How can it be assessed? JAMA. 1988;260(12):1743-8.
3. Donabedian A. The quality of care. How can it be assessed? 1988. Arch Pathol Lab Med. 1997;121(11):1145-50.
4. Klinkhamer P, Bulten H. Chapter 4: Laboratory Guidelines and Quality Control for Cervical Screening. Commission on Laboratory Accreditation Inspection Checklist 2002 edition. Northfield, Illinois: College of American Pathologists. [online] Available from https://www.cancer-network.de/cervical/guidelines/chap4/Chap%204%20of%2017%20Sep%2003.doc [Last accessed March, 2024].
5. Centers for Disease Control and Prevention. (2017) Laboratory quality assurance and standardization programs. [online] Available from https://www.cdc.gov/labstandards/index.html [Last accessed March, 2024].
6. Chandra A, Cross P, Denton K, Giles T, Hemming D, Payne C, et al. The BSCC code of practice—exfoliative cytopathology (excluding gynaecological cytopathology). Cytopathology. 2009;20(4):211-23.
7. Krieger PA, Cohen T, Naryshkin S. A practical guide to Papanicolaou smear rescreens. Cancer Cytopathol. 1998;84(3):130-7.
8. Melamed MR. Quality control in cytology laboratories. Gynec Oncol. 1981;12:S206-S211.
9. Husain OA, Butler EB, Evans DM, Macgregor JE, Yule R. Quality control in cervical cytology. J Clin Pathol. 1974;27(12):935-44.
10. College of American Pathologists. (2002). Commission on laboratory accreditation. Inspection checklist. Northfield: College of American Pathologists. [online] Available from https://www.cihrt.nl.ca/exhibits/June%2024%20Wegrynowski%20Exhibits/P-1755_2004%20(09)%20September_Laboratory%20Accreditation_Anatomic%20Pathology%20Checklist.pdf [Last accessed March, 2024].

CHAPTER 15

Receipt of Surgical Biopsies in the Laboratory and Fixation

INTRODUCTION

All pathology laboratories big and small receive histopathology specimens in various numbers. The duty of every pathologist in the laboratory is to receive this and deliver a written and typed report to the clinician sending it with accuracy and precision to the best of his knowledge. In order to achieve this, the pathologist has to adhere to certain criteria and norms. The objective should be to produce a quality report within a certain period of time (turnaround time) for the client.

RECEIVING FORMALITIES

Laboratories should streamline their schedule to work with these aims:

- All specimens received should be given a laboratory accession number which runs in serial order for histopathology specimens for that particular year, e.g., the first specimen received in the year 2021 would read as 01/2021 and the 45th specimen received would read as 045/2021. This number carries for the specimen in the container (the outer aspect of the container to be labeled with it), block, slide with whatever stain it may be stained, special histochemistry, etc.
- It is the duty of the technician/junior doctor to check that a request for performance of the histopathology examination accompanies each specimen with the name of the requesting clinician, name of patient/age/sex/hospital number/unit number, department, and signature of the clinician. An adequate clinical history and reference biopsy number of any previous biopsies performed with the diagnosis made should be entered in the request form.
- A practice of cutting up a specimen into two or three portions in order to be sent to different laboratories should be thoroughly discouraged and specimens treated in this way not accepted. The clinician should be made aware at the clinicopathological meetings that this practice is detrimental to patient welfare and hampers an optimal result.
- The technician should see that an adequate amount of fixative is added to the specimen in the container; failing which it should be brought to the notice of the pathologist.
- Specimens may be divided into small (endometrium, skin biopsies, cervical punch biopsies, etc.), medium (resected gallbladder, appendix, polyps, etc.), and large biopsies (like hysterectomy specimens, bowel resections, etc.). This gives an idea of the workload and helps in the financial costing in the laboratory.
- A standard time for the cut-up should be fixed on a daily basis so that all capsules with the grossed bits are fed into the automatic histokinette at a particular time routinely for processing.
- The cut-up should always be supervised by the pathologist and in teaching institutions a senior pathologist when a resident is doing it.
- Standard procedures for cut-ups should be adhered to.
- The number of cassettes/blocks given for a particular specimen should have the same numerical number but serial alphabetical blocks labeled A, B, C, etc. so that each block reads as 01A/2021 and 01B/2021 for the first specimen of the year if two bits have been taken.
- Freshly resected specimens on the day of the surgery may directly be taken for cut-up or some laboratories await a day before cut-up so that the specimen is adequately fixed for easy handling. This depends on the practice of the laboratory.
- The place for grossing/cut-up should be a dedicated area in the laboratory with adequate light, continuous

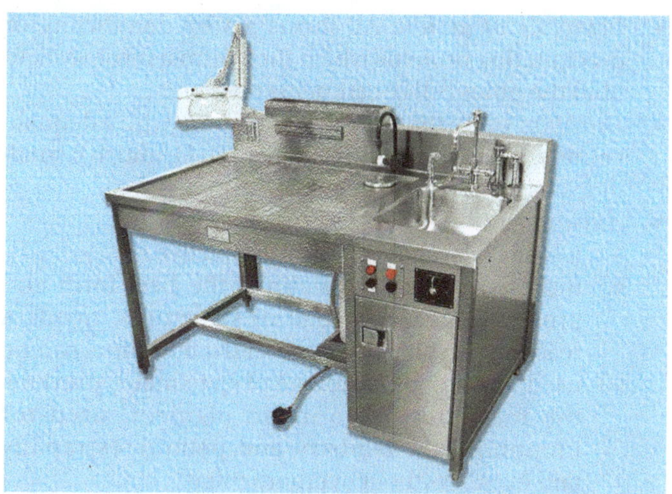

FIG. 1: Grossing station with facility for artificial illumination and running water supply.

running water facility, and a bucket for removal of the waste.

- The stage of the procedure should be cleaned properly and all tissue fragments wiped out before the next specimen is taken so as to avoid floaters of previous specimens.
- **Figure 1** shows a grossing station available commercially; a wooden board and sharp knives instead of this also serve the purpose equally well. Bright window light should be available for grossing.

FIXATION OF SPECIMENS: WHY FIXATION?[1-4]

Fixation is the process by which the tissue cells are fixed in a physical and partly chemical state with minimal distortion and decomposition, keeping it in as life like a manner as possible and thus enabling them to withstand treatment with various reagents used for processing. The process hardens the tissue slightly but does not make it brittle, thereby facilitating easy handling.

An ideal fixative not only stops autolysis and putrefaction of cells but maintains the morphology, is isotonic, enables section cutting and staining with ease, and allows optimal differentiation of various cell types and constituents. It is the basic foundation for the end result under the microscope.

Fixation may be achieved by immersion or perfusion of the specimen. Most laboratories use the *immersion method* for the surgical specimens. Perfusion method is generally used for autopsy specimens and to preserve whole organs for the museum. Perfusion is usually done on organs with a good vascular supply where injection of fixatives into organs, like brain, lung, etc., is done.

General Principles of Optimal Fixation in Routine Practice

- *Essential*: Fresh tissue. Fix as soon as possible (to avoid autolysis).
- Label each tissue container accurately as stated above.
- If fixation is not immediately possible refrigerate the specimen, do not freeze.
- Consider any fresh or incompletely fixed tissue as potentially infectious.
- Do not allow specimens to dry.
- When a specimen is immersed in a fixative, the container should be spacious and large with an adequate amount of fixative. Fixative should penetrate from all sides. Avoid compression or stuffing of the specimen into the container as it will get fixed in the distorted shape. This will make handling difficult.
- Do not place the specimen in a container and then add the fixative.
- An adequate volume of fixative is vital (15–20:1 specimen).
- Cavities should be cut into and opened as well as hollow organs or specimens with natural cavities to allow easy access of fixative. Cotton soaked in fixative may be placed in cavities. If there is a delay in cut-up, large specimens should be cut in the proper way to allow for fixation.
- When perfusion of specimens by fixatives is undertaken, gentle agitation (swirling) of the specimen during early hours of fixation helps.
- When whole specimens are being fixed allow enough for the fixative to penetrate the whole specimen. Make planned cuts to facilitate penetration.
- The thickness of any specimen or tissue slice should not exceed 4 mm or maximum 5 mm if optimal fixation and penetration of fixative is to be achieved in a tissue cassette.
- Initial fixation is best carried out at room temperature (20°C); however, increase in temperature aids fixation.
- Fixatives should be carefully made up from reagents of good quality, fresh if so specified.
- Specimens received in fixative should be checked and the fixative replaced if necessary.
- Fixatives should be changed for each specimen after clearing and washing the container and changing the label as blood, cells, and sometimes fragments of the tissue of the previous specimen may contaminate the fluid and mistakenly represent as fragments of the next specimen if the same fixative in recycled containers.
- Metal lids for fixation containers are best avoided as some fixatives are highly corrosive and react with them (e.g., mercury salts).

- Some fixatives, like Zenker's/Helly's require that specimens should be washed in water prior to processing in order to remove the dichromate salts; and others (picric acid fixatives) require direct immersion in alcohol to remove excess picric acid of the fixatives.
- All fixatives are toxic and irritant and should be handled with care.

TYPES OF FIXATIVES

There are numerous types of fixatives with various advantages and disadvantages, they form a heterogeneous group and classifications can be varied based on composition, function, and action on tissue.

- *A simple way of classifying fixatives is based on their components*:
  - Simple fixative: It contains a single chemical, e.g., formaldehyde (10% formalin), glutaraldehyde (2.5%), and ethyl alcohol (absolute) in cytology.
  - Compound fixative: It contains more than one chemical, e.g.:
    - Formalin based: 10% neutral buffered formalin, 10% formol saline, and 10% formol calcium acetate
    - Mercurial fixatives: Zenker's solution, Helly's solution, B5
    - Picric acid fixatives: Bouin's solution, Gendre's fluid, and Rossman's fluid
    - Dichromate fixatives: Regaud's solution, Moller's solution, and Orth's solution
    - Alcohol containing fixatives: Carnoy's, Clarke's, acetic alcohol formalin (AAF) *(see **Appendix 1** for components of fixatives)*.
- *Other classifications are based on* the tissues on which they act (fluids or microanatomical); their method of functioning (heat fixation, chemical fixation, i.e., denaturation of proteins).

Detail on Important Fixatives

Formalin

It is commercially available as formalin (40% formaldehyde dissolved in water). This is considered as 100% formalin to prepare its various forms.

- *Composition*: *Various forms in use are* 10% formalin used universally in most laboratories, 10% formal saline, 10% formal calcium acetate, *and 10% buffered neutral formalin which is the most superior form. 10% buffered neutral formalin* is considered the best general fixative for pathology specimens (*Composition*: *see **Appendix 1***).
- *Principle of action*: All forms act by denaturing or precipitating proteins which then form a meshwork to hold the other cell constituents together.
- *Duration of fixation time*: 24–48 hours with adequate volume of fixative; slow to penetrate (1 mm/h); small biopsies fix faster.
- *Advantages*:
  - It is easily available and cost-effective.
  - Buffered neutral formalin is the best form and preserves a wide range of structures, needs a reasonably short but optimal fixation time, can be used for long time storage of specimens, prevents the formation of formalin pigment, used for immunohistochemistry and penetrates rapidly and evenly without overhardening.
- *Disadvantages*:
  - All forms are slow in action, can be an irritant and cause allergies.
  - 10% formalin: On oxidation, results in formic acid formation which in areas of hemosiderin gives rise to a brown-black formalin pigment or acid hematin which hampers interpretation after staining.
  - On storage, it becomes cloudy due to formation of paraformaldehyde; this is prevented by adding 11–16% methanol to commercial formaldehyde.
  - 10% formalin causes loss of enzymes and immunological activity, therefore not ideal for enzyme studies or immunohistochemistry (IHC). Buffered neutral formalin is preferred for IHC.
  - Removal of formalin pigment: Treat sections for 30 minutes with a mixture of 200 mL of 75% alcohol and 1 mL of 25–28% liquor ammonia followed by a wash in water (Schridde's method).

Glutaraldehyde

It can be used for electron and routine light microscopy. It is commercially available as 25% or 50% stock solution. A 25% solution is better as polymerization occurs with a 50% solution. It is stable in acid solution (pH 3–5) and at a temperature of 4°C.

- *Composition*: For fixation, it used as 2.5–4% solution made by diluting 25% solution in Sorensen's phosphate buffer at 0.1M pH 7.4, this keeps for 3 months at 0–4°C. Addition of charcoal removes impurities which may collect over time.
- *Principle*: It is a dialdehyde and acts by forming cross linkages by binding to amino acid groups as well as sulphydryl groups.
- *Duration of fixation time*: It fixes small tissue fragments and needle biopsies (in 2–4 hours at room temperature). Larger pieces (up to 4 mm thick) are fixed in 24 hours.

- Excellent primary fixative for electron microscopy, duration of fixation is 1–4 hours depending on tissue size at 0–4°.
- *Advantages*:
  - Better preservation than formaldehyde due to more cross linkage formation
  - Used widely in electron microscopy
  - Causes less shrinkage than formalin
  - Less irritation than formalin
- *Disadvantages*:
  - More expensive
  - Works at low temperature
  - Slow penetration, hence tissues must be small.
  - Not suitable for carbohydrates, i.e., PAS staining and due to background stain.

Osmium Tetraoxide

It is used extensively in electron microscopy, but not in light microscopy.

- *Composition*: It comes in vials of 0.5 and 1.0 G and is used as a 2% solution in distilled water at a pH of 7.4. It takes 2–5 days for the solution to mature.
- *Principle of action*: Osmium tetraoxide cross-links with proteins. It has application in lipid demonstration as it reacts with unsaturated lipids forming monoester and diesters which are not removed by fat solvents. It is stored in a cool and dark place due to its ability of being reduced.
- *Fixation time*: *Flemming's solution—12–24 hours.*
- *Palade's fixative*: 30–90 minutes for tiny fragments of tissue.
- *Advantages*:
  - It rapidly fixes the tissue
  - It stains tissue structure "gray-black" due to its property of being reduced by reactive tissue groups.
  - It is used in demonstrating lipids, has applications in neuropathology.
  - Good nuclear fixatives and for myelin in peripheral nerves.
  - It hardens tissues only slightly
  - *Flemming's fluid* (*see* **Appendix 1**) *and Palade's* buffered osmium tetraoxide fixative are used for electron microscopy.
- *Disadvantages*:
  - Osmium tetraoxide is very expensive.
  - Vapors are very harmful to the eyes and skin.
  - Difficulty in counterstaining after its use.

Mercurial Fixatives

- *Zenker's fixative*:
  - Composition: See **Appendix 1**
  - Principle of action: It acts by precipitating proteins
  - Duration of fixation: Duration of fixation is 12 hours, smaller tissues (<3 mm) are fixed in 2–3 hours.
  - Advantages:
    - It is recommended for congested tissues, reticuloendothelial tissues including lymph nodes, spleen, thymus, and bone marrow.
    - Good for metachromatic staining
    - Zenker's fluid fixes nuclei very well and gives good detail.
    - They are also good for trichome stains and enhance staining with several dyes.
  - Disadvantages:
    - They are not commonly used fixatives; penetration only up to 5 mm.
    - Leaving in Zenker's for 3–4 days makes tissue hard and brittle
    - Their main drawback is that several pigments combine with mercury to produce a brownish-black precipitate. These precipitates can however be removed by placing sections in an iodine solution for 5–10 minutes and then treating them with sodium thiosulfate.
    - The tissues should be washed overnight to remove the excess dichromate, mercurial fixatives do not act on lipids.
- *Helly's fluid (Syn—Spuler's or Maximow's fluid)*:
  - Composition: This fixative has the same composition as Zenker's fluid but differs from it in that 5 mL of formalin is added immediately before use instead of acetic acid.
  - Principle of action: Precipitation of proteins combines with several amino acids
  - Duration of fixation: Zenker's formal (Helly's) is slower than Zenker's fluid; fixation time is 8–24 hours.
  - Advantages:
    - It is excellent for bone marrow, spleen, and extramedullary hemopoiesis and is recommended for blood-containing organs in general.
    - It preserves cytoplasmic granules and is suitable for Giemsa/Leishman's stains.
  - Disadvantages: Same as Zenker's fluid.
- *B-5 fixative*:
  - Composition: See **Appendix 1**
  - Principle of action: It is similar to other mercurial fixatives.
  - Duration of fixation: 8–12 hours
  - Advantages:
    - It is used in bone marrows and on lymph nodes where lymphomas are suspected.
    - Also used in immunohistochemistry.

Picric Acid Fixatives

These require a saturated aqueous solution of picric acid. Aqueous picric acid 2.1% will produce a saturated solution and 5% picric acid is a saturated solution in absolute ethyl alcohol.

- *Bouin's fluid*:
  - Composition: See **Appendix 1**
  - *Principle of action*: It precipitates proteins and forms yellow water-soluble picrates; therefore, tissue should be transferred directly to 70% alcohol after fixation.
  - Duration of fixation: 8–12 hours.
  - Advantages:
    - This fixative keeps well, penetrates rapidly and evenly causes little shrinkage.
    - The acetic acid in this fixative lyses red blood cells and dissolves small iron and calcium deposits in tissue
    - Tissue fixed in it gives brilliant staining with the trichrome methods.
    - It is a good fixative for glycogen as well as connective tissue.
  - Disadvantages:
    - It precipitates protein with yellow discoloration; hence tissues should not be placed in water directly after fixation.
    - Excess picric acid should be washed out of tissue using several alcohol changes. The sections can be treated with a saturated solution of lithium carbonate in 70% alcohol for a few minutes or alternatively treat the sections in ethyl alcohol followed by 5% sodium thiosulfate, then wash in running tap water before staining.
- *Gendre's fluid*:
  - Composition: See **Appendix 1**. Actions are similar to Bouin's fluid but superior to it for carbohydrate and connective tissue.
- *Rossman's fluid*:
  - Composition: See **Appendix 1**. It is similar to Gendre's fluid in action and uses.

Dichromate Fixatives

Dichromate fixatives are Regaud's, Champy's, and Orth's fluids for composition (*see* **Appendix 1**). These may be used as routine fixatives but are particularly good as cytoplasmic fixatives for mitochondria if followed by postchromation for 4–8 days in 3% potassium dichromate.

- *Principle of action*: Chemical fixation by denaturing proteins. Lipids are well-demonstrated, as they are more resistant to extraction by dehydrating and clearing agents after fixation in dichromate fixatives.
- *Advantages*: Demonstration of lipids and cytoplasmic detail like mitochondria in electron microscopy. Chromaffin tissue is well-demonstrated but fluids may be improved for this purpose by the addition of 5% acetic acid to lower the pH. This preserves chromaffin tissue granules.
- *Disadvantages*: Solutions should only be mixed immediately before use as they do not stay. It penetrates evenly and rapidly but has a tendency to overharden tissues and cause excessive shrinkage. The tissues should be washed after fixation and transferred to 70% ethanol to avoid pigment precipitation.
- *Time of fixation*: It is 24 hours and not longer.

Alcoholic Fixatives/Dehydrant Fixatives

Alcoholic fixatives/dehydrant fixatives are not only used in cytology but can also be used for tissues. Some of the fluids for this purpose are Carnoy's fluid, Clarke's fluid, and Newcomer's fluid.

- *Principle of action*: It denatures proteins
- *Advantages*:
  - These solutions produce good general histologic results for hematoxylin and eosin stains.
  - They preserve nucleic acids whereas lipids are extracted.
  - The fixatives penetrates rapidly and gives good nuclear and reasonably good preservation of cytoplasmic elements.
  - They are excellent for smears of cell cultures and chromosome analysis (Newcomer's fluid).
  - Those which contain glacial acetic acid are specially used for hemorrhagic samples. The acetic acid in the fixative hemolyses the red blood cells.
  - Carnoy's fixative is also useful for RNA stains, e.g., methyl green-pyronin stain.
  - All alcoholic fixative preserves glycogen in particular Carnoy's fluid.
- *Disadvantages*:
  - Overfixation in Carnoy's causes excessive shrinkage of cells.
  - Carnoy's fixative must be prepared fresh when needed and discarded after each use as it loses its effectiveness on long-standing, and chloroform can react with acetic acid to form hydrochloric acid (HCl).
  - Tissues fixed in Carnoy's fluid should be placed directly into 100% ethanol, instead of increasing graded alcohols.

Dehydrant-cross-linking Fixatives

Compound fixatives with both dehydrant and cross-linking actions include alcohol-formalin mixtures.

- *Principle of action*: The fixatives denature and precipitate due to disruption of hydrophobic bonds that contributes to the tertiary structure of proteins.
- *Advantages*:
  - It is an excellent fixative for glycogen.
  - Acetic alcohol formalin is an ideal fixative for cellblock preparation.
  - They produce excellent results in the immunohistochemical identification of most specific antigens
  - It penetrates the tissue rapidly; hence, it is used for fixation in immunofluorescence.
- *Disadvantages*: Most alcohol-based fixatives should be prepared not >1–2 days before use.

Postchromation

It is secondary fixation to demonstrate certain morphological details. It is the treatment of tissues with 2.5% or 3% potassium dichromate after normal fixation (used in various fixatives such as dichromate as well as others). It may be carried out either before processing when tissues are left for 6–8 days in dichromate solutions or after processing when sections before staining are immersed in the dichromate solution for 12–24 hours followed in each case by washing well in running water.

This technique is employed to mordant tissues for staining, particularly cytoplasmic organelles, such as mitochondria and chromaffin tissue. It gives improved preservation and staining of these elements. Phospholipids are also more resistant to extraction with postchromation, e.g., as in Weigert's method for myelin; cytoplasmic detail after Zenker's and Helly's fixatives.

METHODS OF FIXATION[1-4]

Heat Fixation

- It is the usual mode of preparing bacteriological smears. After a smear has dried at room temperature, the slide is gripped by tongs and passed through the flame of a Bunsen burner several times. Heat coagulation of proteins makes the smear adhere to the slide.
- It is also used in combination with formal saline in frozen sections. The tissue is placed in 20–40 mL of fluid (10% formal saline) in a beaker and heated to below the boiling point over the spirit flame for 1 minute or until the tissue floats on the surface. It is then cooled immediately and the tissue taken for section cutting. The cryostat has replaced this technique. It can also be combined with the cryostat technique in tissues which take a longer time to freeze fix.
- *Principle of action*: Heat coagulation of proteins
- *Duration of fixation*: A few minutes
- *Advantages*: Rapid fixation; it has application in frozen sections.
- *Disadvantages*: Morphology is not as good as chemical fixation.

Microwave Fixation

It is a now a well-established technique. It is recommended for use not only in fixation but also all steps of tissue processing.

- *Principle*: It provides better fixation due to a homogenous rise in temperature (controlled heating) and due to a diffusion process overcoming the problem of erratic heating by direct flame. Heat denaturation and disulfide bond formation occurs. There is a significant cross-linking of protein molecules with subsequent chemical fixation.
- *Duration of fixation*: 10–15 minutes
- *Advantages*:
  - It can be used for routine histopathology for urgent reports, e.g., in renal transplant and cardiac biopsies.
  - Microwave accelerates staining and has no deleterious effect on special staining, used also in IHC as tissue antigens are better preserved.
  - Microwaved tissues, postfixed in osmium tetraoxide gives good results in electron microscopy.
- *Disadvantages*:
  - Not useful for large volume of histologic material
  - Metallic objects cannot be used.
- *Procedure*: The tissue is irradiated, immersing in formalin solution for a period of 4 minutes, followed by irradiation in buffered formalin for another 4 minutes. The optimal temperature required is 45–55°C.

Freeze-drying and Fixation

Cryostat Sectioning

- *Principle*: The rapid freezing of the tissue sample converts the water into ice. The firm ice within the tissue acts as embedding media to cut the tissue.
- *Most tissues are cut between* –15 and –25°C. Cooling in a cryostat is done by continuous flow liquid helium or nitrogen.
- *Duration of fixation*: 15–20 minutes
- *Advantages*:
  - Rapid diagnosis of lesions and surgical margin assessment
  - Used in enzyme immunocytochemistry and immunofluorescence
  - To stain lipid and certain carbohydrate in the tissue
- *Disadvantages*:
  - Fat containing tissues take a longer time to freeze
  - Morphology is compromised as compared to formalin-fixed tissue.

- *Method*: The OCT medium containing the tissue is placed on the stage provided in the cryostat and a metal weight placed on it. OCT is viscous at room temperature and miscible with H_2O, but freezes into a solid support at –20°C. The frozen tissue is removed and cut in the microtome provided in the cryostat chamber.

Quenching Procedure

- The tissue is cut into thin sections (1 mm thick) and placed in a beaker of isopentane suspended and snap frozen in a flask of liquid nitrogen gas at –150°C (Isopentane is an extremely volatile and extremely flammable liquid at room temperature and pressure). This process is known as quenching. This rapid freezing prevents the formation of ice crystals and preserves the tissue. If only liquid nitrogen is used, it forms vapor bubbles around the tissue, thus producing artifacts around the tissue.
- The tissue is then transferred to the drying chamber where under vacuum and at a higher temperature of –30°C, the ice (tissue water) is removed by sublimation, the water vapor being absorbed by a drying agent such as phosphorous pentoxide. The tissue is impregnated in the embedding medium under reduced pressure as follows:
  - Transfer the dried tissue quickly to a vacuum embedding medium oven containing molten wax. On sinking to the bottom of the bath, the tissue will be impregnated with wax and takes approximately 10 minutes for complete impregnation.

Advantages of Freeze Fixation

- Give better preservation of antigenicity due to nonexposure to the organic solvents and minimal denaturation of proteins
- Used extensively for enzyme studies in neuropathology
- Little shrinkage of tissue

Disadvantages

- Lacks precise morphological detail
- Presents a potential biohazard

Fixation by Perfusion

- *Brain*: Adequate preautopsy intra-arterial embalming is done. Formol saline is perfused for 2 weeks via the middle cerebral arteries. Distortion is prevented by suspending the brain in the fluid by a thread. The brain can then be sliced at 1–2 cm interval after fixation.
- *Lungs*: Inflation with 4% buffered formaldehyde through main bronchi for 1 week, then fixed in neutral buffered formalin as usual.

Special Fixation Procedures for Specific Organs

Most laboratories use 10% formalin as a routine fixative though 10% buffered neutral formalin is ideal. In instances where 10% formalin is routinely used it is a must that small needle biopsies be given special attention for fixation. Outlined below are the tissues that should be fixed as mentioned here.

- *Renal biopsies are sent as multiple cores each for a specific purpose*:
  - Immunofluorescence: Fix the biopsy with the help of OCT medium in the cryostat
  - For electron microscopy: Fix in 2–3% glutaraldehyde
  - For paraffin section: 10% neutral buffered formalin
- *Endoscopic small biopsies of esophagus and intestine (2–3 mm)*: 10% neutral buffered formalin
- *Liver biopsies*: Core biopsy—one core in 10% neutral buffered formalin; second core in 95% or absolute alcohol fixative (alcohol preserves the glycogen)
- *Lymphoid tissue*: Fix in 10% neutral buffered formalin or B5 fixative
- *Muscle*:
  - Small biopsies: Fix in 10% neutral buffered formalin
  - For enzyme studies—frozen, for histochemistry in liquid nitrogen
- *Testicular cores*: 10% neutral buffered formalin, Bouin's fluid or Helly's solution gives good nuclear details to assess spermatogenesis.
- Zenker's and Helly's fixatives, which contain potassium dichromate and mercuric chloride, have also traditionally been used for testis fixation, but they also suffer from significant safety and disposal problems.
- The general trend to use Bouin's fixative as a routine fixative for the testis has certainly improved the general quality of cellular preservation and the resolution of cellular detail, but it presents a number of problems. The presence of picric acid in the fixative however results in safety hazards and disposal problems, requires numerous alcohol rinses for removal before staining, and also results in staining of the working surfaces.
- It has been recently demonstrated that modified Davidson's fluid[5] (*see* **Appendix 1**) provides better preservation of the testes to that of Bouin's fluid, both for routine histology (causes less shrinkage of the seminiferous tubules and superior overall morphologic detail) and IHC staining of testicular antigens in detecting androgen receptor; specific antigenic markers for Sertoli cells, Leydig cells, proliferating cell nuclear antigen, protein gene product 9.5, etc.

- *Endometrium and small biopsies cervix*: 10% neutral buffered formol saline
- *Eyes*:
    - Fixed in the lower compartment of the refrigerator (2–8°C) for 48 hours after the optic nerve is removed. To speed up the fixation, one or two windows are made into the globe after 24 hours.
    - *Davidson's fluid*[6] **(*see Appendix 1*)** is used routinely for the fixation of ocular tissues in several centers. After fixation for 24 hours, tissues should be transferred to neutral buffered formalin for storage.
        - Disadvantage: The odor changes with age as esterification occurs; produces a characteristic odor of ethyl acetate.
- *Bone*: All tissue samples of bone, biopsies, curettings, and resections should be fixed in 10% buffered neutral formalin for up to 5 days. Resections should be sliced into half in the midline longitudinal plane and wrapped in gauze and immersed in a bucket filled with fixative. **Figure 2** shows the types of bone (spongy and cancellous) in resections or amputation.
    - *Cancellous or spongy bone* is found in the epiphyseal region, medullary cavity in diaphysis of long bones **(Fig. 2)**, vertebra, and marrow cavities.
    - *Cortical or outer compact bone*, which is solid and hard, is found in the shaft of long bones (e.g., femur, tibia, and humerus) and external surface of the flat bones (e.g., skull).
        - Cortical bone takes longer to fix and should be immersed in double strength formalin (formaldehyde 37–40%... 20 mL; distilled water.... 80 mL; sodium phosphate monobasic... 4.0 g; and sodium phosphate dibasic 6.5 g).

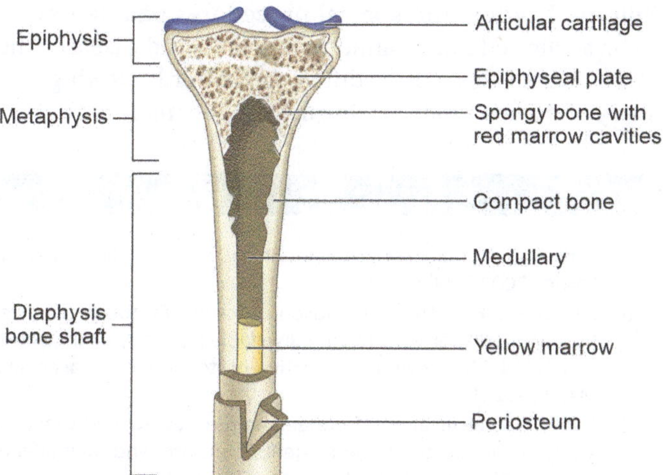

FIG. 2: Shows location of spongy and cancellous bone.

    - All fixed specimens from biopsies and curettings of bone are washed in gently running tap water for 30 minutes. Larger specimens for a period of 1 hour. Further cuts into resections may be made and smaller representative bits taken to fit the tissue cassettes. These bits should be taken from the lesional tissue. The bone is now taken for decalcification before processing.
        - *Decalcification is removal of calcium salts from the bone without altering its cellular structure,* so that the microtome knife can section the tissue easily. Therefore, removal of calcium of bone to enable sectioning by a microtome is the basic principle behind decalcification. This should be achieved without compromising tissue morphology and enabling good stain penetration so that a reasonably accurate diagnosis can be achieved.
        - In most laboratories, decalcification is done using acid solutions:[7]
            - Strong inorganic acids: The most commonly used is nitric acid (5–10%), 3% HCl, Perenyi's fluid, and formalin nitric acid are the other solutions used.
            - The length of time for decalcification is from 24 hours to 2–3 days. Fresh solutions of nitric acid are optimal for usage. It decalcifies heavily mineralized bone.
            - Overdecalcification results in poor nuclear stain and a tendency to destroy antigens and enzymes which may not be demonstrable after the procedure.
            - Decalcification progress should be monitored carefully by a decalcifying endpoint test, i.e., bubble test (see bubble test later).
                - Formic acid:
                    - 8% HCl stock solution:
                        - HCl, concentrated: 80 mL
                        - Distilled water: 920 mL
                    - 8% formic solution:
                        - Formic acid: 80 mL
                        - Distilled water: 920 mL
                    - Hydrochloric acid/formic acid working solution
                    - Combine equal parts of the 8% HCl and 8% formic acid solution.
                - Perenyi's fluid:
                    - 10% nitric acid: 40 mL
                    - Absolute ethanol: 30 mL
                    - 0.5% chromic acid: 30 mL
            - This fluid is slow in action but a good decalcifier for small amounts of calcium.

In addition, it is also used as a softening agent prior to dehydration for dense fibrous tissue. The cellular details are well-preserved and hence subsequent staining is good.

- The disadvantage is that it is slow for decalcifying dense bone and the endpoint of decalcification is difficult to detect.
- Procedure:
  - Specimen should be decalcified in the acid solution 20 times their volume.
  - Change to fresh solution each day until decalcification is complete.
  - Wash specimens thoroughly after this for 1 hour.
  - Specimens should not be crowded in the container. Overdecalcification can damage the specimen, therefore, monitoring by checking for the endpoint is essential.

Endpoint of Decalcification

It is checked for by the following methods:

- Specimen radiograph
- Chemical testing
- Physical testing (less accurate and potentially damages the tissue)

Specimen Radiographs

- *X-ray examination*: It is the most sensitive test for detection of calcium in the bone or tissues as areas of mineralization and tiny calcifications can be easily identified.
- *Chemical test*: It is a simple and a reliable method.

The following solutions are needed to chemically test for residual calcium:

- *5% ammonium hydroxide stock*:
  - Ammonium hydroxide (28%): 5 mL
  - Distilled water: 95 mL
- *5% ammonium oxalate stock*:
  - Ammonium oxalate: 5 mL
  - Distilled water: 95 mL

  Mix equal parts of solution A and solution B.

Procedure

- Insert a pipette into the decalcifying solution containing the specimen.
- Withdraw approximately 5 mL of the decalcifying solution from the specimen and place it in a test tube. Add a piece of litmus paper.
- Add about 5–10 mL of the ammonium hydroxide/oxalate working solution, mix well and allow to stand overnight. Repeat the test every 2–3 days.
- If a precipitate forms, calcium is present, and therefore, decalcification needs to be continued.
- Decalcification is complete when no precipitate is observed on 2 consecutive days of testing.
- Once decalcification is complete, the cassette containing the decalcified tissue is neutralized, washed well in running tap water, and then processed as a paraffin block.

Bubble test: It can be used as a guide to check the progress of decalcification. On adding a strong acid, gas bubbles form on the bone surface as calcium carbonate combines with acid to form carbon dioxide. If the level of calcium carbonate is reduced, the bubbles will not form.

Physical tests: A physical test is done by inserting a sharp instrument such as a razor or scalpel blade and is a rough estimate for checking removal of calcium. However, the disadvantage is occurrence of artificial tears.

CONCLUSION

Routine fixation and special procedures enable tissues to be sectioned and examined in health and disease. The more refined these procedures, the better is viewing and study of tissues, enabling diagnoses to be made.

REFERENCES

1. Culling CF Handbook of Histopathological and Histochemical Techniques, 3rd edition, 1976. Boston, London: Butterworth-Heinemann; 1974.
2. Lynch MJ, Raphael SS. Lynch's Medical Laboratory Technology, 3rd edition. Philadelphia: WB Saunders Company; 1976.
3. Bancroft JD, Gamble M. Theory and Practice of Histological Techniques, 5th edition. London: Churchill Livingstone; 2002.
4. Elghetany MT, Saleem A. Methods for staining amyloid in tissues: a review. Stain Technol. 1988;63(4):201-12.
5. Latendresse JR, Warbrittion AR, Jonassen H, Creasy DM. Fixation of testes and eyes using a modified Davidson's fluid: comparison with Bouin's fluid and conventional Davidson's fluid. Toxicol Pathol. 2002;30(4):524-33.
6. Richmond RS. (1997). Davidson's Fixative Protocol. Science, Products, and Services. [online] Available from https://ihcworld.com/2024/01/25/davidsons-fixative-protocol/[Last accessed March, 2024].
7. Gyle C. Decalcification of bone: literature review and practical study of various decalcifying agents. Methods, and their effects on bone histology. J Histology. 1998;21:49-58.

CHAPTER 16

Processing of Tissues

INTRODUCTION

Processing of tissue is essential in order to make the tissue amenable to section cutting, at the same time retaining its morphology. The salient steps in tissue processing are dehydration, clearing, and infiltration. These steps follow one another and remove all extractable water from the tissue specimens and replace it with a medium such as paraffin wax that solidifies to permit sectioning.

METHOD

Tissue sampling for processing is done in such a way as to be representative of the abnormal lesions seen at grossing. Tissue blocks for processing should be thin, usually 1–2 mm for urgent processing of specimens and 3–4 mm for routine specimens to be processed on an overnight schedule.[1,2] Cassettes in any container should not be packed, so as to allow free passage of fluids to and fro into cassettes for adequate penetration.

Small specimens and tissue fragments, e.g., endometrial biopsies and endoscopic biopsies are wrapped in lens tissue paper before placing them in fenestrated cassettes for processing. The tissues are transferred from reagent to reagent in tissue processing cassettes and a step-by-step processing process occurs which ensures dehydration, clearing, infiltration and embedding.[1-5] The cassettes are metal or plastic containers with perforations. The cassette should include the accession number of the bit marked by soft lead pencil or waterproof ink or computer generated bar code label. All specimens should be adequately fixed before processing.

DEHYDRATION

Alcohols, ethyl or isopropyl, are the usual choice for dehydration. Isopropyl alcohol is cheaper and more easily available; though results are better with ethyl alcohol. Use of alcohol from lower to a higher grade (70–95 to 100%) is the standard norm in dehydration. The volume of a dehydrating agent in each stage should be at least 10 times the volume of tissue to be dehydrated.

Butyl alcohol (Butanol) is slow in action thereby requiring a longer time for immersion. Automatic tissue processors enhance the processing of tissue by application of heat, vacuum, and agitation. Automatic processors also allow stages of sequential processing to be carried out overnight when programmed. Programming can be done for any number of hours to suit convenience, once optimal time requirements are met with—whether for short or overnight long cycles. Tissues may be held and stored indefinitely in 70–80% ethanol without harm.

Duration of dehydration should be kept to the minimum; consistent with the thickness of tissues. Tissue blocks 1 mm thick should receive up to 30 minutes in each alcohol; blocks 4–5 mm thick require up to 90 minutes or longer in each change.

Anhydrous copper sulfate acts as both a dehydrating agent and as an indicator of water content in the last bath of 100% ethanol. A 1–2 cm of anhydrous copper sulfate is layered at the bottom of the bath and covered with filter paper. Anhydrous copper sulfate turns blue if water is present.

Other dehydrants are *acetone and phenol.* Phenol is also a softening agent for tissues, like nail, keratin, etc.

CLEARING

Clearing is replacing the dehydrant with a substance that is miscible with the embedding medium (paraffin) with which the tissue must be impregnated. *The essential requirement of clearing agent is that it should be miscible with both dehydrating agents and impregnating agents.* The clearing agents have the same refractive index as tissues, as a result, when the anhydrous tissue is completely infiltrated with the clearing agent, it becomes translucent and this translucency ascertains the endpoint of clearing.

Xylene is the most commonly used clearing agent in routine paraffin embedding. Xylene clears rapidly and the tissues are rendered transparent. Long-term immersion of tissue in xylene results in tissue distortion; tissues should not be left in it for >3 hours. Prolonged exposure causes the tissue to become brittle and difficult to section. Other clearing reagents *are toluene, chloroform, esters, terpenes, butyl acetate, etc.*

The volume of clearing agent is optimally 30–40 times the volume of the tissue and should not be <10 times. The smaller pieces of tissue are cleared in 30 minutes to 1 hour whereas larger tissues (≥5 mm thick) are cleared in 2–4 hours.

The boiling point of the clearing agent gives an indication of its speed of replacement by the "infiltrating" paraffin wax. Fluids with low boiling point are easily replaced.

INFILTRATION (IMPREGNATION IN WAX) AND EMBEDDING

Impregnation is the process by which the clearing agent is replaced by paraffin wax or its substitute that completely fills all the tissue cavities. This gives a firm consistency which holds the specimen and allows easy handling and cutting of thin sections without any damage to its cellular constituents.

Infiltration is done at the melting point of the wax in use, i.e., 54–64°C, in case of paraffin wax. The volume of the wax should be 25–30 times the volume of the tissue.

Ideally, an infiltrating and embedding medium should be soluble in the processing fluids, suitable for sectioning and ribboning, capable of producing flat section ribbons, molten between 30° and 60°C, translucent and colorless at its melting point, and nontoxic and easy to handle.

Types of Waxes

Paraffin wax: Paraffin wax is a polycrystalline mixture of solid hydrocarbons produced during the refining of coal and mineral oils. It is colorless, or white, partly translucent, odorless and has a wide range of melting points, from 56–64°C. Tissue-wax adhesion depends upon the crystal morphology, and small, uniform-sized crystals provide better physical support for specimens through close packing. Crystalline structure of paraffin wax can be altered by incorporating additives which result in a less brittle, more homogeneous wax with good cutting characteristics. There is consequently less deformation during sectioning. Paraffin wax is routinely used as an impregnating and embedding media. It is cheap, safe, and immiscible with water, provides quality sectioning and is easily adaptable. Tissue blocks can be stored in paraffin wax for a long time without tissue destruction. Low melting point paraffin wax is soft and used for delicate tissues such as fetal and areolar tissues while higher melting point paraffin wax is hard and used for hard fibrous tissues.

If tissues are processed by hand they will require a total of 4–6 hours in three changes of wax whereas with agitation 2–4 hours in two baths will suffice. Following impregnation tissues are embedded in a wax block; this is called *"blocking"* which enables section cutting on a microtome.

Paraplast is a modified paraffin wax; a mixture of highly purified paraffin waxes containing plastic polymers. As a result, it has a greater degree of elasticity and provides excellent tissue infiltration and superior quality, wrinkle free sectioning at 4 μ thickness.

Ester waxes have low melting points (48°C), being hard at room temperature with good adhesive properties. Ester wax is less likely to crumble when cutting hard tissues. It gives good ribbons while sectioning and has good glass adhesion properties.

Water-soluble waxes and polyethylene glycols (PEG) (Carbowax) are media which overcome tissue shrinkage, damage, and distortion inherent in the paraffin wax techniques. In general, they are less elastic, denser, and somewhat harder than paraffin wax.

Advantages of PEG are that it eliminates dehydration and clearing; hence, lipids and neutral lipids are not removed and can be demonstrated in sections; the processing time is reduced; reduces shrinkage and distortion.

Disadvantages of PEG are that they are difficult to flatten without loss of tissue and adhere poorly to slides; solubility in water does not allow sections to float on water.

Short Schedule of Processing Small Biopsies (Total Time: 3–4 Hours)

Minimum fixation time: 3 hours

- Rinse briefly in running water
- Hold if necessary in 80% alcohol

- 95% alcohol, three changes, 15–20 minutes each
- Absolute alcohol, three changes, 15 minutes each
- Equal parts absolute alcohol and xylene, 15 minutes
- Xylene, two changes, 15 minutes each
- Paraffin, three changes, 15 minutes each
- Paraffin under vacuum, 15–20 minutes
- Embed (AFIP, 1994)[4]

Overnight Schedule (for Routine Specimens Using an Automatic Tissue Processor)

Total processing time: 14–16 hours (after adequate fixation)[4]

- 80% alcohol, 1 hour
- 95% alcohol, three changes, 1 hour each
- Absolute alcohol, three changes, 1 hour each
- Xylene, three changes, 1 hour each
- Paraffin, three changes, 1 hour each
- Paraffin under vacuum, 1 hour
- Embed

There are two broad principles of automatic tissue processing—(1) tissue transfer and (2) fluid transfer techniques.

Tissue Transfer Processors

These processors are characterized by the transfer of tissue in cassettes, contained within a metal basket, through a series of stationary reagents arranged in a circular carousel or linear fashion **(Fig. 1)**.[3]

The carousel pattern is the most common model of automatic tissue processing. It is provided with 9–10 reagent baskets and 2–3 wax container positions, each with a capacity for 30–110 cassettes depending upon the model. Fluid agitation is achieved by an oscillatory movement of the tissue basket. Processing schedules are card punched.

Fluid Transfer Processors

In fluid-transfer units, the tissues cassettes remain stationary and processing fluids (from the respective reagent stations) are pumped to and from the stationary container with a tube system.[3] There is a provision for agitation, temperature adjustment, and vacuum pressure in each station. Depending upon the model, these machines can process up to 300 cassettes at any one time. Schedules are microprocessor programmed and controlled.

Vacuum-pressure cycles coupled with heated reagents facilitate effective reduction in processing time as well as improved infiltration of dense tissues.

Manual Tissue Processing

It is undertaken when there is power failure or breakdown of a tissue processor, rapid processing of an urgent specimen, delicate material, hard dense tissues, special diagnostic, teaching or research applications, and small-scale processing requirements.

The main advantage of manual processing over automated methods lies in the flexibility of reagent selection.

Microwave-stimulated Processing

Rapid manual microwave-stimulated paraffin wax processing of small batches of tissues gives excellent results which are comparable to tissues processed by longer automated nonmicrowave methods. Processing is undertaken in a dedicated microwave oven. The main

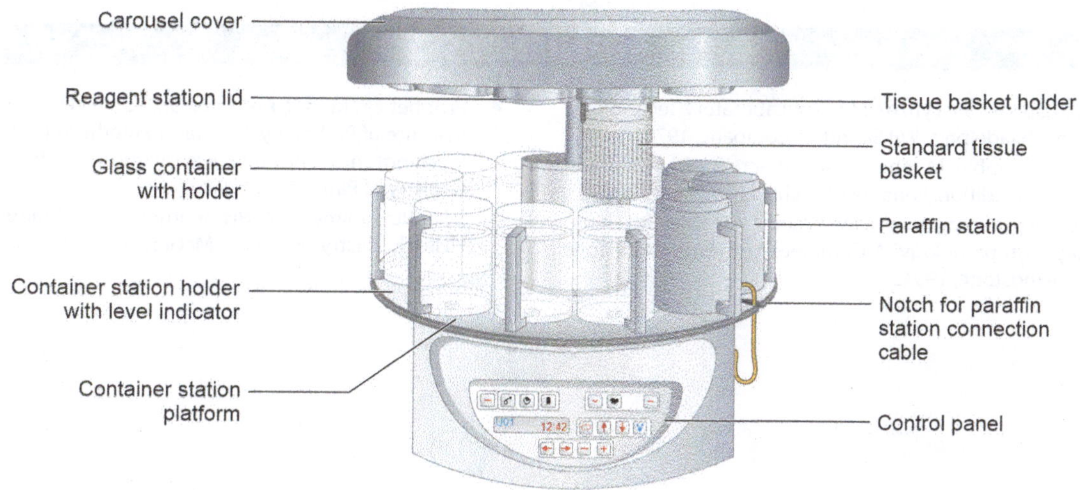

FIG. 1: Automatic tissue transfer processor.

advantage being for rapid results as in renal transplant biopsies.

Processing of Tissues for Electron Microscopy

- The standard protocol for processing of tissues for transmission electron microscopy (TEM), and electron microscopy (EM) involves primary fixation in an aldehyde (usually glutaraldehyde).
- Small 1 mm^3 bits of tissue are fixed in 2.5–3% glutaraldehyde in 0.2M Sorensen's sodium phosphate buffer. EM grade 8% glutaraldehyde available commercially is purchased in 10 mL vials and stored in the refrigerator at 4–5°C
- Postfixation in 1% osmium tetraoxide in sodium phosphate buffer (prepare under hood as vapors are toxic).
- For TEM processing, dehydration is performed by passing the specimen through increasing concentration of an organic solvent, e.g., ethanol.
- Commercially available absolute alcohol contains a small percentage of water which severely restricts infiltration and polymerization of the resin used for infiltration. Hence, it is necessary to complete dehydration in anhydrous alcohol. Ethanol also requires the use of propylene oxide (1,2-epoxypropane) as a transition solvent to facilitate resin infiltration. Propylene oxide is highly volatile, flammable, and forms explosive peroxides and should be stored at room temperature in a flammable solvent facility.
- *Embedding:* The step, following dehydration, is to infiltrate the tissue sample with liquid resin. In routine TEM, synthetic embedding resins are used that are capable of withstanding the vacuum in the electron microscope column and the heat generated as the electrons pass through the section. This requires gradual introduction of the epoxy resin used for infiltration and embedding, beginning with 50:50 mix of transition solvent (propylene oxide) and resin.

Standard Manual EM Processing Schedule for Solid Tissues Cut into 1 mm Block (At Room Temperature) (AFIP, 1994)[5]

- Working phosphate buffer, three changes, 15 minutes each
- Osmium tetraoxide, 1.0% phosphate buffered, 1 hour
- Distilled water, four changes, 5 minutes each
- Uranyl acetate, 1% aqueous, 1 hour (staining)
- 50% ethyl alcohol, 15 minutes
- 75% ethyl alcohol, 15 minutes
- 95% ethyl alcohol, 15 minutes
- 100% (absolute) ethyl alcohol, four changes, 15 minutes each
- Equal parts, 100% ethyl alcohol and propylene oxide, 15 minutes
- Propylene oxide, four changes, 15 minutes each
- Equal parts propylene oxide and epoxyresin, 1 hour
- Epoxy resin, three changes, 1 hour each
- Epoxy resin, 2 hours
- Embed

Use hood when using osmium tetraoxide and propylene oxide.

CONCLUSION

Processing of tissues enables the conversion of fixed tissue into firm material infiltrated with wax thereby enabling its embedding for section cutting. An ideal well-processed tissue is the result of the technician's skill in infiltration and embedding.

REFERENCES

1. Lynch MJ, Raphael SS. Lynch's Medical Laboratory Technology, 3rd edition. Philadelphia: WB Saunders Company; 1976.
2. Bancroft JD, Gamble M. Theory and Practice of Histological Techniques, 5th edition. London: Churchill Livingstone; 2002.
3. Winsor L. Tissue processing. In: Woods AE, Ellis RC (Eds). Laboratory Histopathology: A Complete Reference. New York: Churchill Livingstone; 1994.
4. Prophet EB, Mills B, Arrington JB, Sobin LH (Eds). Armed Forces Institute of Pathology: Laboratory Methods in Histotechnology. Washington DC: Armed Forces Institute of Pathology, American Registry of Pathology; 1994.
5. Lillie RD, Fullmer HM. Histopathologic Technique and Practical Histochemistry. New York: McGraw-Hill; 1976. p. 31.

CHAPTER 17

Embedding

INTRODUCTION

Embedding is the process of surrounding the tissue with a firm substance to hold it in order to enable sectioning. The substance to embed tissue is the same as the one used for infiltration, i.e., paraffin as in paraffin wax embedding. It is the most common medium for embedding, and once having filled all the cavities and spaces in the tissue during infiltration, it will hold it firmly as a block after embedding. Other embedding media are celloidin, ester wax, and water-soluble waxes such as polyethylene glycols.

PARAFFIN EMBEDDING[1-4]

- Soft paraffins have a melting point of about 45°C and are best for tissue such as fetal and areolar connective tissue, hard paraffins have a melting point of 60°C and are used for hard fibrous and bone. Since it is not practical to separate out tissues for hard and soft paraffin routinely; paraffin wax with a melting point of 56°C is recommended for all tissues.
- Specimen orientation is important while placing tissue in cassettes for embedding.
  It is necessary for the technician to know that certain anatomical structures should be placed with specifications while embedding.
- Generally, all tissue bits are placed with the cutting surface flat and face down in the mold **(Fig. 1)**.
- Tubular structures—appendix, vas deferens, fallopian tubes, etc. must be placed so that the knife cuts through the lumen, perpendicular to the long axis **(Fig. 2)**.
- Skin and other epithelium, like intestine, urinary bladder, etc. should be so placed that the section passes through the epithelium as well as subepithelial tissue **(Fig. 3)**. Multiple small bits should be placed such that the epithelium faces the same direction and is in line in all bits.
- Multiple small fragments should be placed one next to the other **(Fig. 4)** and not one above the other.
- Cysts should be embedded with the cut surface down **(Fig. 5)**.

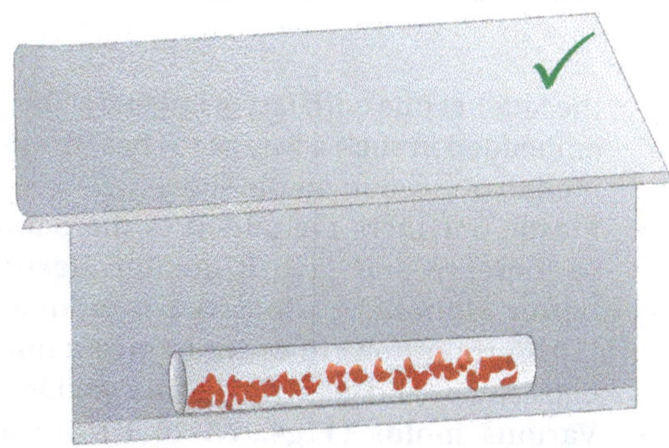

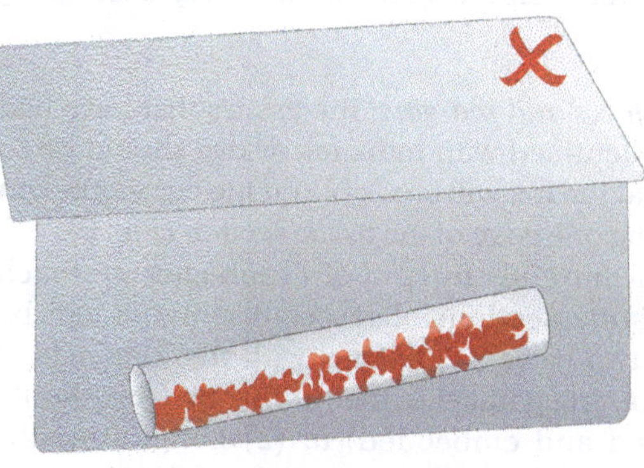

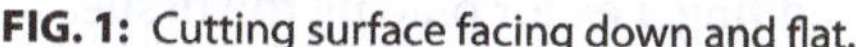

FIG. 1: Cutting surface facing down and flat.

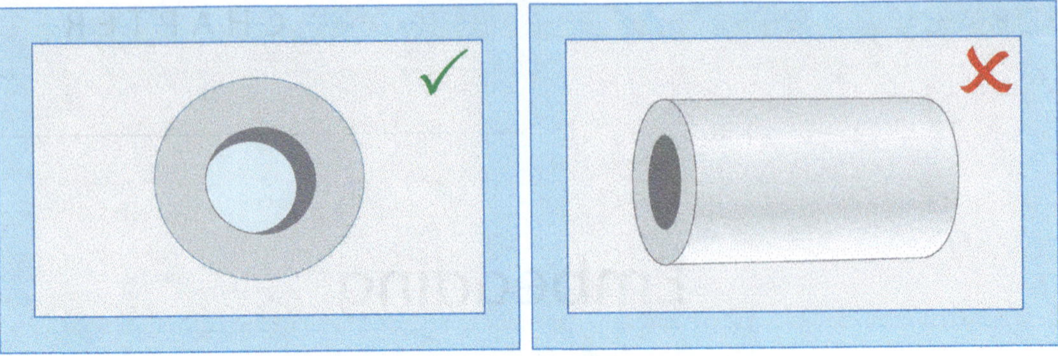

FIG. 2: Tubular structures are placed cut section of lumen facing down.

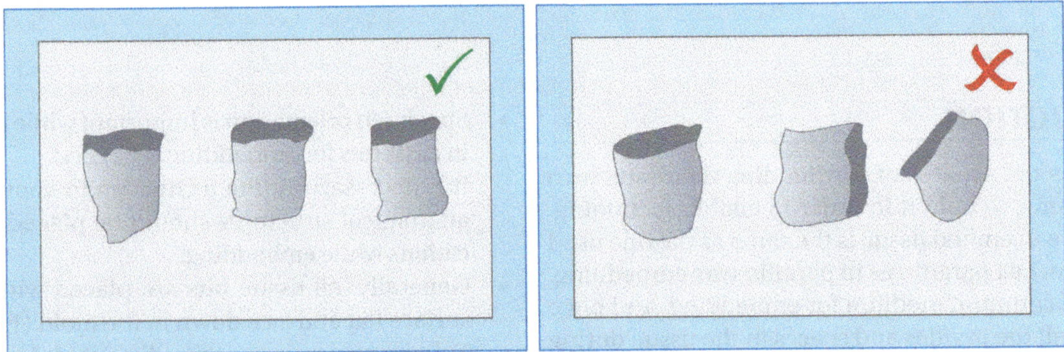

FIG. 3: Epithelia of all bits are in line with each other to facilitate cutting.

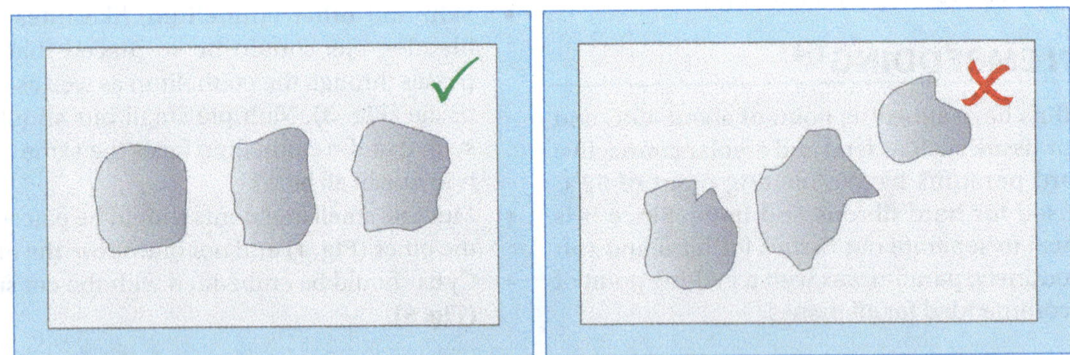

FIG. 4: Each bit should have its cutting surface facing down and not be placed at various levels.

- *Inked surfaces and margins*: The tissues that have had margins identified with India ink or dye should be so placed that the ink will be visible on the cut section on slide, lining one edge of the tissue section **(Fig. 6)**.
- *Resection margins*: In case of esophagus, stomach and intestine sections of resected margins can be taken in two ways: (1) Enface, with the long axis of the bit running parallel to the cut margin (this should be marked and embedded) or (2) Longitudinally, i.e., perpendicular to the cut margin of the intestine. Marking with India ink should be done accordingly (in the latter at one end, i.e., at cut end). The bit should be embedded in such a way as to show the marking of the margin on section on the slide.
- Plastic polymers are added to the paraffin in order to increase and give it greater elasticity. It gives better ribboning. Beeswax is added to paraffin (10% proportion) in order to give a uniform cutting consistency and get wrinkle-free sections.
- Various molds **(Figs. 7A to E)** are available for embedding, i.e., for placing the tissues as stated above within the mold with the cutting surface down and

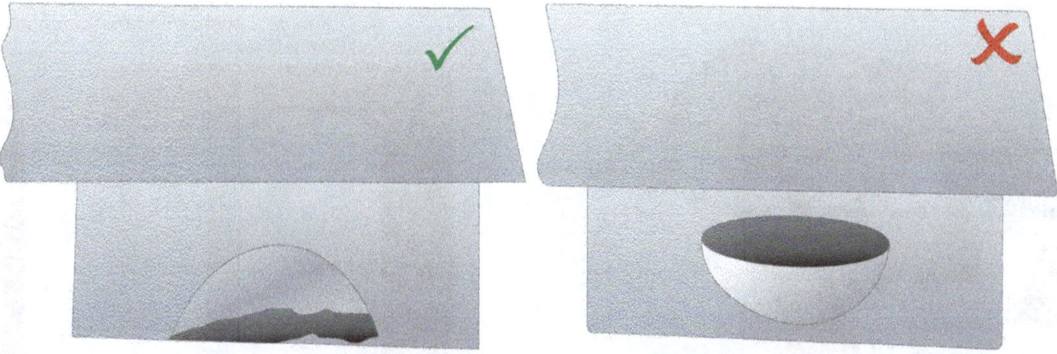

FIG. 5: The cut surface of a cyst should be placed facing down.

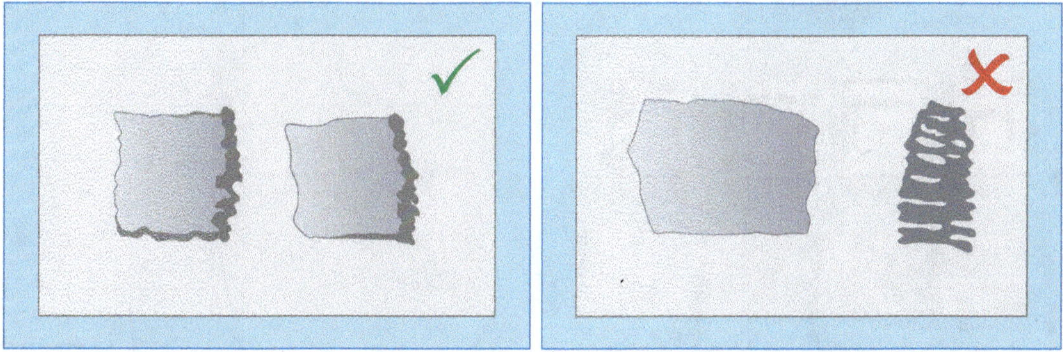

FIG. 6: The marked resection margin should be on one aspect of the bit, so that it appears on the section taken.

pouring liquid paraffin which solidifies in the shape of the mold.

- *Leuckart irons* ***(Fig. 7A)***: These are sturdy, most popularly used and conventional method of blocking. They consist of two L-shaped pieces of heavy brass or metal placed on a base being formed of copper or brass or glass plate. Glycerine is applied to the L pieces and also to the metal or glass plate on which molds are arranged before pouring the molten wax. The tissue is then embedded within the molten wax with proper orientation and labeling. After cooling, the molds are removed resulting in wax cakes.
- *Embedding centers* are machines usually equipped with paraffin dispenser, specimen holding tank, warm plate for specimen orientation in melted paraffin, and a cold plate for transforming the melted paraffin into a solid block with specimen within. These are available as one unit.
- *Multiblock embedding units* allow numerous blocks to be embedded using only one unit and has facility to embed small as well as large blocks.

Technique of Paraffin Embedding

- After infiltration is complete and the tissue ready for embedding the tissue cassette is opened, and the piece of tissue to be embedded taken.
- A mold is selected to match the size of the specimen; there should be sufficient room for the tissue with at least a 2 mm of wax surrounding the tissue.
- The mold is filled with molten paraffin wax. Ovens are available which are sufficiently large to accommodate an enamel jug with a funnel inserted in it for filtering paraffin wax.
- If wax is not filtered, the impurities present may interfere with section cutting. The ovens used for wax embedding should have a temperature ranging from 50 to 65°C, about 5°C more than that of the molten wax.
- Place the selected tissue firmly into the wax with a warmed forceps, flat, cutting surface facing down, with the accession number of the tissue bit.
- Cool the block on the cold plate, a layer of wax forms at the bottom of the mold. Check for specimen orientation.
- Remove the block from the mold.

ALTERNATIVE EMBEDDING MEDIA TO PARAFFIN[1-4]

Alternative embedding media may provide optimum support for tissues where paraffin waxes are unsuited in heat labile tissue, dense, or hard tissue which may not

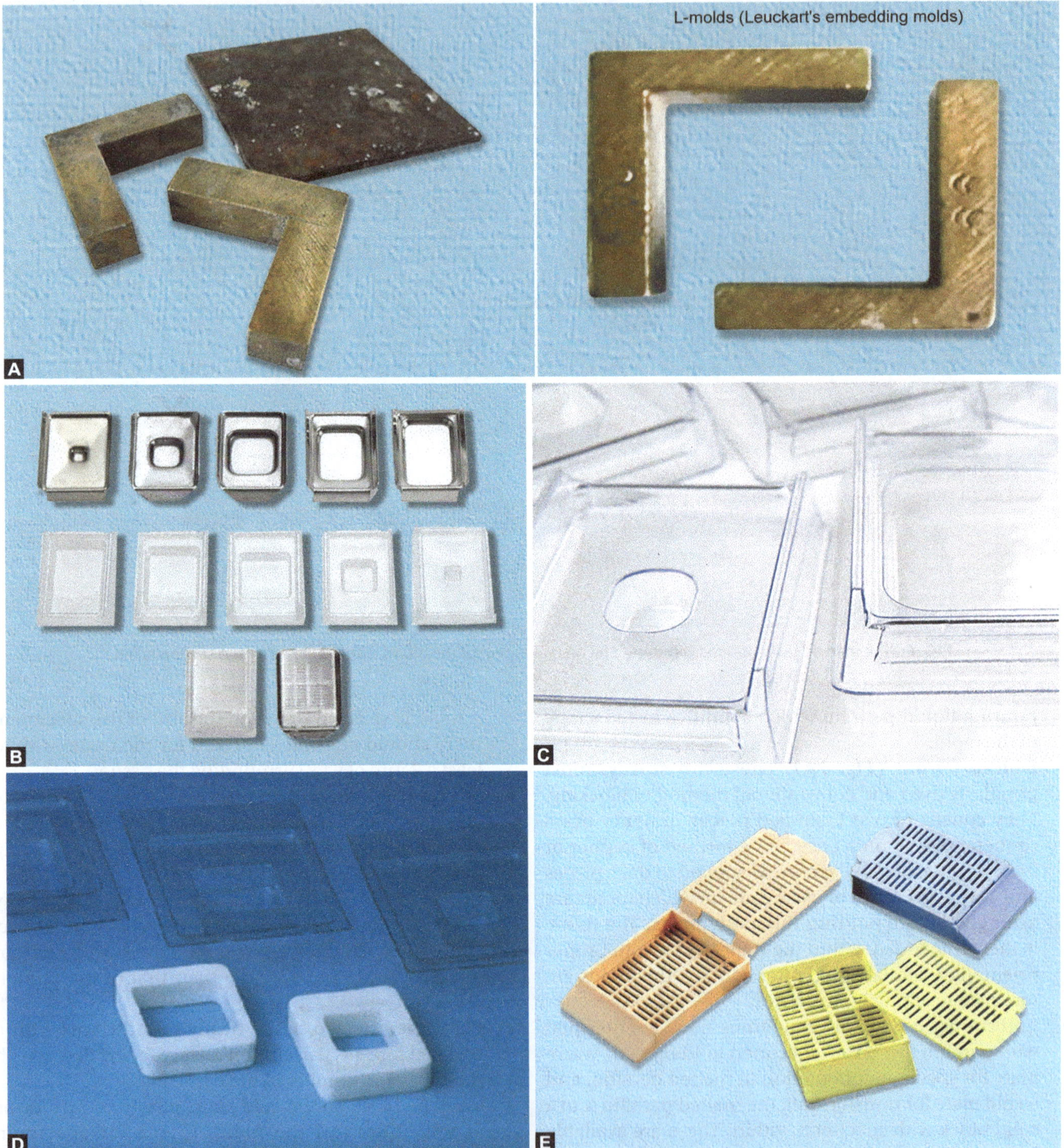

FIGS. 7A TO E: Various molds for embedding of tissues. (A) Stainless steel molds—Leuckart or Dimmock embedding irons, are widely used steel molds; (B to D) steel and plastic molds—nondisposable and disposable; and (E) fenestrated plastic embedding capsules.

have adequate paraffin support, when very thin sections are needed and in whole-organ sectioning of brain or lung.

Types of alternative embedding media are aqueous media, such as agar, gelatin, resin, and celloidin.

- *Agar* is generally used as a double embedding media. The high melting point and low gelling temperature of agar make it ideal for double embedding multiple small tissue fragments.

Agar gel by itself does not provide sufficient support for sectioning the tissue; its main use is in acting as a cohesive agent for small friable pieces of tissue before embedding with paraffin wax.

- *Gelatin* is generally used for whole-organ embedding media and gelatin embedding supports large tissue blocks for sectioning. The low melting point of gelatin (35–40°C) makes it unsuitable for double embedding.
- *Plastic (resin)* finds its utility as an embedding media in electron microscopy but small amounts can be added to paraffin for greater elasticity. The plastic media is a pale liquid media and it polymerizes to a solid during blocking. Resins are readily available, inexpensive, easy to handle, of low viscosity and allow short infiltration times.

  Plastics are classified according to their chemical composition:
  - Acrylic media: Butyl methacrylate and glycol methacrylate—the principle use of methacrylate monomers is its ability to polymerize in the presence of a catalyst, like heat, ultraviolet light or artificial catalysts like benzoyl peroxide (1.5–2.0%) which results in rapid transformation to solids. Methacrylate is readily miscible in ethanol and gives a clear hard block for sectioning. Methacrylate rapidly infiltrates, dehydrates tissue at room temperature, but damages it during polymerization because of marked shrinkage artifact. However, mixes of plastics are devised to overcome these deficiencies. These resins are more suited to hold hard materials such as decalcified bone.
  - Epoxy resin (Araldite): It is a substance which is capable of polymerization to form an irreversible and insoluble three dimensional structure with cross-linking between molecular chains. Its advantages are maintaining the true geometry of the tissue which lends itself to higher resolution work and causes less shrinkage. Long infiltration time is required as the resin has a higher viscosity as compared to methacrylate.
  - Polyester resin: It has the same cutting consistency as that of methacrylate but cutting on long stored blocks becomes difficult, e.g., Vestopal. It is rarely used for microscopy and superseded by other epoxides.
  - Celloidin: It is the purified form of nitrocellulose obtained by treating cellulose with sulfuric and nitric acid. It is supplied as pulpy, cotton-like material and is referred to as gun cotton. In the past, celloidin was used in place of paraffin, as a good support to hard tissues such as bone, uterus as well as for delicate specimens such as eyes, central nervous system tissues, and embryonic tissues. Cellulose does not require heat at any stage of processing and is recommended for and embedding tissues that can be damaged by solutions requiring heat. The working strength is 2%, 4%, and 8%, the solvent being equal parts of ether and alcohol. The advantages are it causes less shrinkage and hardening of the tissues than paraffin because there is no heat involved in the process. Tissues of mixed consistency can be embedded. The relationship of tissue components is well preserved, e.g., layers of the eye.

    The disadvantages are the procedure is time consuming, requiring 7–10 days to infiltrate the specimen. Celloidin attracts water, which prevents the solution from solidifying and causes the block to become too soft for sectioning. Tissues need to be fully dehydrated in absolute ethyl alcohol and treated for 24 hours in a mixture of ether-absolute alcohol before embedding. The block requires storing in 70–80% alcohol and the knife and block must be kept moist with 70–80% alcohol. It is also extremely difficult to obtain sections thinner than 10 μm. The cutting of serial sections of celloidin-impregnated tissue is difficult as ribbons are difficult to get.

    There are two methods of embedding in celloidin: (1) dry method and (2) wet method; the latter being more popular.
  - Low viscosity nitrocellulose (LVN): LVN has a lower molecular weight than celloidin but can be used instead of it. At 20% concentration in ethyl alcohol, it forms a solution.

    It is insoluble in water but soluble in most hydrocarbon solvents and forms a harder block than celloidin, thus permitting easy sectioning.
    - Sections have a tendency to crack when embedded in pure LVN; hence, a small amount of celloidin (1%) is added to give elasticity to the block or 95% alcohol as solvent instead of absolute alcohol.
    - The average time for impregnation is 6–11 days.
    - LVN is an explosive and not handled near fire places.

DOUBLE EMBEDDING AND DOUBLE INFILTRATION METHODS[1,2,4]

Double embedding is the process by which tissues are first fully impregnated by a supporting medium, such as agar, celloidin, or nitrocellulose, then infiltrated by another different media such as wax in which they are also embedded. The main use of this method is for cutting sections of delicate tissue and preparing sections from blocks of tissue of varying consistency, e.g., eyes wherein the retina can easily detach with single media embedding.

- *Agar-paraffin wax double embedding*: Double embedding in agar-paraffin is useful for minute and friable tissue fragments such as curettings and endoscopic biopsies, which could easily be lost during processing. It facilitates embedding and orientation of tissues. This method provides additional support to hard tissues and makes microtome sectioning easy.
  The fixative is passed through Millipore filter using suction so that the fragments collect on top of the filter in the filter tube. Molten agar is slowly poured onto the filter, allowed to solidify and then the excess agar is trimmed off. The agar block plus the filter paper is embedded in the paraffin wax. The filter paper provides no difficulty in sectioning the block.
- *Agar-ester wax double infiltration*: Double infiltration of tissues in agar and wax aids thin serial sectioning of the tissues at 0.5–1.0 μm. The fine crystalline nature and hardness of ester wax improves tissue-wax adhesion and provides adequate support for thin serial sectioning.
- *Nitrocellulose-paraffin wax double infiltration*: It combines the plasticity and support provided by nitrocellulose with convenient handling and sectioning. Methyl benzoate is used as a solvent for nitrocellulose. Tissues may be infiltrated with a thick nitrocellulose solution; the resulting block is hardened in chloroform or toluene and then embedded in paraffin wax.
  Sections of double-embedded tissues may tend to wrinkle or curl on the water bath. Floating on 95% ethanol facilitates section flattening.

CONCLUSION

In order to visualize tissue components, the tissue has to be held firmly in a medium which will enable section cutting and this purpose is served by the embedding media such as paraffin. Mixing paraffin with various waxes depending on the tissue to be embedded, and also using other synthetic media enables tissues of varied texture to be sectioned and examined for their microanatomical detail.

REFERENCES

1. Lynch MJ, Raphael SS. Lynch's Medical Laboratory Technology, 3rd edition. Philadelphia: WB Saunders Company; 1976.
2. Bancroft JD, Gamble M. Theory and Practice of Histological Techniques, 5th edition. London: Churchill Livingstone; 2002.
3. Prophet EB, Mills B, Arrington JB, Sobin LH (Eds). Armed Forces Institute of Pathology: Laboratory Methods in Histotechnology. Washington DC: Armed Forces Institute of Pathology, American Registry of Pathology; 1994.
4. Lillie RD, Fullmer HM. Histopathologic Technique and Practical Histochemistry. New York: McGraw-Hill; 1976. p. 31.

CHAPTER 18

Microtomes and Section Cutting

INTRODUCTION AND PRINCIPLE

The secret of microtomy lies mainly in acquiring personal skills to manipulate the microtome and this essentially proves true the phrase "practice makes perfection".

Microtomy is derived from the Greek words "mikros" meaning "small" and "temnein" meaning "to cut"; and is defined as sectioning of tissue with precision instruments designed for cutting it into sections thin enough for examination under the microscope.

The first microtome was invented by Cummings in 1770. Most instruments then were hand models and the first table model was introduced in 1840.

There are two different modes of operation in a microtome, first is where the microtome knife or cutting knife is movable and the block stationary. The second is knife being stationary and the block mobile. Modifications of these principles have resulted in different models.

- *With a movable knife (block stationary)*: The best example of this is the freezing microtome and the sliding microtome.
- *With a stationary knife (block moves)*: Here, the objects move along a vertical plane, e.g., rotary microtome, the most widely used microtome; and the rocking and sledge microtome, where the object holder moves around a horizontal axis.

TYPES OF MICROTOMES[1]

Rotary Microtome (Fig. 1)

The rotary microtome was invented by Minot in 1885–1886 in Germany and independently by Pfeiffer in 1886 in the United States.

It is the most commonly used microtome in the laboratories. The microtome is so named due to its action by a rotating handle having a rotating handle which moves 360°.

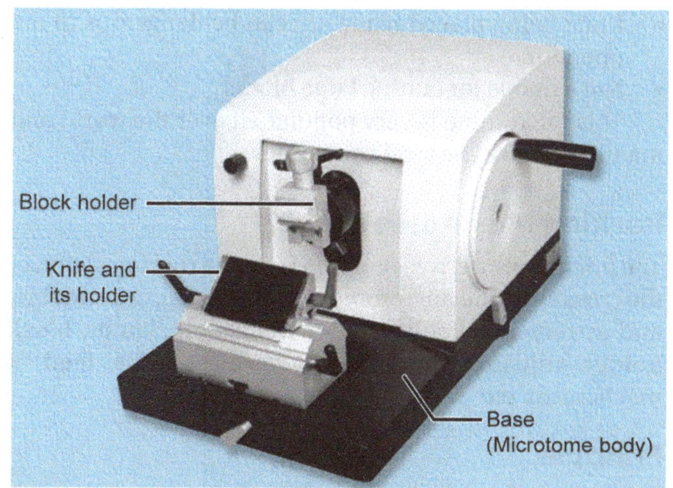

FIG. 1: Rotary microtome.

Principle

The rotary action of the hand-wheel (360°) advances the specimen and activates the cutting. During this rotation, it moves the block holder up and down advancing it across a static knife blade, thereby cutting the section. The specimen in the block holder moves vertically down through the cutting surface and returns to the starting position in one rotation; being advanced by a micrometer screw. The thickness of the sections is adjusted between 3 and 10 μ.

Manual, semiautomated, and automated models are available. A single motor operates the coarse and fine adjustments of the manual one; two motors, one for coarse and one for fine, operates the automated one. The autocut microtome (semiautomated) has a motor which can be operated and controlled. With suitable accessories, the machine can cut thin resin sections of 0.5–2.0 µm.

Advantages

- Stable (no vibrations) and easy to adapt to all types of tissues (hard, fragile, and fatty)
- Ability to cut thin (2–3 µm) sections
- Cutting angle and knife angle can be adjusted.
- Suitable for cutting small tissues embedded in paraffin wax and celloidin.
- Technological advances in the automation have improved the section quality, increased productivity, and occupational safety.

Disadvantages

- Complex design
- Initial cost relatively high
- Knife being placed blade up; can be dangerous to the operator.
- Not suitable for cutting large blocks

This microtome is very popular all over the world and manufactured by several companies.

Rocking Microtome (Fig. 2)

The microtome derives its name from the rocking action of the cross arm. The microtome is old in design, dependable, and extremely reliable. It has a knife with clamps, block holder, adjustment screws, operating handle, feed in mechanism, etc.

Principle

The knife is fixed and the block of tissue moves through an arc and strikes against the knife by means of a ratchet wheel operated micrometer screw thread. The turning of the ratchet wheel gives a forward push to the block which moves. Steady backward and forward movement of the handle gives good ribbons. Due to the arc-like movement, the sections are cut in a slightly in curved plane.

Advantages

- Excellent for serial sectioning (60–90 sections ribbons)
- Small blocks can be easily cut.
- The instrument is cheap, reliable, and easy to maintain.
- In emergency, it can be adapted for frozen sections after freezing the tissue.

Disadvantages

- Does not give flat sections because of the arc-like rocking movement
- It is light in weight, and cutting hard tissues results in vibrations.
- The blocks cannot be used with other microtomes due to the curved surface.

Rotary Rocking Microtome (Fig. 3)

It is slightly more robust than the rocking microtome and presents a flat surface of the tissue block. The tissue block is taken away from the knife in the upward stroke. It can be used for paraffin sections and has application in cryostats.

The Minot microtome, named after the inventor professor Minot, is a good example with a stationary knife and movable block and can be used for paraffin sectioning.

Advantages

Cuts flat sections.

Sliding Microtome (Fig. 4)

This type of microtome was first developed by Adams in 1798.

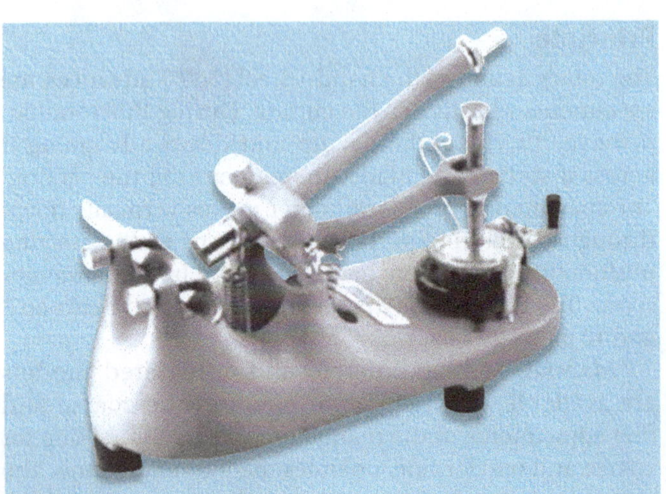

FIG. 2: Rocking microtome.

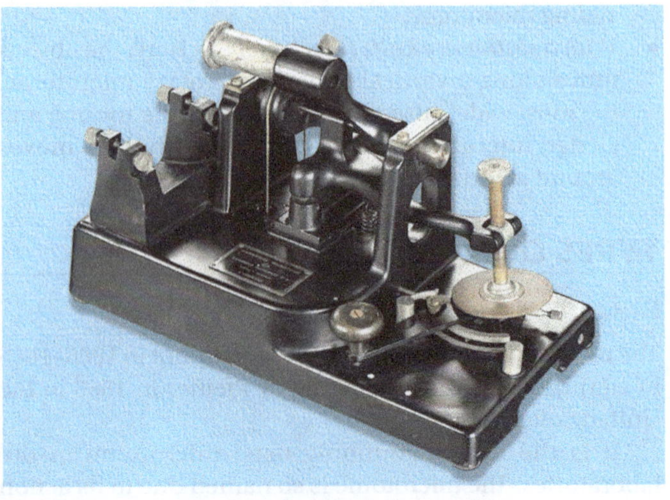

FIG. 3: Rotary rocking microtome.

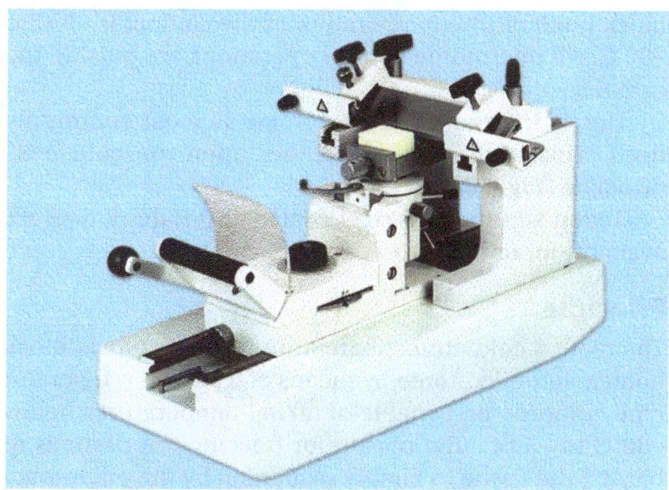

FIG. 4: Sliding microtome.

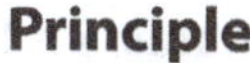

Principle

Two types of models exist, one where the knife is static and the other where the knife moves horizontally against a fixed part which is designed for cutting large sections.

Advantages

- Used for cutting celloidin-embedded tissues
- Ideal for brain sectioning, i.e., whole-organ sectioning
- Simple design with no complex moving parts
- Large and serial sections can be cut.
- Knife is large and does not need frequent sharpening as a greater cutting edge is available.
- Easy to operate and maintain

Disadvantages

- The sliding knife tends to jump on striking hard tissue
- Difficult to sharpen the long knife

Sledge Microtome (Fig. 5)

This type of microtome was designed to cut sections of very large blocks. It is similar to a sliding microtome. The block holder is mounted on a steel carriage which slides backward and forward on guides; against a fixed horizontal knife. Usually a wedge-shaped knife is used.

Advantages

- The microtome is heavy, consequently stable, and not subject to vibrations.
- Large and hard tissues can be cut.
- Used in freezing microtome and for celloidin-embedded tissues

Disadvantages

The microtome is much slower to use as compared to other microtomes (unless much practice of the instrument is made).

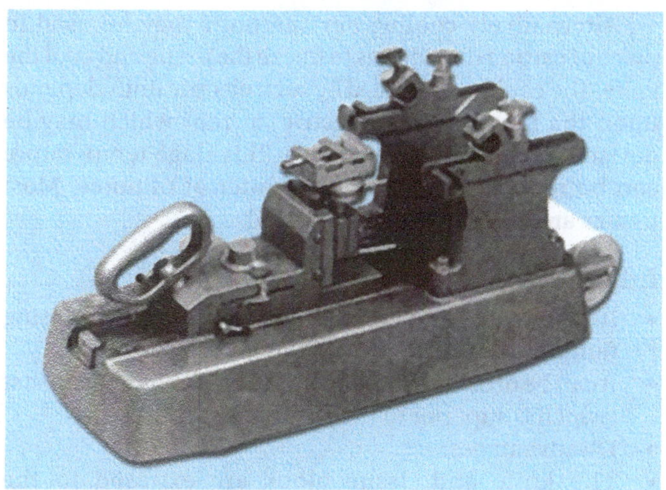

FIG. 5: Sledge microtome.

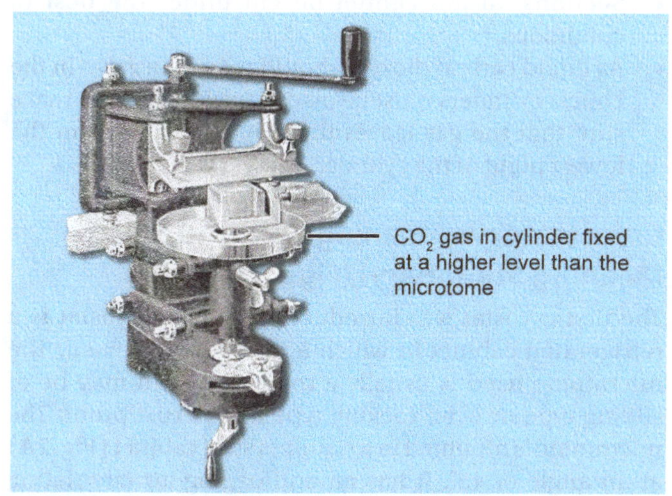

FIG. 6: Freezing microtome using carbon dioxide (CO_2) gas.

Freezing Microtome (Fig. 6)

The simple old type of freezing microtome is a machine that is clamped to the edge of a bench and is connected to a cylinder of carbon dioxide by means of a specially strengthened flexible metal tube. It consists of a central pivot with an attached horizontal arm which moves around the pivot. On this arm, two clamps hold a wedge profile microtome knife also held in a horizontal position **(Fig. 6)**. The specimen (block holder) is mounted juxtaposed to the knife.

Principle

The object is mounted on a block holder (chuck) also known as freezing stage with a centrally advancing screw. The block holder is perforated and attached to a feed pipe carrying carbon dioxide gas which can be sprayed on to the tissue for freezing. The knife moves over the block around a horizontal axis when once the tissue hardens **(Fig. 6)**.

Alternatively cooling devices/units may be used in place of carbon dioxide gas to freeze the tissue and cool the knife. The cooling produced by such electric units depends upon the flow of direct electric current which may be devised to regulate temperature. This stage temperature can be reduced to –36°C in a matter of minutes. Most tissues are cut between –20 to –25°C.

Advantages

- It is used in the demonstration of fat as processing fluids are not used.
- It can be of diagnostic use when affordability of cryostat (which is superior to this) is not possible.
- Disadvantages:
- The knife and tissue block are exposed to the atmosphere temperature and conditions after freezing.
- No serial sectioning possible
- Sections <8 µm cannot be cut under the best of conditions.
- As liquid carbon dioxide should reach the valve in the chuck, cylinders must be placed upside down to make sure that the gas leaves the cylinder valve from the lowest point of the cylinder.

Cryostat (*Cryo* Meaning Cold and *Stat* Meaning Stationary) (Figs. 7A and B)

The first cryostat was introduced in 1959. Cryostat is a refrigerated cabinet in which a microtome is fixed. The microtome used is usually a rotary type but may be of sliding type or even rocking type and is rust proof. The microtome is mounted in a stainless steel cabinet **(Fig. 7A)** at an angle of 45°. It has an antifogging air circulating system, a drain for defrosting and a shelf for 4-6 metal block holders. The temperature of the cabinet is –5°C to –30°C. All microtome control operations are outside the cabinet.

Harris international microtome is most commonly used. This unit operates on the "open top-cold box" principle **(Fig. 7B)**.

Teflon and stainless steel-coated disposable knives are available for use in cryosectioning.

Principle

To create a cold atmosphere around tissue block, block holder, and microtome by means of a special refrigerator type compressor, capable of taking temperatures below –30°C to –50°C. The reason for freezing the tissue is to harden the tissue to enable sectioning by the microtome knife. The coolant used is usually Freon 22.

Advantages

- Used extensively for rapid diagnosis, fat stains, and enzyme histochemistry in neurological applications as well as in fluorescent microscopy
- Both the knife and tissue are maintained at same low temperature.
- Capable of slicing sections as thin as 1 µm
- Serial sectioning is possible.
- Automatic defrosting and sterilization
- Antifogging air circulatory system

Disadvantages

- Constant supervision and maintenance of temperature is required.
- The whole instrument should be kept in air-conditioned room to prevent excessive cryostat compressor functioning.

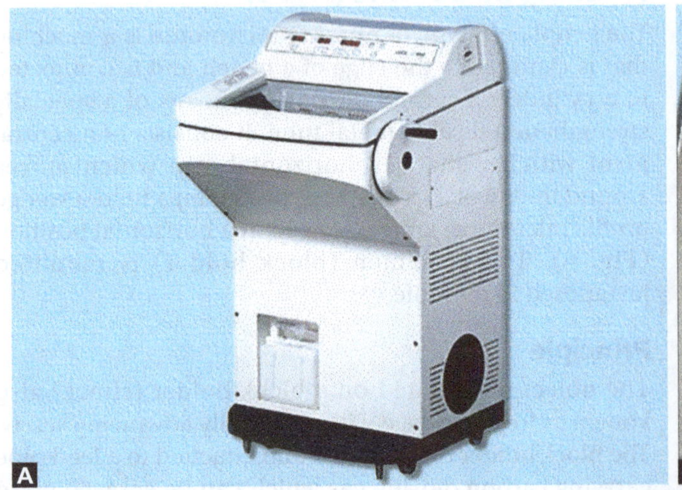

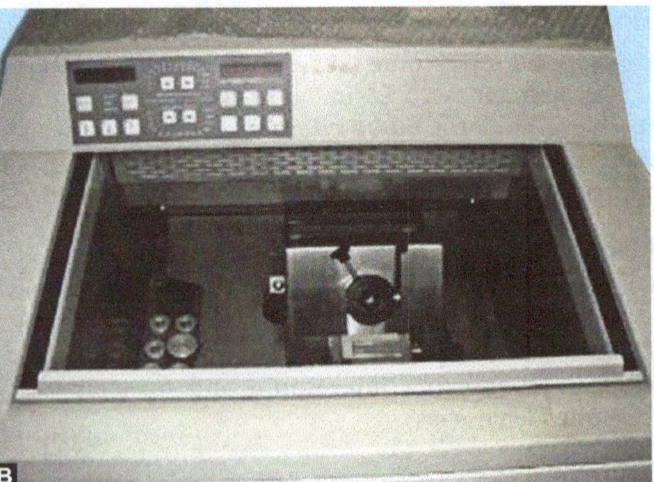

FIGS. 7A AND B: Cryostat: (A) Microtome is mounted in a stainless steel cabinet; and (B) Open top-cold box of cryostat.

- Lubricants of special type with a low congealing point have to be used. This prevents the lubricants solidifying at a cooler temperature within the chamber.
- Freeze artifacts seen as holes in the tissues
- If the temperature is too low, the tissue becomes hard and crumbles and becomes difficult to cut (In such cases, warm the tissue by pressing the thumb over the tissue).
- Difficulty in sectioning fixed tissue
- High cost of the instrument
- Morphology not clear

Microtomes for Ultrathin Sections

The ultramicrotome was produced by Richards in 1956. It is used for cutting semithin (1 µm or slightly thinner) sections for optical (light) microscopy in order to scan the area or ultrathin sections (40–80 nm) almost exclusively for electron microscopy. The thickness of an ultrathin section can be estimated by the color that the section reflexes from its surface. This color may reflect as gray (<60 nm), silver (60–90 nm), pale gold (90–120 nm), dark gold (120–150 nm), and purple (150–190 nm). Tissues are extremely small, rarely >0.5 mm in size, and the greatest dimension of the block is <0.1 cm. Glass or diamond knives are used to cut sections and these are collected in a receptacle **(Fig. 8A)** made around each knife-edge with waterproof sticky tape to contain distilled water. The water acts as a floatation bath on which the section cuts are floated and can be picked up later and placed on a grid **(Fig. 8B)**.

Two types are in use today:

1. Mechanical
2. Thermal advance
3. With a combination of the two, i.e., mechanical and thermal advance

Both types are extremely sensitive to atmospheric temperature variations and both types are used with either glass or diamond knives. In order to achieve even sections, both microtomes are operated by an electric motor.

The principle is similar to a regular microtome with movement on a micrometer screw which advances the specimen for cutting. In the thermal advance type, the advance is produced as a result of the heat generated between the block and the knife at the time of cutting.

Variations and combination of both A and B are available. In general, the mechanical type system is used for semithin sections and the thermal advance system for ultrathin sections.

MAINTENANCE OF A MICROTOME[2,3]

After use every time, microtomes should have all paraffin and other residues on it brushed or wiped away. All moving parts especially the sliding surfaces, the tooth-wheel, the axle, and the ratchet must be oiled with one or two drops of thin lubricant oil, e.g., three-in-one oil.

Depending on its use, microtome advance on the geared wheel and pawl movement should be checked. One movement of the toothed wheel after a 360° rotation of the axle should indicate a block advance or knife advance (as the case may be) of 1 µm.

MICROTOME KNIVES[2,3]

Knives are made of different types of material.

- *Metal*:
  - Standard steel
  - Razor blades
  - *Disposable knives*: Made of steel
- *Nonmetal*:
  - Glass knives
  - Diamond knives

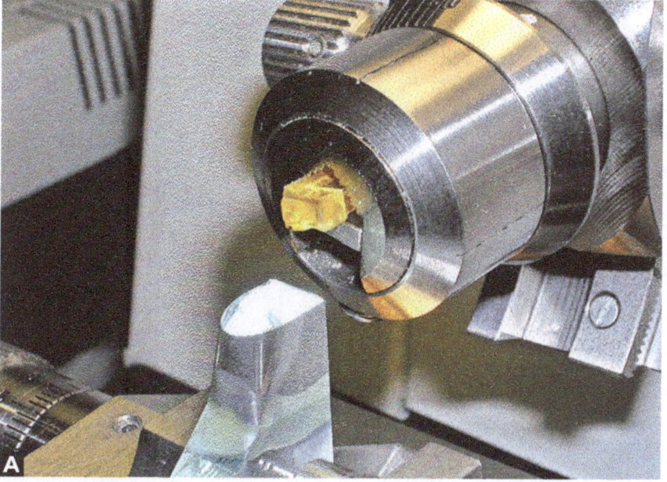

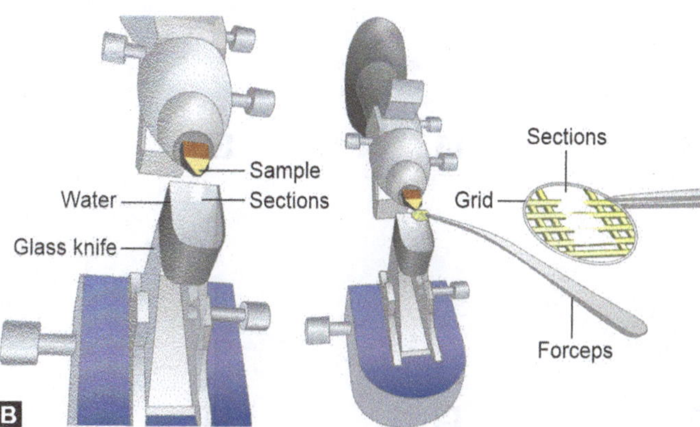

FIGS. 8A AND B: (A) Ultramicrotome with block and receptacle; and (B) Process of cutting and placing on grid.

Metal

Standard steel knives are made of high-grade steel with a high carbon content (e.g., tantalum) tempered from the tip inward for one-third of width. These knives are available in 120 mm, 180 mm, 210 mm, and 260 mm lengths and cut fine sections. Hardness of knives is measured by "Vickers scale hardness." In the Vickers hardness test, the surface of the knife is indented by a diamond under a standard force of about 5–120 kgf (kilogram-force) for 15 seconds. Vickers hardness test is calculated by dividing the applied force by the surface area of the indentation. This method is accurate and used for all metal knives.

Actual hardness of the cutting edge may vary between 400 and 900 on the Vickers hardness scale (VHS). The hardness of the knives should be of such a nature as to hold a good sharpening for a long duration of time. It is important to use knives of required hardness as per the "Vickers Scale".

Types of metal knife edge **(see Figs. 9A to F)**:

- *Very concave* **(Fig. 9A)**: It is used for fresh specimens and soft celloidin-embedded specimens.
- *Plano-concave* **(Fig. 9B)**: It is flat on one side and concave on the other side with varying degree of concavities. The more concave is used for soft paraffin sections with the sledge, rotary, and rocking microtome and the less concave ones are used for harder celloidin-embedded tissue.
- *Wedge-shaped* **(Fig. 9C)**: It is plain on both sides. Its size varies from 100 to 350 mm in length with varied masses. It is used in routine paraffin sections, frozen sections, and all types of microtomes.
- *Wedge and plane* **(Fig. 9D)**: It is used for most paraffin-embedded sections, hard celloidin, and some plastics (diamond knives).
- *Knife with bevel* **(Fig. 9E)**: In practice, there is always a final bevel at the cutting edge. This bevel may be symmetrical on both sides, or not. The final bevel helps with sharpening and resharpening. An imaginary line drawn through the centre of the cross section of the knife, forms an angle with a line drawn parallel to the line of motion; this forms the knife angle or the angle of edge **(Fig. 10)**.
- *Knife with chisel edge* **(Fig. 9F)**: The relative blunt edge makes it a sturdy knife.

Razor Blades on Steel Knives

Regular shaving razor blades are fixed with a clamping device to standard steel knives. The razor blade edge projects slightly over the cutting edge of the standard knife and acts as the cutting edge. The advantage of this is that a constant sharp cutting edge is available and the blades can always be discarded when blunt. No honing needs to be done. The principle disadvantages include fracture of the blade incurred as a result of cutting hard tissue.

Disposable Knives

Disposable knives are made of steel and coated with special polytetrafluoroethylene (PTFE), which allows ribbons to be cut easily.

Two types of disposable knives are available:

1. Low-profile knives
2. High-profile knives

Stainless steel disposable blade holders are available for *high-profile* and *low-profile* disposable blades, which can be fixed on all types of microtomes.

The *high-profile disposable microtome blade* is made of good quality heavy gauge steel as compared to other brands, avoids vibration of the blade, best used for cutting

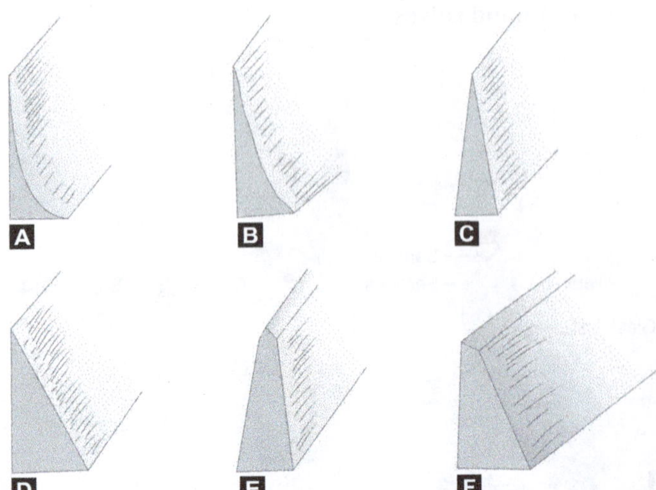

FIGS. 9A TO F: Types of metal knife edge.

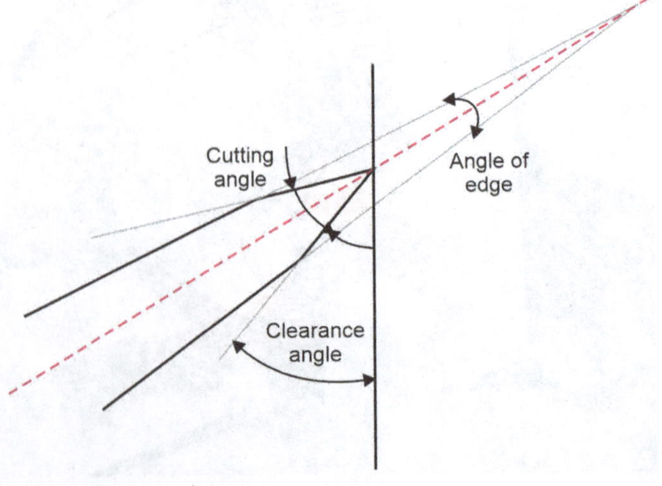

FIG. 10: Knife and cutting angles: The angles of the metal microtome knife in relation to a paraffin tissue block.

through extremely hard or fibrous tissue. These ultrasharp and high-quality microtome sectioning blades offer sharp edges for distortion and chatter-free sections. They are available in packs which dispense blades directly into blade holders (easy to fit and handle); and safe storage compartments with space provided for used blades.

The *low-profile disposable microtome blades/triple facet microtome blades* are manufactured from high carbon stainless steel. The blades fit the standard low-profile blade holders to be used with them and best used to cut delicate and thin tissue bits; also supplied in a dispenser pack with storage compartment for the safe discard of spent blades.

Advantages of Disposable Knives

- A damaged or dull cutting edge may be replaced by a new, perfect edge within seconds without time consumption and lengthy process of resharpening.
- Honing is not required.
- It can be used as long as it has a sharp edge.
- Gives improved quality of sections.
- Corrosion and heat resistant
- Its hardness can be compared to that of standard steel knives.
- Easily available and discardable

Disadvantages of Disposable Knives

- Relatively expensive
- Not as rigid as other microtome knives, tendency for minor vibrations

Parts of Metal Knife (Fig. 11)

There are four parts of metal knife.

1. The heel of the knife is where the handle can be attached at one end.
2. The toe is the diametrically opposite end.
3. The cutting edge
4. The back

Angles of a Metal Knife (Fig. 10)[2,4]

The angles of importance in a knife are bevel angle (cutting angle), wedge angle (knife edge angle), clearance angle, angle of inclination, and stropping (upper and lower facet) angle.

- *Bevel angle (knife edge angle)*: Angle formed between the cutting facets where they meet at the cutting edge. The angle usually varies between 18 and 30°, the smaller the bevel angle the sharper is the knife. Too small a bevel angle results in the elastic distortion of the edge.
- *Wedge angle*: It is the angle formed when an imaginary extension of the sides of the knife meet at a point, also known as the blade angle (in **Fig. 10** it is called 'angle of edge') and is around 15°.
- *Stropping angle (upper and lower facet angle)*: It is the angle between the surface of the block and the upper facet and lower facet respectively of the knife.
- *Angle of inclination*: Angle formed between the surface of the block and the line bisecting the bevel angle. If the angle is too large, the sample in the block can crumble and the knife can induce periodic thickness variations in the sections (some authors extend this up to the upper facet when it is known as "cutting angle").
- *Rake angle*: It is 90° minus angle of upper facet of knife.
- *Clearance angle*: Angle between the surface of the block and the lower straight edge of the knife. It may be only 2–5°. It is essential in order to prevent friction between the knife and the block. A low clearance angle gives less compression to the tissue block and

A and B
Note the space for the attachment of the knife handle (arrow). This area is called the heel. The other end of the knife is called the toe

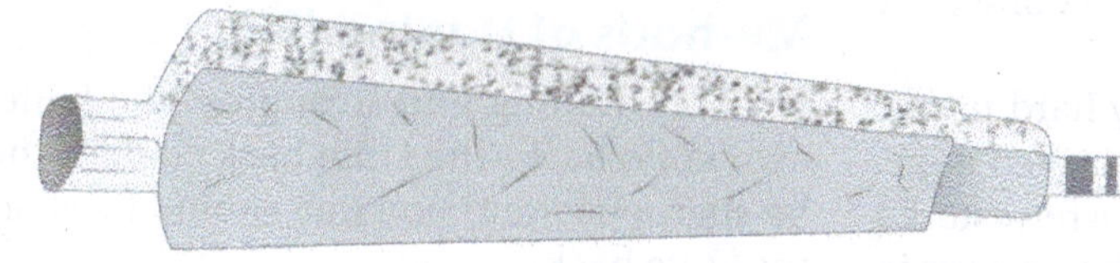

FIGS. 11A TO C: (A and B) Knife with knife back; and (C) Handle.

produces a smooth plastic flow during sectioning. This is a crucial angle for sectioning and can be adjusted easily. Once the right angle is found it can be used throughout and rarely needs to be changed frequently for that particular blade.

Nonmetal Knives

These knives are small and used almost exclusively for ultramicrotomy.

- *Glass knives*: The knives are made from specially made glass strips (e.g., Ralph type) of adequate thickness (0.5–1 cm). These strips are cut at an angle to produce a cutting edge by means of a special instrument called the knife maker. The knives are used for both semithin (1 μm) and thin silver gray sections (60–100 μm). Such knives once dull are discarded.
- *Diamond knives*: These are used in electron microscopy for sectioning epoxy resin blocks. They have a cutting edge of 3 mm that has a longer life span. Though made of industrial diamonds, these knives cost a considerable amount and cannot be sharpened. They tend to fracture if mishandled or if processed hard tissue is sought to be cut by them.

MAINTENANCE OF MICROTOME KNIFE[2,3]

The most important part of the microtome knife is the cutting edge and this edge must always be maintained in good condition in order that ideal sections are obtained. All knives are sharpened at the factory whereby a bevel is obtained with a cutting edge. By usage, these knives develop irregularities and breaks. These irregularities and breaks must necessarily be removed by a process of honing (sharpening) and stropping whereby a smooth finish is given to the already honed cutting surface.

Owing to the brittleness, steel knives should not be dropped or placed on the table with the cutting edge downward. Both these may result in chipping and even breakage of the knife. The knife should be cleaned in xylene or toluene before or after use.

Sharpening of Metal Knives

Sharpening of metal knives includes both honing and stropping. By the honing procedure crude nicks are removed from the knife edge and stropping is done after honing to refine the honed edge further.

After prolonged use or after cutting very hard tissue, the cutting edge becomes damaged, with a jagged edge. A straight cutting edge and a correct bevel must be restored by grinding the knife on a hone. Honing is the process in which all the nicks and irregularities in the cutting edge of the knife are removed to make the cutting edge straight and sharp.

Honing is done by the use of hand-hones or electrically operated hones. In order to hone a hard steel knife, the hone should be even harder and for this purpose either naturally occurring stones or artificially produced material like plate glass or carborundum may be used. Hones are actually known as sharpening stones and have wide abrasive properties.

Naturally occurring hone stones: They are known as oil stones because oil is used as a lubricant. The finer the grain in the stone, the harder is the hone.

- Arkansas stone is a hard pale yellow white stone and has a polishing effect with medium fineness.
- Yellow Belgian glass stone and green Belgian glass stone
- Belgian black vein stone—best used for manual sharpening

Lubricants are used in most sharpening techniques because they act as a coolant, prevent the extreme edge of the knife losing tamper, and prevent the stone's pores to be blocked by knife's metal particles.

Two types of lubricants are used:

1. Aqueous lubricants, e.g., glycerol, soap solution, vegetable oil, and liquid detergent (10%)
2. Nonaqueous lubricants, e.g., three-in-one oil, oils thinned with paraffin oil, or liquid paraffin is recommended.

Artificially produced hones are used with an abrasive powder, a suspension of which is made in water. The average size of the powder particles for grinding is 20 μm (not >40 μm) and for polishing is 4 μm (not >8 μm).

The carborundum is an artificial stone having a coarse surface and is useful for badly nicked knives.

Plate glass: It is available as 1/4″ to 3/8″ thick with a length of 14 inches and width of 2 inches. It is used with abrasive powders, is cheaper than other hones, easy to use and clean, and readily available.

Abrasive powders include diamond powders, carborundum (silicon carbide), aluminum oxide, iron oxide, and ceric oxide. These are available as various-sized particles and have applications in both sharpening and polishing of knives.

Methods of Honing (Fig. 12)

For both honing and stropping, the knife must have its own knife back. The knife back enables the bevel edge to be sharpened and no knife should be sharpened without the knife back.

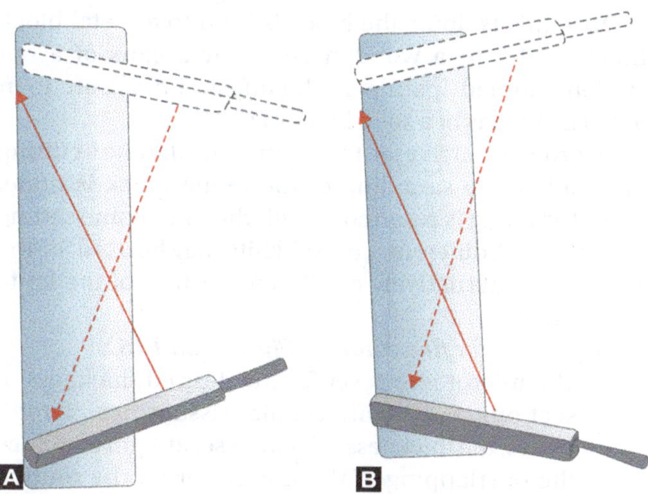

FIGS. 12A AND B: (A) Honing: Note that the movement is from heel to toe. The cutting edge is leading. (B) Stropping—movement of toe to heel, cutting edge toward the operator.

- The knife handle is fitted to the knife if it is sharpened by hand but in machine sharpening no knife handle is required.
- A small quantity of light oil is applied to the hone and smeared over the surface.
- The movement for honing is with the hone being placed on a table, the knife moves with cutting edge forward in apposition to the honing surface; heel of the knife is leading.
- The knife is placed at the end of the hone nearest to the operator with the cutting edge facing away from the operator.
- The knife is pushed diagonally from heel to toe. The direction of the movement is such that one entire cutting surface is honed in one upgoing strop: Turned over on its back and moved across the hone to its original position (figure of eight movement).
- In general, 20–30 such strokes are sufficient to hone a knife for an ordinary use.
- Each knife cutting edge should be examined with a microscope using incident light at a magnification of hundred. A thin white light should be seen (von Mohl's criteria) **(Fig. 13)**.

Precautions while honing:

- Lubricant must be used.
- The blade must be kept vertically flat because if the knife edge is raised slightly during honing will cause the edges flat.
- After the honing is complete, the knife edge should be wiped and moistened with xylene.
- *Care of a hone*: The hone is to be kept covered when not in use, wrapped in a soft cloth, and kept in a box with a lid to preserve its surface.

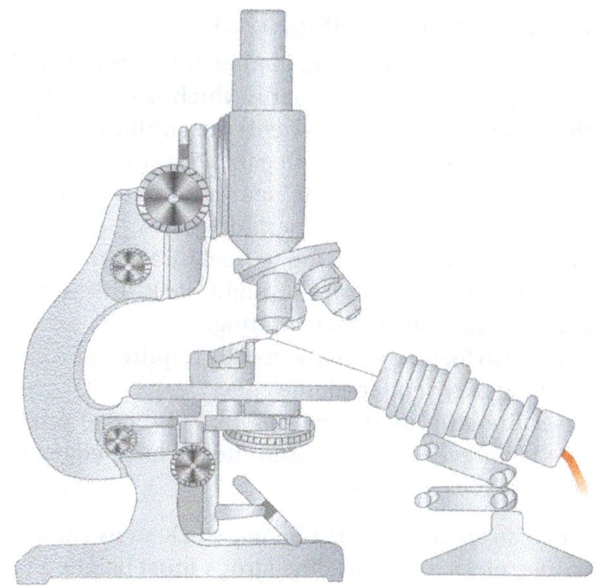

FIG. 13: Examination of knife edge under 10× after honing and stropping.

Automatic Hones

Automatic hones are designed for safe, quick, and convenient on-site use for resharpening of microtome knives. These have a compact and portable structure. The knife is fitted to a holder which allows the cutting edge to be in contact with a plate made of metal or glass. The knife automatically turns over the plate at regular intervals from edge to edge, till the honing is complete.

Semiautomatic Hones

Semiautomatic hones have a manual feed of the knife but are again time saving and easy to manipulate. The manual feed results in an uneven knife edge. After use all hones must be washed with warm soap water, thoroughly rinsed with water and dried. This maintenance leaves the hone free from metal particles and prolongs its life.

Stropping

This is the final technique for sharpening the knife before cutting sections. It is done to polish the honed cutting edge and removes the fine nicks. Stropping removes the buffs formed during honing. The knife edge cannot be sufficiently sharp to cut good sections directly from honing or sharpening. Stropping must follow honing.

Strops are made of horse leather especially got from horse rump area and are 18 inches × 3–4 inches mounted on a solid wooden block.

Types of strops are:

- *Rigid/fixed*: It is preferred as it is easy to manipulate.
- Flexible/hanging—with one end fixed.

Method of Stropping (Fig. 12B)

- Since the strop is made of leather, it is cuttable and so to strop a movement is made which is the reverse to that of honing (i.e., toe to heel) the cutting edge of the knife given no chance to slice into the strop.
- The knife is placed on the near end of the strop with cutting edge toward the operator.
- The knife is drawn in a toe to heel direction. Then the knife is turned over and brought back. This action is exactly opposite to that of honing.
- Twenty to forty strokes are usually required and excess stroking may spoil the knife edge.
- After the stropping is complete, knife edge must be oiled to prevent rusting. Examine the knife edge under microscope.

Care of a strop: Strops must be wiped clean as sand/dust can cause nicks in a knife. The strops must be oiled (with thin oil) before use and regularly at intervals of 1 year and dressed with a fine carborundum powder available through the makers of such microtome knife strops.

SECTION CUTTING[2,3,5,6]

Sectioning tissues is an art and takes much skill and practice. This is done on microtomes. Histotechnologists are considered as artists of the laboratory. Successful sections require:

- Properly prepared material with the supporting medium matching the specimen. This means that the tissue should ideally be well fixed, well processed and infiltrated, and embedded by the right type of wax to minimize artifacts in the sections. Common artifacts include tears, "Venetian blinds", holes, folds, etc.
- *A proper microtome*: A well-maintained microtome is rarely responsible for poor quality sections. It is only the choice of a microtome that matters to suit the requirement, e.g., for routine use, a rotary microtome is best and for full-organ sections, a sliding/sledge microtome, etc.
- *A skilled operator*: It must be able to recognize and correct difficulties as they arise; as the saying goes "practice makes one perfect".

Paraffin Section Cutting

Trimming of paraffin blocks: Once tissues have been blocked excess paraffin on all aspects of the block of tissues should be removed to leave approximately 3 mm of paraffin around it. Somewhat more paraffin should be available at the back of the block.

Once this is done, the block is fixed to a metal block object holder or a wooden chuck by means of a hot wooden handled spatula. Both knife and block are then cooled by means of a solid block of ice.

In order to arrive at the optimum plane of cutting where adequate sampling of the tissue block is done, coarse trimming is resorted to with the microtome setting at 20–25 μm. A different "coarse" knife may be used for the purpose or alternatively a different portion of the knife may be used.

- *Procedure (for fine cutting)* ***(Figs. 14 and 15)***:
    - The microtome is set for the desired thickness of sections. For highly cellular tissues, e.g., lymph nodes, the thickness selector is set at 4 μm to reduce the overlapping of the nuclei; for all the routine tissue 5–6 μm thickness is adequate **(Fig. 14)**.
    - The correct position of the properly embedded blocks in the microtome **(Fig. 16)** will result in the final preparation of the entire surface which should be free of tears, lines, folds, or cellular distortion. If the block is not parallel to the knife, readjust the block holder screws.
    - The knife tilt angle is optimized for each microtome and blade type. Both the block and the knife should be wiped dry.
    - Blocks should be properly trimmed to expose the tissue.
    - Cutting is then performed by using regular even and gentle strokes. Rapid wheel movement should never be done as often this generates static electricity with sections tending to fly away, crumble, roll, or curl.

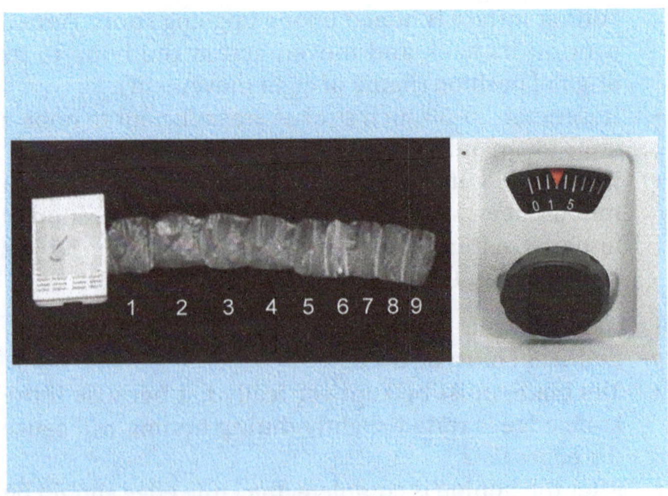

FIG. 14: Micron setting adjustment on a rotary microtome.

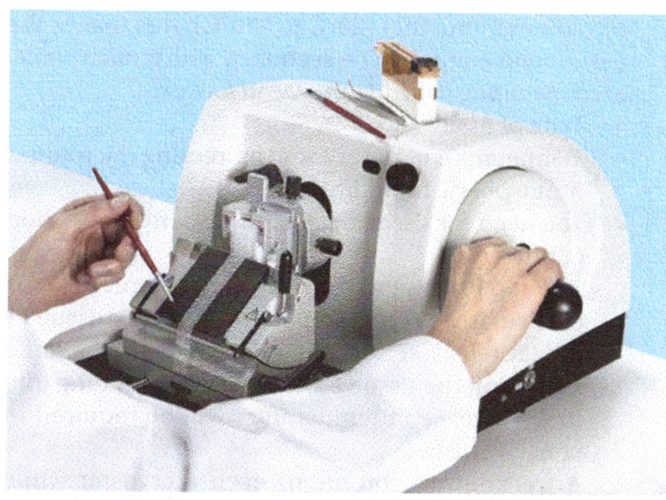

FIG. 15: Advancement of handle by one rotation moves the block through the desired thickness of microns (rotary microtome).

- To obtain ribbons, the tissue should be small and the block able to generate sufficient heat and pressure to wield together the edges of the paraffin sections that are cut.
- Whether single sections are made or ribbons, these sections should be placed on a water bath whose temperature is 5–8°C below the melting point of the wax used to process and block the tissue. Transport of single sections may be done by means of an artist's brush. Hold on to the free end of the section/ribbon, after about six continuous sections have been cut; with a pair of forceps, free the attached end and float the ribbon onto the bath. With this, the sections unfold themselves and flatten out. A brush may be used to facilitate the straightening. It may be necessary to add hot water with a dropper pipette to deal with the wrinkles on individual section. A dissecting needle or any other pointed instrument should never be used since these are likely to produce holes in the section.
- Ideally spread sections or ribbons may now be transferred to clean new histology glass slides. The slides are gently held beneath the section in the water bath picked up with a gentle sweep. Many authors believe that a direct transfer may be done without treating the slides with egg albumin as the tissue protein in the section itself is sufficient to ensure section adhesion to the glass slides. Others feel that egg albumin smearing on slides plays a positive role in tissue adhesion. When egg albumin is used only a minute amount is applied to the slide and spread. If excess amounts are applied, these stain eosinophilic with the hematoxylin-eosin stain and obscure clear viewing of the tissue section.
- After section cutting, the block is removed and its cutting surface sealed with molten wax. This ensures that tissue will not dry or become hard and brittle and facilitates resectioning of the blocks, weeks, months, and years later.
- The use of adhesives promotes the growth of bacteria and fungi in the water bath. Daily cleaning of the water bath with Clorox, soap, and water is recommended to prevent such contamination.
- See **Appendix 2** for errors in section cutting, their cause, and rectification.

• *Other requirements during paraffin section cutting*:
  - *Block holders*: Metal or wood chuck
  - *Water bath*: This is a thermostatically controlled bath with the inside colored black for floating the cut sections. It is rectangular and 10–12 inches in size and 3–4 inches deep; the temperature being set at 45°C, i.e., about 8° below the melting point of wax. It is colored black on the inside for better viewing of sections.

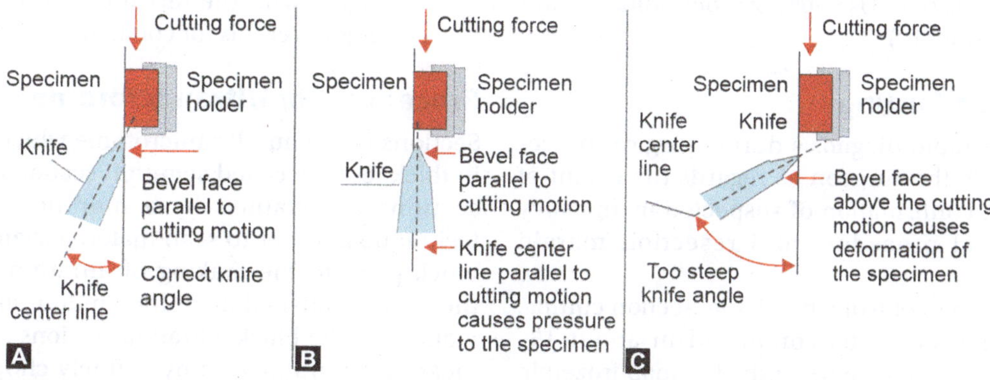

FIGS. 16A TO C: How angles (in particular cutting angle) affects cutting of sections.
Courtesy: Leica Systems.[4]

- *Forceps and fine paint brushes*: The former help in the pickup of paraffin ribbons while sectioning and both can be of help in the removal of section folds and creases as sections are floated in the water bath.
- *Slide warmer*: Hot stage method is used for drying sections on slides. It consists of an electric hot plate which is maintained at a temperature of 45–50°C. The slides with the sections are placed on the hot plate for 30–40 minutes; or alternatively placed in an oven at 50–60°C for 2 hours. This helps in section drying, melting of the excess paraffin wax, and fixing of tissues to the slides.
- *Drying ovens* are available with an inbuilt fan, especially designed for drying tissue sections on slides.
- *Albuminized slides/adhesives for coating slides (optional)*: A thin smear of the adhesive is applied to glass slides as mentioned above, before sections are picked up from the water bath. This attaches the tissue sections firmly onto the slide enabling them to withstand harsh treatment by acid and alkali solutions while staining as in ammoniacal silver solutions. Albuminized slides and adhesives are also used for cryostat sections.
- *Mayer's egg albumin-glycerol*:
  - Whites of fresh eggs: 50 mL
  - Glycerol: 50 mL
  - Distilled water: 50 mL

    Mix well and filter through several layers of gauze or coarse filter paper and add a crystal of thymol to prevent the growth of molds.

    OR
  - Stock:
    - Egg albumin flakes (commercially available): 5 g
    - Distilled water: 100 mL
    - Add one crystal of thymol
- *Working solution*: Use 50% of stock solution and 50% glycerine (IP)

Frozen Section Cutting

- It is done for rapid diagnosis during surgical procedures to guide the surgeon as regards the extent of surgery, e.g., confirmation of suspected malignancy before radical procedure and resection margin clearance.
- The entire process of fixing the tissue, section cutting, and reporting has to be completed in about 15–20 minutes. The tissue to be studied is snap frozen in a cold environment (–20°C to –70°C); this makes the tissue solid enough to be sectioned with a microtome.

Section cutting depends on several factors:
- Type of tissue
- Temperature of the cryostat or freezing microtome
- Atmospheric humidity
- The need for tissue fixation prior to frozen section cutting
- The type of tissue may cause problems. This is particularly so with adipose or fibrofatty tissue as the fat released from the cells results in the knife sliding off the tissue block rather than cutting into it. A decrease in temperature will be required to congeal the fat.
- A freezing microtome or even a cryostat while opening or closing is exposed to the atmospheric humidity. During use, the atmospheric water crystallizes, these crystals in themselves acting as a knife resulting in the shattering of sections.
- *Common temperatures used in the cryostat are as follows*:
  - Common carcinoma: –18°C to –20°C at atmosphere humidity of 30%. Sometimes lower temperatures may be needed.
  - Adipose tissues and sarcomas: –22°C to –25°C at atmosphere humidity of 30%.
  - These are approximate values and will vary depending on other factors.
- Atmospheric humidity plays a great role in frozen section cutting. In order to decrease or prevent water crystallization altogether, a freezing mixture is used the principle of which is to reduce the freezing point of the tissues by prior impregnation.
- Commercially available freezing mixtures are provided by cryostat manufacturers, e.g., optimum cooling temperature (OCT) mixture.
- A drop of the freezing mixture is placed on the freezing stage, next place the tissue over this, cover it again with the mixture and place the cryostat weight over this for cooling.

Procedure for Ultramicrotome

Sections cut in an ultramicrotome which measure 1 μm in thickness are called semithin sections. Such semithin sections are stained by a modified toluidine blue technique in order to scan material available in a tissue block prior to the making of ultrathin sections. Once the user is satisfied as to the amount and adequacy of material in the block, ultrathin sections are made. Tissue meant for ultramicrotomy is finely chopped with each tissue for blocking measuring not >0.1 cm (1 mm) in greatest dimension and the blocks are prepared in resin. Processing of these needs a special procedure and is dealt with in the section on processing.

CONCLUSION

Microtomy and section cutting is an art which improves greatly with experience. The hand that rules the microtome is the secret behind the reporting pathologist!

REFERENCES

1. Leica Biosystems. Histology: Clinical microtomes. [online] https://www.leicabiosystems.com/en-in/histology-equipment/microtomes/ [Last accessed March, 2024].
2. Shariff S. Laboratory Techniques in Surgical Pathology. Bengaluru: Prism Books Pvt Ltd.; 1999.
3. Thomas JA, Shariff S. A Compendium on Microtomy and Special Stains (Silver Jubilee Manual). Department of Pathology, Bangalore: St John's Medical College; 1991.
4. LabCE.com. (2018). Instrumentation for Microtomy: Knife Angles. [online] Available from https://www.labce.com/spg605385_instrumentation_for_microtomy_knife_angles.aspx [Last accessed March, 2024].
5. Culling CF Handbook of Histopathological and Histochemical Techniques, 3rd edition. Boston, London: Butterworth-Heinemann; 1974.
6. Prophet EB, Mills B, Arrington JB, Sobin LH (Eds). Armed Forces Institute of Pathology: Laboratory Methods in Histotechnology. Washington DC: Armed Forces Institute of Pathology, American Registry of Pathology; 1994.

CHAPTER 19

Hematoxylin and Eosin Stain

INTRODUCTION AND APPLICATIONS

The single universally used stain in all laboratories is the hematoxylin and eosin (H&E) stain.

The H&E stain has several applications in the laboratory; it is done on all paraffin-embedded tissue in histopathology as a routine, rapid H&E for frozen sections, fine-needle aspirates, and on all cytology fluid samples.

In the past, stains and their components were made by the laboratory technician; in particular, the hematoxylin stain was made batch after batch and kept for ripening; taken to use when ready. Commercially available reagents were uncommon and worked out expensive, and most laboratories made their stains for better financial gains. Presently however the trend has changed and laboratories find it easy to order rather than prepare their stains, the cost of the stain being met with by the patient in whose bill it is included!

WHAT IS HEMATOXYLIN?[1]

- Hematoxylin stain dye is a natural one and extracted from the heart wood of a tree *Haematoxylum campechianum* originally grown in Mexico. Oxidation of the hematoxylin produces hematin, which is the actual dye used for staining. Natural ripening and oxidation is by sunlight when hematoxylin solutions are allowed to stand for several days, take about 4–5 months before the stain is ready for use. Once prepared, this is superior and lasts much longer on slides compared to the artificially ripened stain. Chemical methods for ripening are done with sodium iodate as the oxidizing agent, resulting in the use of hematoxylin in about a few weeks to a couple of months. Other oxidizing agents include mercuric oxide and potassium permanganate.
- Addition of the mordant improves the ability of the hematin to attach to the tissues. A mordant is a substance (metal ion), which forms a complex with the stain or dye and aids in attaching the stain to the tissues during staining by forming a tissue-mordant-dye complex which is insoluble in aqueous and alcoholic solvents. Hematoxylins are typically classified by the mordant used in their staining. The type of mordant also influences the final color of the stained components. The most common mordant used in routine histology is *aluminum ammonium sulfate (alum)*. This mordant causes the nuclei to stain reddish in color, which then changes to the more familiar dark blue color when the sample is exposed after staining to a weak basic solution (bluing).
- A lake is the name given to a complex formed between a mordant and a dye, which then attaches to the substrate. The combination of hematoxylin with mordant is known as hematoxylin lake (blue black), lakes with different metals have different hues, e.g., aluminum lakes are purple to blue, iron lake is blue black, copper lake is blue green to purple, tin lakes are red, lead lakes are dark brown, etc. (see **Appendix 3** for types of hematoxylins).

Hematoxylin and Eosin Stain[2-6]

Indications: Universal stain on all tissues which brings out good nuclear and cytoplasmic detail.

Technique: Paraffin-embedded tissue.

Fixative: 10% formalin.

Principle: Oxidation of the hematoxylin produces hematin, which is the actual dye used for staining. Addition of the mordant improves the ability of the hematin to attach to the tissues. Mordants strengthen the positive ionic charge of the hematin. This aids the bonding of the hematin to the (negatively charged) anionic tissue component, which is the nuclear chromatin.

- *Progressive staining* occurs when the hematoxylin is added to the tissue without being followed by a differentiator to remove excess dye. This stains the nuclei only and because there is no differentiation step, some background staining can occur, especially with charged or treated slides, e.g., Mayer's hematoxylin. Enhancement of blue color occurs while washing the slides in running water.
- The *regressive staining* is accomplished by overstaining in a neutral solution and then removing the excess stain from the other constituents with acid ethyl alcohol or some other differentiating agents. The excess stain is removed selectively until the right intensity is obtained, e.g., hematoxylin staining followed by differentiating in acid alcohol which removes the excess hematoxylin from the nucleus as well as the dye from unwanted sites such as cytoplasm, e.g., Harris hematoxylins.
- Eosin is the most commonly used counterstain that distinguishes and stains the cytoplasm. It is typically pink. The *eosins* are the most suitable and convenient stains to combine with alum hematoxylins to demonstrate the general histological architecture of a tissue, the pink hue contrasting against the nuclear hematoxylin blue. The eosins are acid xanthene or phthalein dyes. The name "eosin" is derived from the peculiar pale pink color resembling dawn pink. The most frequently used stain among this group is eosin Y, which may be used with both water and alcohol. The addition of a small amount of acetic acid sharpens the staining of the eosin. Eosin with phloxine added enhances the red color with H&E staining.

Procedure (using Harris hematoxylin and watery eosin Y as cytoplasmic stain):[7]

- Deparaffinize with xylol, 2 minutes each; two changes
- Absolute ethyl alcohol, 5 minutes
- 95% ethyl alcohol, 5 minutes
- 80% ethyl alcohol, 5 minutes
- 60% ethyl alcohol, 5 minutes
- Bring sections to water
- Harris hematoxylin, 15 minutes
- Rinse with tap water
- Differentiate with 1% hydrochloric acid (HCl) in 70% ethyl alcohol
- Wash with tap water
- "Bluing" with running tap water or alkaline solution, 10–20 minutes
- Stain with watery eosin, 15 seconds
- Depending on the color required, rinse in water, 1 minute
- 80% ethyl alcohol
- 95% ethyl alcohol, 2 minutes
- Absolute alcohol, two changes
- Xylene, two changes. Following the eosin stain, the slide is passed through several changes of alcohol to remove all traces of water, then rinsed in several baths of xylene which "clears" the tissue and renders it completely transparent.
- Mount with Entellan [Merck/DPX (dibutyl phthalate in xylene)]

Results

- *Nuclei:* Blue to blue black
- *Cytoplasm and other substances*: Pink

Advantages

- Simple procedure
- Cost-effective particularly if hematoxylin is prepared in the laboratory itself
- Pleasing colors
- Most histological structures are visualized and the stain is used as a first time "look" into tissues in all laboratories.

Disadvantages

- Too much cannot be read into the H&E stain; ratification with special stains must be done.
- Deparaffinization is important and should be adequate. Residual paraffin prevents the dyes from penetrating the tissues, thus giving an uneven stained appearance. Some of the paraffin melts and is removed when slides after being cut are kept in an incubator for a period of 20–30 minutes, the remaining is removed by changes in xylene till the entire paraffin film around the section clears up.

Dehydration after staining is very important to help preserve the stains in the slide. Remember all stains used are water soluble and any retained water in the final stages of dehydration will lead to "fading" of the stain after a few weeks or months.

Note: The differentiation in staining allows to selectively remove stain from tissues to the optimal level for a pleasant viewing. In the case of hematoxylin, 1% HCl (for rapid differentiation) and acetic acid (for slower, more controlled differentiation) are most commonly used. While HCl has historically been the standard, milder acids provide gentler dye removal in automated staining. Staining methods that include a destaining or differentiation step are referred to as "regressive" stains.

Bluing reagents, such as Scott's tap water, are used to change the hematoxylin from red to the traditional blue color. These basic solutions chemically alter the dye to produce the color change. Bluing is also achieved with a buffer solution like tap water where the pH itself causes the water to be basic enough to allow for the bluing of nuclei; other bluing substances are lithium carbonate or ammonia water.

Mild acidity is critical to the shelf-life of hematoxylin. Without it, the alkalinity of the tap water rinse will not raise the pH for the dye lake to precipitate, and the color will change from cherry red to purple red. Adding small amounts of acetic acid to the hematoxylin periodically will aid in maintaining appropriate pH and can extend the life of the stain.

Mounting: The coverslip is always applied before the section has a chance to dry and a high-quality mountant is used.

Put a drop of mountant next to the section. Align (arrow left in **Fig. 1**) the edge of coverslip onto the side of the slide, lifting it away from the section, then gently lower the other end of the coverslip by means of a tooth of a forceps allowing its weight to fall on the section as shown (dotted arrow), ensuring there are no air bubbles between the two.

The long-term storage qualities of the mountant must be known because crystals can appear in poor quality mountant, sometimes after a long period (months or years). Generally, mountants are colorless and completely miscible with the dehydrant or clearing agent.

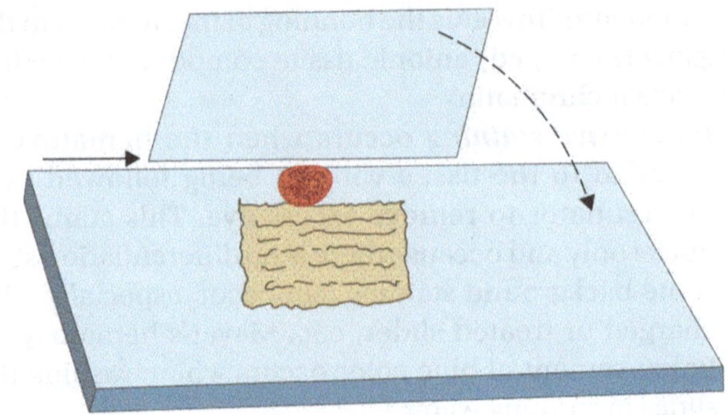

FIG. 1: Method of mounting.

***Appendix 3** gives the composition of the various hematoxylins and their preparation techniques.*

CONCLUSION

Hematoxylin and eosin stain has been used for decades for the recognition of various tissue types and the morphologic changes that form the basis of contemporary disease diagnosis. The stain has not been replaced over years because it works well with several fixatives and displays both cytoplasmic and nuclear detail. Hematoxylin stains nucleic acids a deep blue-purple color and eosin stains the cytoplasm a contrasting pink. Extracellular components and nucleoli stain varying shades of pink. The stain is ideal in the diagnosis of malignant cells due to its characteristics of staining the nucleus.

REFERENCES

1. Shariff S. Laboratory Techniques in Surgical Pathology. Bengaluru: Prism Books Pvt Ltd.; 1999.
2. Lynch MJ, Raphael SS. Lynch's Medical Laboratory Technology, 3rd edition. Philadelphia: WB Saunders Company; 1976.
3. Bancroft JD, Gamble M. Theory and Practice of Histological Techniques, 5th edition. London: Churchill Livingstone; 2002.
4. Lillie RD, Fullmer HM. Histopathologic Technique and Practical Histochemistry. New York: McGraw-Hill; 1976. p. 31.
5. Leica Biosystems Knowledge Pathway. [online] Available from www.leicabiosystems.com [Last accessed March, 2024].
6. Kumar GL, Kiernan JA. (2010). Education Guide: Special Stains and H&E, 2nd edition. [online] Available from https://www.agilent.com/cs/library/technicaloverviews/public/08066_special_stains_eduguide.pdf [Last accessed March, 2024].
7. Prophet EB, Mills B, Arrington JB, Sobin LH (Eds). Armed Forces Institute of Pathology: Laboratory Manual of the Armed Forces. Washington DC: Armed Forces Institute of Pathology, American Registry of Pathology; 1994.

CHAPTER 20

Special Stains

INTRODUCTION

Special stains performed in the laboratory are the histochemical and immunohistochemical reactions which help to identify tissues and tissue antigens respectively, which may not be clear by the routine hematoxylin and eosin (H&E) stains. These special stains will be dealt with here.

HISTOCHEMICAL REACTIONS

Histochemical reactions are a result of ionic interaction between groups of opposite charges in tissues; the result of a colored interactive product; and precipitation of salts of a metal like silver from a solution, such as methenamine silver solution.

Special stains for the following substances in histochemistry will be covered:

- For epithelial mucins and glycogen
- Connective tissue stains
- Varied silver stains apart from those for connective tissue
- Stains for microorganisms—bacteria and fungi
- Pigment stains, stains for minerals, etc.

STAINS FOR MUCINS AND MUCOSUBSTANCES[1]

Mucins in simple terms are secretions of epithelial cells of the gastrointestinal (GI) tract, respiratory tract, and female genital tract. They are composed of a central protein core with several attached chains of carbohydrates or polysaccharides. The latter may account for 60–80% of the molecular weight of the molecule. The protein core consists of amino acids serine and threonine. A structurally distinct feature of mucins is the presence of tandem repeats of specific amino acid sequences within the protein molecules, based on which mucins are categorized into distinct families (MUC1, MUC2, MUC3, etc.), depending upon differences in the sequence and size of the tandem repeats. There are several other glycoprotein molecules that share structural similarities with the mucins and often are confused with mucins, e.g., proteoglycans which are high molecular weight glycoconjugate complexes that are found in high concentrations within the extracellular matrix and connective tissues. In older literature, these proteoglycans were referred to as connective tissue mucins. However, the structure, (particularly the protein core of the proteoglycans), is different and distinct from that of mucins.

Epithelial Mucins[2]

Epithelial mucins are characterized based on the chemistry and composition of the carbohydrate component of the mucin. The charged or "acid" mucins contain carbohydrates with carboxylate (COO-) or -sulfonate (SO_3) groups, i.e., they are negatively charged. The acid mucins are found widely distributed throughout the GI and respiratory tract. They are composed of three estimable fractions—the carboxylated mucosubstances, the weakly sulfated mucosubstances, and the strongly sulfated mucosubstances. They are composed of *hexosamine and acid groups*—glucuronic acid, iduronic acid, or sialic acid, identifiable at pH 2.8 and under. All of these acid mucins are Alcian blue (AB) positive.

The neutral mucins lack acidic groups and thus carry no charge, they consist of *hexosamine* and *hexose units* and *lack free acid groups*, (they are identifiable at pH 5 and over). The neutral mucins are found in the surface epithelia of the stomach, Brunner's glands of the duodenum, and the prostatic epithelium. They are periodic acid–Schiff

(PAS) reaction positive and Alcian blue negative. *The histochemical reactivity of mucins is dependent largely upon the carbohydrate composition of the mucins.*

Identification of Different Types of Mucosubstances[1-4]

Sometimes it becomes necessary in day-to-day practice to identify precisely the type of mucosubstances being secreted by a particular type of epithelium or even a neoplasm. For instance, pleural mesotheliomas are chiefly identified by their capacity to secrete acid mucosubstances, chiefly sulfated and sometimes nonsulfated in types; whereas, adenocarcinomas are known to secrete neutral mucosubstances. The types of intestinal metaplasia in the stomach which is associated with the secretion of sulfomucosubstances predisposes to malignancy. In the cervical epithelium, the presence of sialic acid has been thought to increase the viscosity of mucus. Also, normal cervical mucosa secretes chiefly neutral mucins but cervical carcinoma is associated with the secretion of acid mucins. This is also the case in the prostate.

The single universal stain for mucosubstances irrespective of whether these are neutral or acidic is the *mucicarmine stain.* (Its propensity to stain acid mucins is supposed to be better than neutral mucin.) The PAS tests neutral mucosubstances chiefly, and the Alcian blue tests the acid mucosubstances at pH 2.8. The Alcian blue may be used at different molarities too with the addition of varying quantities of magnesium chloride, to estimate the amount of carboxylated, weakly sulfated, and strongly sulfated acid mucosubstances.

Mucicarmine Stain

Introduction

Carmine was first extracted for use in 1849 from cochineal insects, and the active form was carminic acid, a natural dye. This was extensively used in the past in the staining of mucins but presently has been overtaken by other stains. Its main application was in the identification of signet ring cell carcinoma of the stomach. The technique is still widely popular in demonstrating the capsule of the fungus *Cryptococcus neoformans*.

Indications

- Stains all epithelial mucins both normal and in neoplasia.
- Demonstrates very well capsule of the fungus *Cryptococcus neoformans*.

Principle

The active dye molecule in the mucicarmine stain is a chelate complex formed between cationic aluminum ions and carminic acid, the reaction conferring an overall positive charge to the large carmine complex and allowing it to bind to the acid substrates of low density such as mucins by electrostatic attraction (to the anionic groups of acid mucins). Neutral mucins on the other hand demonstrate little or no staining due to a lack of anionic sites while the acid mucins stain strongly.

Control

The small intestine and appendix.

Fixative

For about 10% buffered formalin.

Technique

On 4 μm thick paraffin sections.

Procedure

- Bring solutions to water.
- *Stain nuclei with alum hematoxylin*: 10 minutes
- Wash in running water.
- *Differentiate in 1% acid alcohol*: 5 minutes
- Wash well in tap water
- *Stain with mucicarmine solution*: 20–30 minutes
- Wash in running water
- Bring to mountant and coverslip

Results

- *Mucosubstances*: Pink to red
- *Nuclei*: Blue

Stain Components

- *Carmine (CL 75470) (BDH)*: 1 g
- *Aluminum hydroxide*: 1 g
- *Aluminum chloride*: 0.5 g
- *Ethyl alcohol*: 100 mL
- Dissolve carmine and aluminum hydroxide in ethyl alcohol. Mix by shaking and then add aluminum chloride. Boil for 3 minutes. Cool and make up to 100 mL with the 50% alcohol. Store at plus 4°C.

  The mucicarmine solution usually keeps for 6 months or so at 4°C.

Advantages

- It stains all types of mucosubstances irrespective of their being neutral or acidic in type but has a positive predilection to stain acid mucosubstances.

- To stain mucin secreted by epithelial cells in most intestinal carcinomas.
- Useful in staining encapsulated fungi, e.g., *Cryptococcus.*

Disadvantages

- Rarely used these days for epithelial mucins as Alcian blue and PAS are better.
- Ehrlich's hematoxylin should be avoided as certain mucins will take this stain and consequently not take up the mucicarmine stain.

Alcian Blue Stain

Introduction

Alcian blue is the most popular method for the demonstration of acid mucins. It was introduced by a chemist known as Haddock in 1948; who described its composition as being copper phthalocyanine (CuPc) dye.

Routinely used is Alcian blue 8GX or GS. (ICL, merck, sigma, fluka, and chroma).

Other dyes of importance are:

- Alcian green 2GX stains acid mucin as bright green.
- Alcian green 3BX stains acid mucin as blue-green.
- Alcian yellow stains acid mucin yellow.
- The various types of acid mucins can be categorized into three types as described further.

Carboxylated Mucosubstances

- *Sialomucosubstances (nonsulfated)*: These sialomucins contain a sialic acid moiety which is an acetylated derivative of neuraminic acid. It reacts with Alcian blue at a pH of 2.5 and above. These mucosubstances are:
  - Enzyme labile: Found in goblet cells of peripheral airways of lungs, and intestine, mucous cells of the submandibular salivary gland. They are enzyme labile, i.e., sialidase labile.
  - Hyaluronic acid containing mucosubstances (nonsulfated): Enzyme labile containing hyaluronic acid is found in connective tissue, synovial fluid of joints, and pleural mesotheliomas (enzyme hyaluronidase dissolves this).
  - Enzyme resistant (nonsulfated sialidase and hyaluronidase resistant) is found in gastric pyloric glands and mucous glands of major bronchi.

Weakly Sulfated Acid Mucins

These are sialomucins and are usually epithelial in origin and present in a wide range of cell types and mucous glands, e.g., bronchial submucous glands and in colonic goblet cells. They are PAS positive and stain with Alcian blue at pH 1.0 and above. Sulfated sialomucosubstances are also found in prostatic carcinoma and malignant synovioma.

Strongly Sulfated Acid Mucins

Comprise of chiefly connective tissue mucosubstances, such as chondroitin sulfate, heparan sulfate, and keratan sulfate. They are also found in epithelia such as bronchial mucus glands (sulfomucins) and a minor fraction in the intestinal goblet cells. They are so designated "strongly" because of their ability to stain with Alcian blue at pH levels of 0.5 and below. They are largely PAS-negative.

Indications

In normal tissues, it helps to demonstrate cells containing mucin in order to illustrate the normal histological structure, e.g., glandular elements of organs, such as prostrate and salivary glands. It stains acidic epithelial mucins such as sialomucins and sulfomucins of the large intestine. It stains proteoglycans/hyaluronic acid components of connective tissue and cartilage. Cervical epithelium in malignancy secretes sialic acid.

In diseases is useful to identify types of mucin so as to assist in the histological diagnosis of certain neoplasms or otherwise:

- Pleural mesothelioma characterized by its production of hyaluronic acid.
- Intestinal metaplasia in the stomach predisposing to malignancy secretes sialo and sulfomucosubstances (Alcian blue positive); in contrast neutral mucins of gastric mucosa and Brunner's glands are not reactive with the Alcian blue.
- All myxoid stromal tumors show positive staining with Alcian blue, therefore, it is useful in identifying mucin-secreting degenerating tumors, e.g., myxomas and neurofibromas.
- It is helpful in the diagnosis of mucin-secreting tumors, such as ovarian tumors and low-grade appendiceal mucinous neoplasms (LAMNs).
- Staining of mucin may be useful in autoimmune diseases and hereditary diseases like discoid lupus erythromatosus (subcutaneous tissue); it can be used to demonstrate myxoid degeneration in the dermis in myxedema; in Hurler's disease, hereditary arthro-osteochondrodysplasia, osteogenesis imperfect, etc.

Principle

The standard Alcian blue stain at pH 2.5 stains all acidic mucins. All acidic mucins whether carboxylated or sulfated will ionize at a pH of 2.5 to produce anionic groups (COO and SO_3). These tissue polyanions form electrostatic bonds with the positively charged (cationic dyes) resulting in alcianophilia. The specificity of Alcian blue is partly due to its large molecular size thus staining acidic substrates of low density.

Control

The small intestine, appendix, or colon (large intestine contains sulfomucins which are more strongly acidic as compared to sialomucins of the small intestine).

Fixative

For about 10% neutral buffered formalin, Bouin's solution.

Technique

The technique includes 4 μm paraffin sections.

Procedure

- Bring sections to water.
- Stain with Alcian blue solution to the required depth of staining for 5–10 minutes.
- Wash in tap water.
- Counterstain with an alum hematoxylin for 5 minutes or nuclear fast red (Kernechtrot) for a few seconds as a nuclear stain. [Makeup nuclear fast red (Merch; BDH) using 0.1 g in 100 mL of 5% solution of aluminum sulfate with the aid of heat. Cool, filter, and add one crystal of thymol.]
- Wash in tap water.
- Bring to the mountain and coverslip.

Result (Fig. 1)

- *Acidic mucosubstances*: Light blue to dark midnight blue
- *Nuclei*: Hematoxylin—blue purple
- Nuclear fast red—red

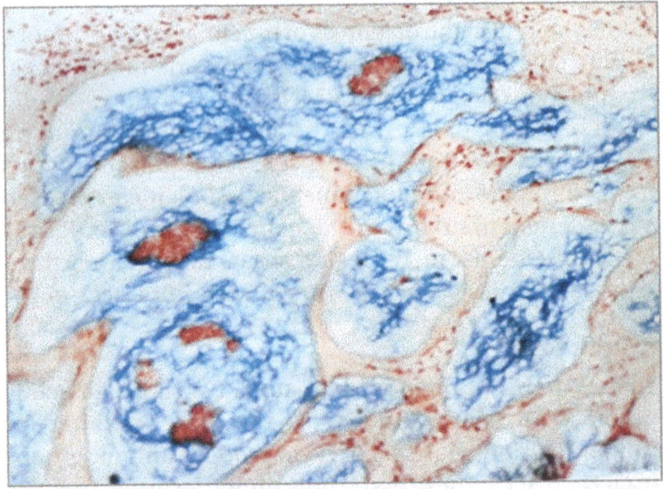

FIG. 1: Bright blue stain of extracellular acid mucin. Alcian blue stain ×100.

Stain Components

- *Alcian blue (8GX) powder*: 1 g
- *3% acetic acid*: 100 mL

Advantages

Even prolonged exposure to stain at pH 2.8 will not "force" other substances to be stained by this stain.

Disadvantages

- If an alum hematoxylin is used for an excessive period of time, this stain may obscure the blue tinge of the Alcian blue.
- Alcian blue is carcinogenic.

Alcian Blue with Varying Electrolytic Concentration

Introduction and Indications

- Separates out carboxylated and weakly and strongly sulfated acid mucins.
- Useful method for separating the acid mucins in order to detect only carboxylated acid mucins as hyaluronic acid in malignant mesotheliomas and nonsulfated or sulfated sialomucins as in intestinal metaplasia or colonic carcinoma.

Principle

Critical electrolyte concentration (CEC) is the point at which the amount of an electrolyte such as magnesium chloride in Alcian blue solutions is sufficient to prevent staining with Alcian blue **(Table 1)**. This is due to the successful competition of electrolyte cations of the salt with dye cations for binding sites on tissue polyanions.

Make Alcian blue solution as detailed earlier, then add magnesium chloride in the quantities given below per 100 mL prepared Alcian blue solution.

TABLE 1: Shows varying strength of magnesium chloride added to get Alcian blue stain at varying electrolyte concentration.

Molarity	Magnesium chloride	Substances tested
0.06 M	1.2 g	Carboxylated and weakly sulfated mucosubstances
0.3M	6.10 g	Weakly and strongly sulfated mucosubstances
0.5 M	10.15 g	Strongly sulfated mucosubstances
0.7 M	14.20 g	Strongly sulfated mucosubstances
0.9 M	18.30 g	Strongly sulfated mucosubstances and keratan sulfate

Control

This is the same as for the method of Alcian blue staining.

Fixative

For about 10% formalin/10% buffered neutral formalin.

Technique

This includes routine paraffin-embedded tissue.

Procedure

- Dewax sections and bring sections to water.
- Stain in various molarities of Alcian blue solution overnight at room temperature.
- Wash in water and counterstain in 0.5% aqueous neutral red, for 2–3 minutes.
- Rinse in absolute alcohol.
- Clear in xylene and mount as desired.

Results

Staining with Alcian blue will be retained or lost according to the type of acid mucin present (see last column in **Table 1**).

Advantages

- Simple to perform.
- Helps to identify various components of acid mucins.

Disadvantages

Weighing of magnesium chloride should be accurate for optimal results.

The Periodic Acid–Schiff's Reaction (Schiff's Leucofuchsin)

Introduction

The PAS technique is the most versatile and widely used of the techniques for the demonstration of mucins, glycoproteins, and carbohydrates. It stains both acid and neutral mucins. The reactivity of the PAS technique is not based on the presence of acidic groups but instead on the structure of the monosaccharide units. It has varied applications in the demonstration of carbohydrate moieties throughout the body in health and disease.

Indications

The salient ones are as follows:

- To demonstrate glycogen, neutral mucosubstances, basement membranes of skin pigments; such as lipofuscin; lipids such as cerebrosides; fungi such as *Candida albicans*, *Histoplasma capsulatum*, *Cryptococcus*, and *Blastomycosis;* actinomycosis and bacteria, macrophages with organisms in Whipple's disease and Russell bodies.
- Glomerular basement membranes
- Intracytoplasmic globules in hepatocytes in $\alpha 1$ antitrypsin deficiency.
- Trophoblasts in the placenta and β cells in the pituitary.
- It is also useful in lysosomal storage disorders such as Neimann's Pick disease, Gaucher's disease, and glycogen demonstration in glycogen storage disorders.
- To differentiate between myeloblasts and lymphoblasts, in the diagnosis of acute lymphoblastic leukemia (ALL) (block staining) and acute erythroid leukemia (AML)-M6.
- Amyloid, cartilage matrix, colloid, corpora amylacea, and ocular lens material.
- *Glycolipids*: Gangliosides, mainly gray matter composed of fatty acids, i.e., cerebrosides and globoid cells of Krabbe's disease.
- *Adenocarcinoma*: PAS and mucicarmine are used to identify mucin-producing tumors, e.g., salivary and pancreatic tumors.

Principle

The principle is to release the dialdehydes from carbohydrates by oxidation with periodic acid and the subsequent combination of such aldehydes with "Schiff" reagent to give a substitute dye which is red in color (this dye is not basic fuchsine) but localized to the site of the aldehyde release.

Control

Use skin, aorta, or normal liver for positive PAS staining.

Fixative

For about 10% neutral buffered formalin is preferred; 10% formalin.

Technique

On paraffin sections 4–5 µm.

Procedure

- Bring sections to water.
- Rinse in distilled water.
- Oxidize with 1% periodic acid for 5 minutes.
- Rinse in distilled water.
- Use Schiff's reagent for 10 minutes.
- Sulfite rinse (optional) (two rinses; 1 minute each)
- Wash in tap water for 10 minutes; this intensifies the color reaction.
- Stain the nuclei with alum hematoxylin for 5 minutes.
- Wash in tap water.
- Bring to mountant.

Note:
- The tap water wash at step 7 is necessary to develop the positive red color. Within limits, the longer the wash the darker the color.
- Originally, it was recommended that the Schiff's reagent be washed off with dilute sulfurous acid (the sulfite rinses). Since water recolors Schiff's reagent, it was believed that a water wash could lead to false positive results. It is now known this is not the case, provided the Schiff's reagent is removed quickly and the sections do not stay in the water (contaminated with it) for extended periods.

Results (Fig. 2)

- *PAS-positive material*: Magenta pink to red
- *Nuclei*: Blue

Stain Components

- The periodic acid 1% solution
- *Periodic acid*: 1 g
- *Distilled water*: 100 mL

Periodic acid is the most common substance to be used for oxidation. One of its superior properties is that it will not further oxidize the resulting aldehyde. Thus, standardization is easier; however, four important rules must be observed when periodic acid is used:

1. Oxidation time must be limited to a maximum of 10 minutes.
2. Oxidation should not be carried out at >20°C.
3. The periodic acid solution should have a pH of 3–5.
4. Prepared solutions must be kept at 4°C in a refrigerator.

Schiff' Reagent

Basic fuchsin (pronounced as fook-sin) when treated with sulfurous acid results in a colorless product called *Schiff's reagent*. Basic fuchsin is not a pure dye and consists principally of pararosaniline and magenta II. Pararosaniline is present in combination with acetone or chloride and is consequently unstable. For this reason, when basic fuchsin is treated with sulfurous acid it forms the Schiff's reagent. This substance in combination with two aldehyde molecules produces a reddish-purple complex. This color is not due to basic fuchsin and may vary in intensity depending on the various aldehydes present in the tissue examined.

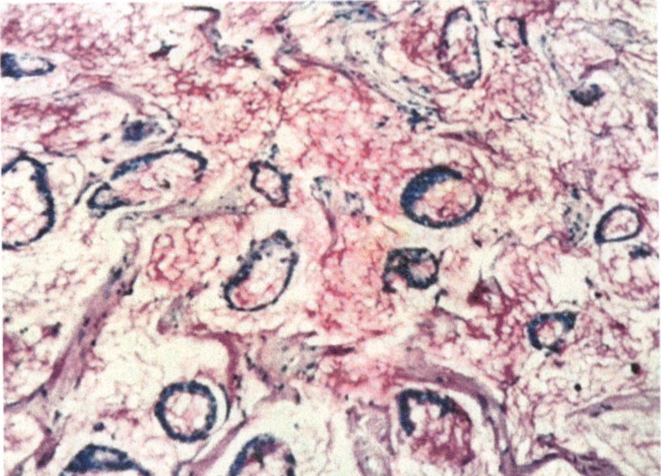

FIG. 2: Periodic acid-Schiff (PAS) positivity in colloid carcinoma. Cells are immersed in pools of mucin. PAS-positive ×100.

- *Basic fuchsin*: 1 g
- *N. hydrochloric acid*: 20 mL
- *Sodium metabisulfite*: 1 g
- *Activated charcoal*: 2 g
- *Distilled water*: 200 mL

Boil the distilled water. Allow to cool to 80°C, add basic fuchsin. Filter at 50°C and add hydrochloric acid. At 25°C, add sodium metabisulfite. Store in the dark for 48 hours. Add activated charcoal. Shake for 1 minute. Now, filter it. This filtrate should be clear.

(Sodium metabisulfite in the presence of HCl releases sulfurous acid with resultant SO_2 which in turn reacts with basic fuchsin to form Schiff's reagent.) The activated charcoal absorbs the excess sulfurous acid.

Testing for the Activity of Schiff's Reagent

- Pour a few drops of Schiff's reagent into 10 mL of concentrated formalin. If the reagent is active, the solution turns reddish pink rapidly. If the blue color develops after some time, the solution is breaking down.
- *Sulfite rinse*: Rinse should be prepared fresh each day.
- Sodium metabisulfite, 0.5% aqueous.

Advantages

Widely used in all techniques for the demonstration of glycoproteins, carbohydrates, and mucins (neutral mucins).

Disadvantages

- The temperature for oxidants to act should not exceed 25°C as it is likely to oxidize other substances besides aldehydes.
- *Safety*: Basic fuchsin (in Schiff's reagent) is a known carcinogen. It is advisable to wear gloves, goggles, particle masks, and laboratory coats while preparing the solution. Avoid contact and inhalation of hydrochloric acid as it is a strong irritant to the skin, eyes, and respiratory system.
- *The two most important rules for the preservation of Schiff's reagent are*:
  i. A deep brown-black bottle to prevent oxidation from taking place. (If the solution should ever turn pink, discard it).
  ii. A 4°C temperature.

Combined Alcian Blue–Periodic Acid-Schiff Reaction

Introduction

The combination of the Alcian blue and the PAS techniques is used to distinguish neutral mucins from acid mucins. In most protocols, sections are stained with the standard Alcian blue (pH 2.5) method followed by the PAS technique. The Alcian blue at a pH of 2.5 will stain all acid mucins a deep blue. The subsequent application of the PAS technique will stain the neutral mucins bright magenta against the blue acid mucins. Tissues or cells that contain both neutral and acidic mucins may demonstrate a purple coloration.

Indications

Some substances may require the demonstration of both acidic and neutral mucosubstances at the same time in the very same section. The best example of this is to detection of intestinal metaplasia in gastric biopsies. The metaplastic epithelium takes on a blue-purple hue in contrast to gastric mucosa which stains magenta pink. Therefore, it is routinely used in GI biopsies.

In carcinomas of the cervix and prostate, the neoplasms secrete acidic mucins and the normal epithelium secretes neutral mucins.

Principle

See individual stain.

Control

Intestinal metaplasia in gastric mucosa is a known case.

Fixative

For about 10% neutral buffered formalin; 10% formalin.

Technique

On paraffin sections 4–5 μm thick.

Procedure

- Bring sections to water.
- *Stain with Alcian blue solution*: 5 minutes.
- Wash in tap water.
- *Oxidize with 1.0% periodic acid*: 5 minutes.
- Wash in distilled water.
- *Use Schiff's reagent*: 8 minutes.
- *Wash in tap water*: 10 minutes
- Bring to mountant.
- If a nuclear stain is required, this may be used after stage 7.
- Use alum hematoxylin for 3 minutes or nuclear fast red for a few seconds.

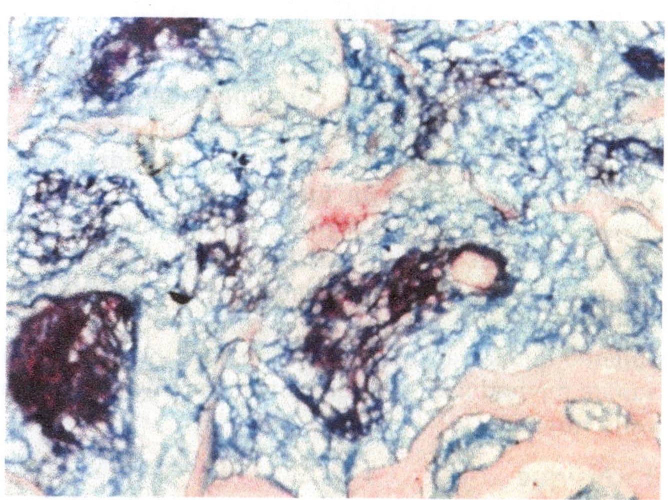

FIG. 3: Acid mucins are blue, purple color indicates a combination of acid and neutral mucins.

Results (Fig. 3)

- *Acid mucosubstances*: Blue
- *Neutral polysaccharides*: Magenta pink to red.
- *Mixture of acid and neutral mucosubstances*: Purple
- *Nuclei*: Red (nuclear fast red) and blue (alum hematoxylin)

Stain Components

- Alcian blue (CI 74240) 1 g; 3% acetic acid 100 mL
- 0.5–1% periodic acid (see PAS technique)
- Schiff's reagent
- Alum hematoxylin

Gomori's Aldehyde-fuchsin Stain for Sulfated Mucins

Introduction

Sulfated acid mucosubstances can be identified from nonsulfated acid mucosubstances by the following methods:

- Gomori's aldehyde-fuchsin method
- High iron diamine (HID) technique
- Aluminum sulfate method and Alcian blue with varying electrolyte concentrations

Indications

To detect sulfated acid mucosubstances.

Principle

The aldehyde-fuchsin stain has a great affinity for sulfated mucosubstances. An initial oxidation occurs followed by a variable time in a solution consisting of basic fuchsin, concentrated hydrochloric acid, and paraldehyde for the reaction to occur.

The value of aldehyde fuchsin in identifying mucins is greatly increased when aldehyde fuchsin and Alcian blue are combined. This combined technique will give color separation of sulfated and nonsulfated acid mucosubstances. The differentiation depends on the greater affinity of aldehyde fuchsins for sulfated groups than for carboxyl groups as prior staining with aldehyde groups blocks the sulfated mucosubstances and subsequently staining with Alcian blue demonstrates the carboxylated acid mucosubstances. The other stains for sulfated mucins are the HID technique; the aluminum sulfate method and Alcian blue with varying electrolyte concentrations.

Technique

On 5 μm thick paraffin sections.

Fixation

Routine formalin fixation.

Control

Normal segment of colon (sigmoid region of middle and lower crypt).

Procedure

- Deparaffinize sections and take down to 70% alcohol.
- Stain with aldehyde fuchsin for 20 minutes.
- Rinse well in 70% of alcohol, then in water.
- Stain with Alcian blue for 5 minutes.
- Wash, dehydrate, clear, and mount.

Results (Fig. 4)

- *Strongly sulfated mucins*: Deep purple
- *Weakly sulfated mucins*: Purple
- *Nonsulfated acid mucins*: Blue

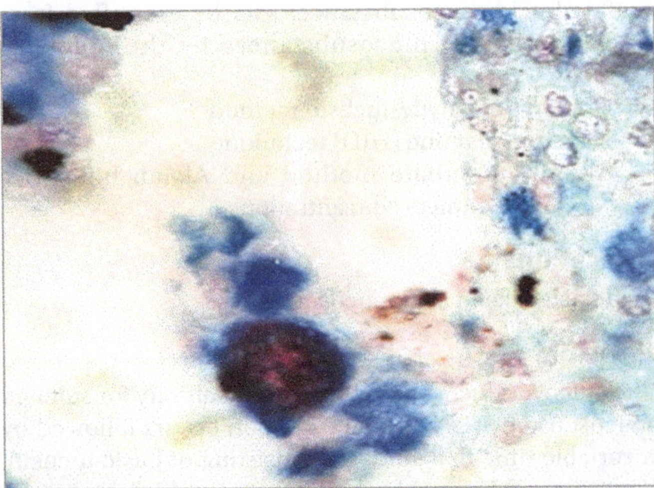

FIG. 4: Strongly sulfated intracellular mucin stains purple against nonsulfated acid mucins (blue). Gomori aldehyde fuchsin (GAF) ×100.

Stain Components

Gomori's aldehyde fuchsin solution.

Formula

- Dissolve 1 g of basic fuchsin in 100 mL of 60% alcohol.
- Add 1 mL of concentrated hydrochloric acid and then 2 mL of paraldehyde (use fresh paraldehyde solution)
- Allow to "ripen" by standing for at least 2 days at room temperature (solution develops a blue color) and store at 4°C.
- Alcian blue solution
- 1% Alcian blue in 3% of glacial acetic acid.

High Iron Diamine

Introduction

Aluminum sulfate demonstrates only sulfated mucins and is a confirmatory technique for the presence of this group of acid mucins.

Principle

High iron diamine is currently the standard method for detecting highly acidic sulfated mucins. A mixture of diamine salt is oxidized to form a black cationic chromogen, which bonds with sulfate ester groups. By counterstaining with Alcian blue, a clear color distinction is made between the groups of acidic mucins (sulfated from carboxylated mucins).

Indications

This specifically detects highly acidic sulfated mucins.

Control

Normal segment of colon (sigmoid region of middle and lower crypt).

Fixative

For about 10% buffered neutral formalin; 10% formalin.

Procedure

- Deparaffinize and bring sections to distilled water.
- Treat section in HID solution for 18–24 hours.
- Wash well with water.
- Stain with Alcian blue solution for 5 minutes.
- Wash in water.
- Stain nuclei with neutral red for 2–3 minutes.
- Wash, dehydrate, clear, and mount.

Results (Fig. 5)

- *Sulfated mucins*: Black-brown
- *Carboxylated mucins*: Blue
- *Nuclei*: Red

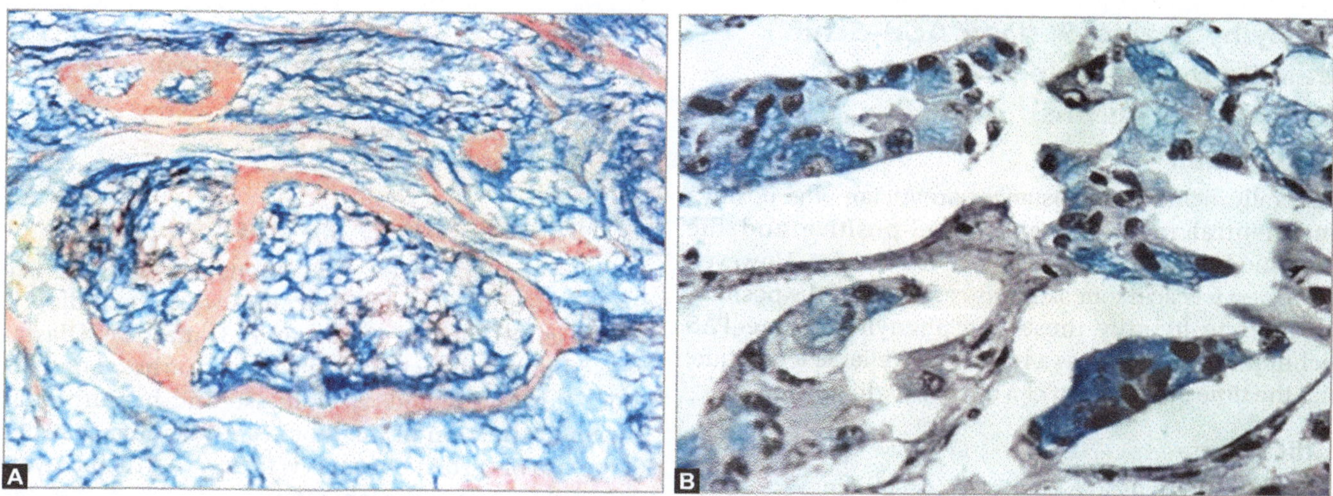

FIGS. 5A AND B: Extracellular (left) and intracellular (right) black-brown stain of sulfated mucins. The blue stains show carboxylated mucin. High iron diamine (HID) ×100 and 400 respectively.

Stain Components

HID Solution

- *N,N dimethyl-meta-phenylenediamine dihydrochloride*: 120 mg
- *N,N dimethyl-para-phenylenediamine dihydrochloride*: 20 mg
- *Distilled water*: 50 mL
- *Ferric chloride (60% solution)*: 1.4 mL

Dissolve the two diamine salts simultaneously in the distilled water then add the ferric chloride solution.

- *Nuclear stain*: 0.5% neutral red
- Alcian blue solution (as mentioned earlier)

Aluminum Sulfate Method

Introduction

Aluminum sulfate demonstrates only sulfated mucins and is a confirmatory technique for the presence of this group of acid mucins.

Principle

A 0-03% solution of basic dye (nuclear fast red, methylene blue) in 5% aluminum sulfate produces a highly specific staining reaction for sulfated mucopolysaccharides. This is a highly specific method of staining sulfated mucopolysaccharides and is due to the attachment of the metallic ion (aluminum) to the dye on one side and the tissue on the other as a result of the electrostatic charge.

Control

Normal segment of colon (sigmoid region of middle and lower crypt).

Fixative

For about 10% buffered neutral formalin.

Technique

On paraffin sections.

Procedure

- Dewax and hydrate sections.
- Stain in above diluted solutions, 5–30 minutes.
- Rinse in water.
- Differentiate in 70% alcohol till the tissue background is colorless (usually 20–30 seconds).
- Dehydrate in graded alcohols.
- Clear in xylene.
- Mount in polystyrene or other mounting media.

Results

- *Sulfated mucins*: Blue
- *Nonsulfated mucins and nuclei*: Red
- A mixture of sulfated and nonsulfated acid mucins tends to stain a purple color

Stain Components

For about 0–1% stock solutions of the various dyes are prepared by dissolving the requisite amount of the dye in boiling 5% aluminum sulfate, filtering, and cooling. This stock solution is further diluted to 1 in 3 with a cool 5% aluminum sulfate solution. Aqueous solutions of the dyes are also prepared in a similar fashion and diluted with water before use.

Phenylhydrazine–Periodic Acid–Schiff Stain (to Detect Periodic Acid–Schiff Positive Acid Mucins)

Introduction

Generally, acid mucosubstances are Alcian blue positive and neutral mucosubstances PAS-positive and the combined AB-PAS reaction detects both these. However, at times, a few acid mucosubstances are also PAS-positive. In order to identify these, the phenylhydrazine–PAS technique is used. This is a reasonably reliable technique, and the time of treatment can be safely adhered to.

Indications

To specifically detect PAS-positive acid mucins.

Fixation

Routine

Principle

Phenylhydrazine condenses preferentially with periodate-treated aldehydic groups of neutral mucosubstances alone, thus blocking any further subsequent reaction with Schiff's reagent. The PAS positivity of the acid mucosubstances is unchanged.

Technique

Paraffin-embedded sections.

Procedure

- Deparaffinize sections and take them down to distilled water.
- Treat all sections (test and controls) with a periodic acid solution for 2 minutes.
- Wash well in distilled water.
- Treat the test and control sections with the phenylhydrazine solution for 1 hour (at room temperature) and the negative control sections with distilled water for the same period of time.
- Wash well in distilled water then treat all sections with Schiff's reagent for 8 minutes.
- Wash in running tap water for approximately 10 minutes followed by nuclear staining with hematoxylin in the conventional manner.
- Dehydrate, clear, and mount in either a natural or synthetic resin.

Results

- *Neutral mucins*: Negative
- *Acid mucins*: Magenta

Stain Components

1% aqueous periodic acid; 5% aqueous phenylhydrazine hydrochloride

Formula

The formula for 5% aqueous phenylhydrazine hydrochloride:

- *Phenylhydrazine hydrochloride*: 5 g
- *Distilled water*: 95 mL

Enzyme-digestion Methods

There are chiefly three types of enzymes that are used for mucosubstances identification work, including (1) sialidase, (2) hyaluronidase, and (3) diastase. Diastase is used in the detection of glycogen. Carboxylated acid mucins are detected by sialidase and hyaluronidase enzyme extraction of the mucins. A potential drawback to the use of certain enzymes is their cost which prevents their routine use in the laboratory.

Sialidase or neuraminidase extracted from the vibrio cholera group of organisms or clostridium digests sialomucosubstances. The digestion is followed by staining with Alcian blue to know whether or not digestion has occurred. Should digestion be followed with the combined Alcian blue-PAS techniques, it is seen that the sialidase-labile mucosubstances lose their Alcian blue reactivity and give a positive PAS reaction instead, that is they change their staining result from blue to magenta. A few sialic acid-containing mucosubstances are not digested by sialidase. In such substances, if sialidase digestion is preceded by deacetylation the sialidase resistant sialomucosubstances are rendered labile to the enzyme.

The commonly used hyaluronidase is bovine testicular in origin which digests in addition to hyaluronic acid and chondroitin sulfate A and C. The digestion procedure is followed by Alcian blue staining. hyaluronidase digestion has applications in confirming the presence of malignant mesothelioma which secretes hyaluronic acid.

Use of Metachromasia in Mucin Stains

Both sulfated and carboxylated mucins are metachromatic. Dyes used to demonstrate metachromasia include toluidine blue, thionine, azure A, safranin, and Bismarck brown.

Glycogen

Introduction

Glycogen is a polymer of glucose. It is an important storage carbohydrate in man and its presence is frequently tested for in cells like the hepatocytes. As it is rapidly broken down after the death of tissue, rapid fixation after removal at biopsy is necessary to demonstrate it. It is soluble in water and insoluble in alcohol. In the process of fixation and gradual penetration of fixative, aggregates of glycogen are seen in only certain areas of the cell giving a stream-like effect to the section (of a liver) called "streaming artifact."

This usually cannot be avoided. Formal saline fixation proves adequate as formalin tends to bind glycogen to protein, thus retaining it to a certain extent; fixation in ethyl alcohol is also known to preserve glycogen better.

PAS with Diastase Method (for Removal of Glycogen)

Indications

- Glycogen (PAS-D) is positive in Ewing's sarcoma while it is negative in lymphomas.
- It is tested for in the liver in glycogen storage disorders.
- In detecting fungi such as *Aspergillus* and bacteria, such as actinomycosis.

Principle

Glycogen can be selectively removed by digestion with specific enzymes, e.g., Malt diastase which causes the loss of PAS reactivity. The diastase (or amylase) acts on glycogen to depolymerize it into smaller sugar units (maltose and glucose), that are washed out of the section.

Control

Liver section

Common Fixatives

They have no inhibitory effect on diastase action.

Technique

On 5 µm thick paraffin sections.

Procedure

- Bring sections on two separate slides to water.
- Treat one (suitably marked) with 0.1% malt diastase in distilled water for 30 minutes. Alternatively, saliva can be used as it contains sufficient diastase to digest glycogen.
- Wash in running tap water.
- Stain the untreated section (control) and the treated section (test) with the PAS reaction.

Result

If glycogen is present, the diastase-treated section will not stain with the PAS reaction. On the other hand, the untreated section (control) will stain positively. If both do not stain it would mean glycogen is not present. If both do stain, the positivity of the reaction is due to mucosubstances not digestible by diastase.

- *Glycogen*: Negative
- *Nuclei*: Blue

Best Carmine Technique for Glycogen (Best, 1906)

Indication

This is a highly selective stain for glycogen.

Principle

This staining technique demonstrates glycogen by hydrogen bond formation between OH groups on the glycogen, and hydrogen atoms of the carminic acid. Fibrin, mast cell granules, and neutral mucin stain weakly with this method.

Control

Liver

Fixation

Fixed in 10% neutral buffered formalin.

Technique

Standard paraffin-embedded sections.

Procedure

- Dewax test + positive control sections and rinse in 100% alcohol then 80% alcohol
- Duplicate sections may be treated with diastase if desired.
- Stain nuclei of all sections well using one of the iron hematoxylin solutions, e.g., Weigert's iron hematoxylin.
- Treat with carmine solution for 10 minutes.
- Transfer slides quickly to a Coplin jar of differentiating (Best's) solution.
- Wash in alcohol (not water), clear, and mount.

Results

- *Glycogen*: Bright red
- *Neutral mucin, mast cells, and fibrin*: Weak red
- *Nuclei*: Blue

Stain Components

- *Carmine stock*: 60 mL distilled H_2O + 2 g carmine (CI 75470), 1 g potassium carbonate, 5 g potassium chloride. Boil gently in a large conical flask for 5 minutes. Cool, filter, and add 20 mL of concentrated ammonia water. Allow it to ripen at room temperature for 24 hours. Store in a dark container at 4°C. This will keep 1–2 months.
- *Carmine working solution (make fresh each time)*:
    - Stock solution of 15 mL
    - Ammonia concentrated solution 12.5 mL
    - Methanol 12.5 mL (staining time to be increased as stock solution ages).

- *Best's differentiator*:
  - Methanol: 40 mL
  - Ethanol: 80 mL
  - Distilled water: 100 mL

Connective Tissue Stains[2-6]

Connective tissue is the tissue that connects, separates, and supports all other types of tissues in the body. It consists of a cellular portion in a surrounding framework of a noncellular substance. The cell types of connective tissue include fibroblasts, mast cells, histiocytes, adipose tissue, reticular cells, osteoblasts, osteocytes, chondroblasts, chondrocytes, and blood-forming cells. The intercellular substance is usually composed of both amorphous (nonsulfated and sulfated mucopolysaccharides) and forms elements, such as collagen fibers, reticular fibers, and elastic fibers.

Collagen fibers are the most common type of intercellular fibers and are found in abundance in most of the tissues of the body. They can be categorized into various types and occur individually as in loose areolar tissue, arranged in an open weave pattern, or as large bundles of fibers clumped to form a structure of tensile strength, e.g., tendons. Viewed under polarized light collagen fibers are birefringent.

Introduction

Collagen of both the mature and immature variety stains varying shades of pink with routine H&E methods. In certain instances, such as neoplasms, it would be necessary to define the collagenous nature of a pink substance that is found interlaced within cellular material. It is for this reason that collagen stains are used, and the most commonly used ones are the van Gieson Stain and the Masson's trichrome stain.

van Gieson Stain

Of all these stains, van Gieson stain is a relatively insensitive stain that stains only mature extruded collagen (does not stain reticulin, i.e., precollagen) and cannot differentiate with great ease from such mature extruded collagen and maturing collagen. It still remains a popular stain as a first line of differentiation between collagen and muscle.

Indications

- Specific for collagen-red by van Gieson and green/blue by Masson's trichrome, depending on the counter stain. Differentiates leiomyoma from fibroma and schwannoma and leiomyosarcoma from fibrosarcoma.
- Peutz-Jeghers polyp, to demonstrate the central core of smooth muscle.
- To demonstrate fibrous stroma of endometrial polyp.
- To show (delineate) the extent of fibrosis in a given tissue.
- To differentiate amyloid from collagen (van Gieson stains amyloid khaki color and collagen as red)
- The van Gieson stains bile a bright green and helps to differentiate hepatocellular carcinoma with intracellular pigment from metastatic adenocarcinoma in the liver with no pigment.
- Van Gieson is used as a counterstain in the Von Kossa stain (mineralized bone black and osteoid red) and Verhoeff's stain (elastic tissue black and background yellow to red)

Principle

Aniline (meaning: Synthetic) dyes (e.g., acid fuchsin) have a strong affinity to adhere to collagen fibers in an acid environment. This affinity is taken advantage of by using these dyes in the various collagen stains.

The van Gieson is a mixture of picric acid and acid fuchsin. It is the simplest method of differential staining of collagen and other connective tissue such as smooth muscle. When using combined solutions of picric acid and acid fuchsin, the small molecules of picric acid penetrate the entire tissue rapidly but are only firmly retained in the close-textured red blood cells and muscle. The larger molecules of fuchsin solution displace the picric acid molecules in the collagen fibers which have larger pores and allow the larger molecules to enter thereby giving a red stain to these.

The acid most commonly used in a stain such as van Gieson, is picric acid which not only provides an acid environment but also acts as a suitable contrast color for noncollagenous stained areas therefore, the combination used in the van Gieson stain is called the picrofuchsin stain. It should be remembered that when such an acid requirement is necessary the nuclear stain, hematoxylin, should be of the "iron" type which will not be affected by the acid environment.

Control

Artery or skin.

Fixation

Fixed in 10% neutral buffered formalin.

Technique

Paraffin sections 5 μm thick

Procedure

- Bring sections to water.
- Rinse in distilled water.
- Stain with Weigert's hematoxylin (freshly prepared) for 10 minutes.

- Wash in distilled water.
- Stain in van Gieson's solution for 1–3 minutes.
- Dehydrate in 95% alcohol.
- Do not use water.
- Clear and mount.

Results (Fig. 6)

- *Collagen*: Red
- *Muscle and other noncollagenous tissue*: Yellow
- *Nuclei*: Dark blue

Stain Components

- Acid fuchsin 1% aqueous solution—2.5 mL
- Picric acid saturated aqueous solution—97.5 mL
- Besides acid fuchsin; other aniline dyes are aniline blue (spirit soluble), aniline blue (water soluble), methyl blue, and indigo carmine.

Advantages

The advantages include ease of performance and simplicity of use.

Disadvantages

- Immature (young) collagen does not stain with van Gieson.
- Iron hematoxylin should be used as the nuclear stain.

Masson's Trichome Stain (Modified Mallory: Masson 1929)

Introduction

The first account of a triple stain was by H Gibbs in 1880 followed by BW Richardson in 1881. It is a more sensitive stain than the van Gieson stain. Masson's trichrome and Mallory's trichrome both not only differentiate between collagen and muscle, particularly smooth muscle but pick up immature collagen too.

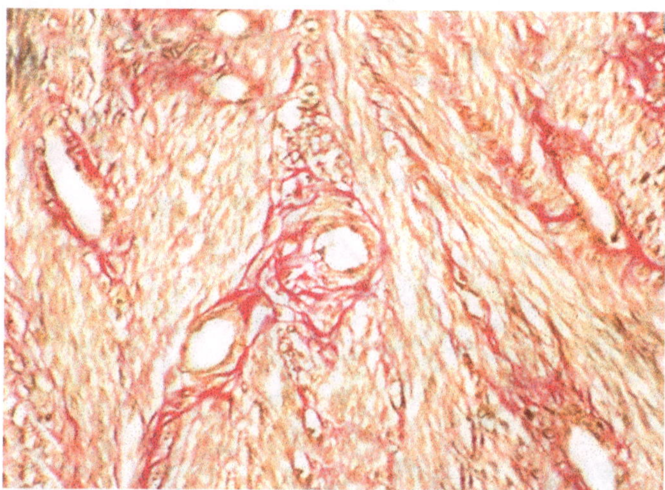

FIG. 6: Collagen stains red and separates sheets of muscle fibers (yellow) in a leiomyoma. Van Gieson ×100.

Indications

The indication is the same as for van Gieson. This has an application in early fibrosis of the liver and single collagen fibers around hepatocytes are picked up.

Principle

As opposed to the van Gieson stain (which is a single unit stain) Masson's trichrome uses a combination of Biebrich scarlet-acid fuchsin. This combination, when used, stains both the collagen and muscle red. With the use of the counterstain which may be either light green or aniline blue, the collagen stains an intense green (with light green) or a shade of blue (with aniline blue). By implication, three dyes are employed (trichrome) one of which is a nuclear stain. The principle in trichome staining is that a smaller dye molecule will penetrate and stain a tissue element (acid fuchsin), but whenever a larger dye molecule (counter stain) can penetrate the same element, the smaller molecule will be replaced by it. Heat influences the penetration of the larger dye molecules. Erythrocyte protein produces a dense network.

With the smallest pores between the protein elements, muscle cells fall next with medium-sized pores, and collagen has the least dense network and is seemingly quite porous (largest pores). The largest dye molecules (aniline and light green) will therefore penetrate only collagen (which is porous), leaving muscle and erythrocytes unstained.

Control

Artery or skin.

Fixation

Fixed in 10% neutral buffered formalin.

Technique

Paraffin sections 5 µm thick; routine fixation.

Procedure

- Bring the solution to water.
- Rinse in distilled water.
- If tissue is fixed in Bouin's or Zenker's solution, proceed to step 4. If not, mordant in Bouin's fixative for 1 hour at 56°C or overnight at room temperature.
- Wash in running water until the yellow color disappears, after which rinse in distilled water.
- Expose to iron hematoxylin solution for 10 minutes.
- Wash in running tap water for 10 minutes and rinse in distilled water.

- Expose to Biebrich scarlet-acid solution for 15 minutes (solution can be reutilized)
- Rinse in distilled water.
- Treat with phosphomolybdic acid-phosphotungstic acid solution for 10–15 minutes.
- Aniline blue solution for 5–10 minutes or light green for 5 minutes.
- Rinse in distilled water.
- Acetic acid solution 1% for 3–5 minutes.
- Dehydrate and mount.

Results (Figs. 7A and B)

- *Collagen (mature)*: Blue or green depends on the counterstain
- *Collagen (newly formed)*: Red
- *Muscle (irrespective of skeletal or smooth)*: Red
- *Keratin; red cells*: Red
- *Nuclei*: Blue

Stain Components

Biebrich Scarlet–Acid Fuchsin Solution

- *Biebrich scarlet aqueous 1%*: 90 mL
- *Acid fuchsin aqueous 1%*: 10 mL
- *Glacial acetic acid*: 1 mL

Phosphomolybdic Acid–Phosphotungstic Acid Solution

- *Phosphomolybdic acid*: 5 g
- *Phosphotungstic acid*: 5 g
- *Distilled water*: 100 mL

Counterstain–Light Green Solution

- *Light green*: 5 g
- *Glacial acetic acid*: 2 mL
- *Distilled water*: 250 mL

Heat water, and dissolve light green. Filter and add the acetic acid.

Counterstain–Aniline Blue Solution

- *Aniline blue*: 2.5 g
- *Acetic acid*: 2 mL
- *Distilled water*: 100 mL

1% Acetic Acid Solution

- *Glacial acetic acid*: 1 mL
- *Distilled water*: 100 mL

Advantages

- It is a better differentiator than van Gieson stain for muscle fibers and collagen.
- Liver biopsies to assess early fibrosis and the degree of fibrosis; to know the stage and progression of the disease in hepatitis B and C viral infections, alcoholic liver disease, chronic biliary disease, and cirrhosis of the liver.
- Routine kidney biopsies.

Elastic Tissue Stains

Introduction and Applications

Elastic fibers are strongly eosinophilic by the H&E stain and when arranged compactly as in the arterial elastic laminae are easily identified due to their refractivity. They differ from collagen by their insolubility in organic and inorganic solvents (collagen is soluble in 2% acetic acid).

Indications for Elastic Stain

- *Malignant hypertension*: To demonstrate hyalinization of blood vessels and reduplication of lamina elastic interna.

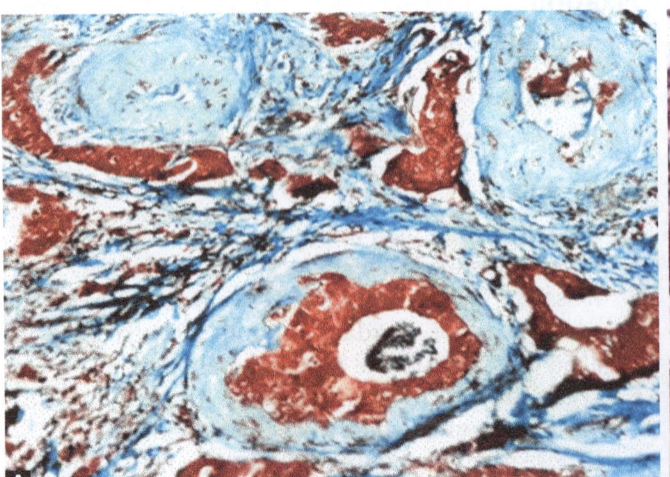

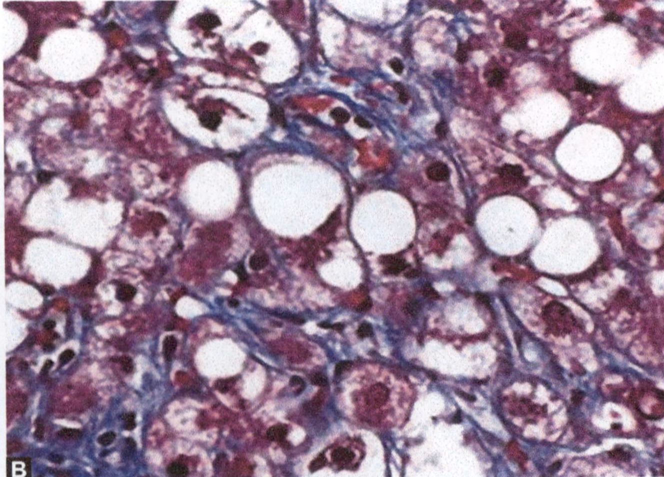

FIGS. 7A AND B: (A) Collars of blue collagen (counter stain aniline blue) around mammary ducts. The rest of the tissue shows red and (B) Section shows blue fibers, collagen type I around hepatocytes, i.e., early fibrosis of a fatty liver picked up by the Masson's trichrome stain.

- *Malignant nephrosclerosis*: The arcuate arteries and other renal blood vessels show reduplication.
- *Arteriovenous malformations*: To demonstrate elastic fibers in the arterial segments.
- *Aneurysms*: To differentiate true and false aneurysms.
- *Breast lesions*: Periductal elastosis in infiltrating carcinoma, central elastosis in radial scar.
- *Skin lesions*: To demonstrate the elastic degeneration of the skin e. Solar elastosis, pseudoxanthoma elasticum, elastofibroma.
- *Marfan's syndrome*: To demonstrate the depletion and fragmentation of the elastic lamina and vascularity of the media and adventitia.
- *Giant cell arteritis*: To show the disruption of elastic lamina.
- In almost all its applications to the staining of vessels as well as elsewhere, the elastic stain is best combined with the van Gieson stain.

Several methods are used for the demonstration of elastic fibers. Some of the popular ones are:

- Verhoeff's method (the most popular method)
- Weigert's resorcin fuchsin
- Gomori's aldehyde fuchsin
- Orcein

The *principle* behind these stains is not well understood.

The *Verhoeff's stain consists of* overstaining of tissues with a combination of iodine–ferric chloride–hematoxylin (Verhoeff's iron hematoxylin) followed by ferric chloride differentiation. Elastic fibers have disulfide bridges, these are connected to anionic sulphonic acid derivatives which combine with basic dyes. The differentiation is accomplished by using excess mordant (2% of ferric chloride) which breaks the tissue mordant dye complex. The dye is attracted to a larger amount of mordant (ferric chloride) in the differentiating solution and is removed from the rest of the tissue. Elastic fibers have a strong affinity for the iron hematoxylin complex formed by the reagents in the stain and will retain the dye longer than other tissue elements that are decolorized.

The technique allows for any fixation, it is easy to prepare, quick to perform, and is most consistent, giving an intense black staining of the coarse elastic fibers, although the inner fibers are less well demonstrated. The results are permanent and show little fading even after several years.

Orcein is a naturally occurring vegetable dye that is now synthesized and stains elastic fibers in an acidic solution. In the resorcin-fuchsin, aldehyde fuchsin, and orcein methods a hydrogen-ion bonding between the stain molecule and the substrate may be responsible for the staining of elastic tissue.

Verhoeff's–van Gieson Stain for Elastic Tissue

Principle

Discussed earlier.

Control

Medium-sized blood vessel.

Fixation

Fixed in 10% neutral buffered formalin.

Technique

Paraffin sections 5 µm, (fix firmly to slide with egg albumin); routine fixation of tissues.

Procedure

- Bring sections from alcohol to distilled water.
- Expose to Verhoeff's elastic tissue for 15 minutes.
- Wash in distilled water.
- Differentiate in 2% ferric chloride—only a few minutes, check under a microscope, and if differentiated too far, restain.
- Place in 5% sodium thiosulfate for 1 minute (removes excess iron).
- Wash in tap water for 5 minutes.
- Counterstain with van Gieson stain for 1–2 minutes.
    - Differentiate in 95% alcohol (does not use water).
    - Clear and mount.

Results (Fig. 8)

- *Elastic fibers*: Blue black to black
- *Nuclei*: Blue to black

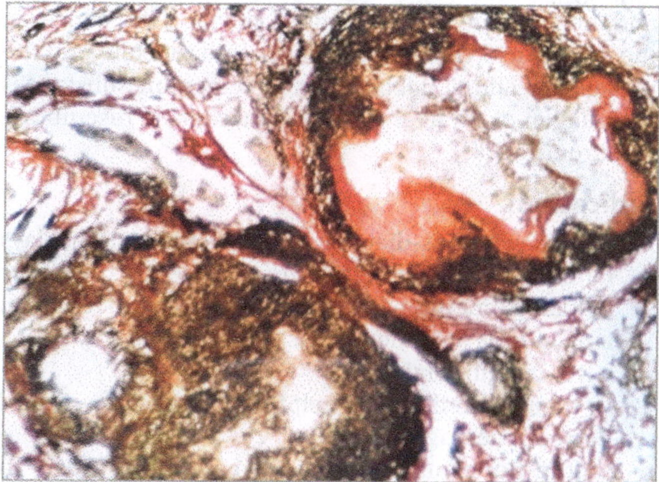

FIG. 8: Dense elastosis as wavy black bundles around ducts in breast carcinoma, collagen stains red. Periductal and stromal elastosis is a known feature in breast carcinoma. Verhoeff-van Gieson ×100 stain.

- *Collagen*: Red
- *Other tissue elements cytoplasm and muscle*: Yellow

Stain Components

Elastic Tissue Stain

Dissolve 1 g of hematoxylin in 22 mL of absolute alcohol on an open dish on a hot plate. Cool, filter, and add 8 mL of a 10% aqueous solution of ferric chloride and 8 mL of iodine solution (2 g of iodine plus 4 g of potassium iodide dissolved in 100 mL of distilled water).

For better results, make up fresh solutions just before use.

Ferric Chloride Solution

- *Ferric chloride*: 2 g
- *Distilled water*: 1,000 mL
- *Sodium thiosulphate solution*:
  - Sodium thiosulfate: 5 g
  - Distilled water: 1,000 mL

Advantages

Outlines elastic fibers clearly.

Disadvantages

Remember to directly in alcohol without using water.

Reticulin Stain

Introduction

Reticulin is a procollagen and finer than collagen, stains black with reticulin stain, and is unstained with collagen stain. Collagen fibers on the other hand are coarse, doubly refractile, and stain red with a collagen stain like van Gieson; and yellow, lavender, or brown on silver impregnation. Reticulum and collagen are basically similar and though there may be minimal chemical differences in the amino acid content of collagen and reticulin and the presence of additional bindings or cementing substances in collagen, such as a mucopolysaccharide resembling hyaluronic acid.

Indications

- In kidney lesions-diabetic glomerulosclerosis displays laminated argyrophilia of the K-W lesions; chronic lobular glomerulonephritis shows a tangle of reticulin; amyloidosis of kidney shows a diffuse pale gray with a silver reticulin stain.
- In the liver, reticulin is helpful in early cirrhosis and detects creeping in fibrosis.
- In the bone marrow, reticulin detects fibrosis in myelofibrosis; metastatic carcinoma shows reticulin-free areas.
- *In vascular tumors* hemangiopericytoma shows pericytes with radiating reticulin fibers external to the basement membrane in contrast to hemangio-endothelioma with reticulin around tumor cells within the basement membrane. Outlines vascular pattern in angiosarcoma.
- Reticulin stain helps to differentiate follicular hyperplasia and follicular lymphomas as in the latter the reticulin around the follicle is compressed. Lymphomas produce loss of follicular pattern. The absence of reticulin fibers is seen in metastatic carcinoma. This application of reticulin stain in lymph nodes is rarely used these days as immunomarkers have replaced the utility value of reticulin in lymph node pathology. Angioimmunoblastic lymphomas and T-cell lymphomas are typically rich in high endothelial venules well outlined by the reticulin stain.
- In ovarian tumors, granulosa cell tumors groups of cells are surrounded by reticulin while in thecomas, individual cells are surrounded by reticulin fibers.
- Tumors of the nervous system arising from meso-dermal tissues show abundant reticulin, e.g., gliomas, meningeal tumors, and sarcomas. Astrocytomas are characterized by the pattern of angiogenesis.
- In paraganglioma, the reticulin stain reveals the typical cell nests or organoid (zellballen) pattern.
- In endometrial stromal sarcoma, the individual cells are surrounded by reticulin with an enhanced vascular pattern.
- A chicken wire pattern of vascularity is characteristic of myxoid liposarcoma and oligodendroglioma.
- Absence of reticulin fibers may be helpful in the diagnosis of epithelial neoplasia and Ewing's sarcoma of bone.

Principle of Staining

The staining procedure for reticulin is an impregnation method. The aldehyde groups of the carbohydrate of reticulin fibers reduce the colorless silver complex to a dark brown oxide of silver which is precipitated in particulate form on reticulin fibers.

The methods of the foot, Bielschowsky–Maresch, Perdrau–Da Fano, Wilder, Gordon and Sweet's, Gomori and Lillie, all use silver oxide or hydroxide in ammonical solution.

The del Río-Hortega, Foot, and Laidlaw variants use an ammonical solution of silver carbonate. The precipitated silver carbonate is dissolved in ammonia water to give ammonium silver carbonate.

So, ammonium silver carbonate (Laidlaw's method) or ammonium silver oxide or hydroxide (other method, e.g.,

Foot's) are complexes reduced to a dark brown silver oxide by reticulin fibers and subsequently reduced to black metallic silver by formalin.

Reticulin Stain–Bielschowsky's Method–Foot's Modification

Technique

Paraffin sections 5 µm thick, usual fixatives; preferable to fix sections on albuminized slides.

Procedure

- Bring sections to water.
- *Treat with 0.5% aqueous sodium thiosulfate*: 5 minutes (Skip if mercurial fixatives are not used)
- Wash in distilled water.
- *Treat with 0.25% potassium permanganate solution*: 5 minutes
- Wash in distilled water.
- *Treat with 5% oxalic acid*: 15 minutes
- Wash in distilled water.
- *Treat with silver nitrate solution*: 30 minutes
- Wash in distilled water quickly.
- *Expose to Foot's silver oxide solution*: 20 minutes
- A quick wash in distilled water.
- *Treat with 5% formalin (AR)*: 2 minutes
- Wash in distilled water.
- *Treat with gold chloride solution*: 3 minutes
- *Fix in 5% sodium thiosulfate solution*: 2 minutes
- Dehydrate, clear, and mount.

Treatment with gold chloride can be deleted for routine purposes due to its expense.

Results (Figs. 9A and B)

Reticulin: Dark violet to black

If nuclear stain such as nuclear fast red or hematoxylin is used between steps 11 and 12, then nuclei stain red or blue.

Stain Components

Solutions

Foot's silver oxide solution: Add 20 drops of 40% sodium hydroxide to 20 mL of 10% silver nitrate. Dissolve the brown precipitate by adding strong (28%) ammonia water drop by drop with constant shaking until only a few granules remain. About 2 mL (theoretically 1.7 cc) is required. Dilute to 80 mL with distilled water. Use once. This solution should be freshly made in clean glassware.

This solution gets reduced by the aldehyde groups of reticulin in tissue to a lower oxide (which is dark brown in color).

Potassium permanganate solution

- *Potassium permanganate*: 0.25 g
- *Distilled water*: 100 mL
- Potassium permanganate is used for presilvering for purposes of oxidation. Acidified potassium permanganate is used by Gordon and Sweet (1936). For about 4% chromic acid or 0.5% periodic acid may also be used.

Oxalic acid solution

- *Oxalic acid*: 5 g
- *Distilled water*: 100 mL

Oxalic acid is used for bleaching to remove potassium permanganate.

Silver nitrate solution

- *Silver nitrate*: 2 g
- *Distilled water*: 100 mL

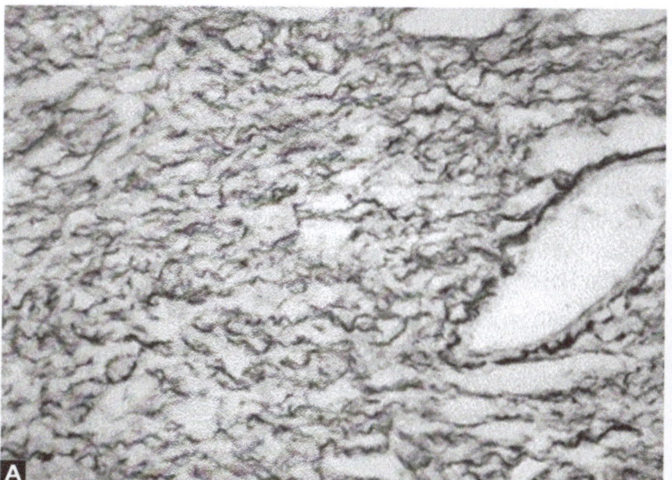

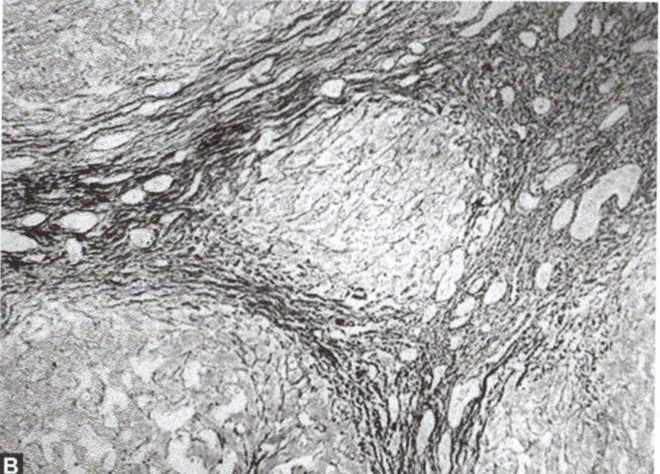

FIGS. 9A AND B: (A) Reticulin stain ×100 shows reticulin fibers encircling tumor cells in a hemangioendothelioma and (B) Reticulin stain ×100 done on a liver section to show pseudonodule formation, separated by reticulin fibers.

This is used as a "sensitizer" instead of which uranium, ferric chloride, or iron alum may also be used. These sensitizers are used as mordants as they also have an oxidizing effect.

Formalin solution

- *Neutral formaldehyde (AR) 37–40%*: 5 mL
- *Distilled water*: 95 mL

Formalin reduces the lower oxide (brown in color) to metallic silver oxide (black). Sodium sulfite or hydroquinone can also accomplish this.

Gold chloride solution

- *Gold chloride solution 1%*: 1 mL
- *Distilled water*: 9 mL

Though gold toning may be avoided due to cost it is a useful step. In untoned sections, the background is yellowish because of colloidal metallic silver, which is annoying to the eye. Toning removes the silver and replaces it with gold chloride. This is reduced to metallic gold by sodium metabisulfite or thiosulfate giving a pale gray background that is pleasing to the eye.

Toning is essential and has applications in the differentiation of woven bone from lamellar bone as it polarizes well. Toning also enhances counterstaining if such a counterstain as nuclear fast red is used.

Sodium thiosulphate solution: Sodium thiosulfate in this stain has two uses. In the first step, it removes excess of mercury if mercurial fixatives are used. In the last step; however, it removes excess of unreduced silver or gold prevents further oxidation and does not permit any further reaction. It also reduces gold chloride to metallic gold.

Advantages

Done well, it outlines all reticulin fibers and aids in diagnosing several disease conditions.

Disadvantages

- Several precautions have to be taken while doing the stain and in the preservation of the solutions.
- The high alkalinity of silver solutions tends to be traumatic to sections and may result in detachment of the section from the slide. This may be overcome by:
  - Fixing sections on albuminized slides.
  - Keeping sections before staining in the incubator at 60°C for at least 2 hours in order to fix the albuminized sections.
  - Celloidinizing the sections by using 1% celloidin after deparaffinizing and blotting the excess.
- Sections should be cut from well-processed tissue, well spread and of uniform thickness.
- Foot's silver oxide solution should be well filtered using Whatman's filter paper No. 1 to avoid precipitation of silver on the sections.
- The atmosphere should be dust-free as any dust particles will precipitate silver.
- Always use distilled water throughout the staining procedures.
- All glassware, especially that used in the preparation of silver solutions, should be washed in 10% nitric acid and then washed in several changes of distilled water.
- A silver flask or a silver-paper coating of containers for silver solutions may be used to avoid oxidation. These solutions should be colorless and not black or brown at the time of usage.
- Use alcohol alone for dehydration to get good results.
- *Explosive hazard*: In the preparation of the commonly used silver impregnation solutions various chemical reactions occur. With aging or exposure of ammonical silver solutions to air or light, shiny black crystals of explosive silver compounds, e.g., "fulminating silver," silver nitride is AgN_3 and silver azide (AgN_3) are formed.
- Violent explosions may occur while removing a stopper, throwing a solution down a sink, or even.
- When holding it up to light. In order to avoid this:
  - All ammonical silver solutions should be prepared fresh just before use.
  - Any used solutions should be inactivated by adding an excess of sodium chloride solution or dilute hydrochloric acid.

Phosphotungstic Acid Hematoxylin (Mallory-1900)

Introduction

Phosphotungstic acid hematoxylin (PTAH) stains several structures—demonstrates gliosis in the central nervous system, striations in tumors of skeletal muscles, and fibrin deposits in lesions. Muscle is stained blue-black to dark brown, and fibrin and neuroglia stain deep blue.

Indications

To stain connective tissue, muscle fibers, and glial tissue.

Phosphotungstic acid hematoxylin stains ependymomas while it does not stain choroid plexus papillomas, providing a means of differentiating the two.

Principle

The mechanism by which two-color staining is achieved from a mixture of hematin and phosphotungstic acid is obscure. The excess phosphotungstic acid in the solution binds all available hematein to form a "blue lake" pigment. This lake stains the muscle cross striations, fibrin, nuclei, and other tissue elements blue. The rest of the phosphotungstic acid stains the other elements like collagen red brown.

Control

Normal muscle tissue.

Fixation

For about 10% of buffered neutral formalin.

Technique

Paraffin-embedded tissue.

Procedure

- Bring sections down to water.
- Mordant in 4% iron alum for 0.5–1 hour.
- Wash well in distilled water.
- Oxidize in freshly made 0.25% o (w/v) potassium permanganate solution, for 5 minutes.
- Wash in water.
- Decolorize in 5% (w/v) oxalic acid solution for 5–10 minutes or until colorless.
- Wash for 2 minutes in running tap water and then rinse in distilled water.
- Stain overnight or for 12–14 hours in Mallory's PTAH stain.
- Blot off excess stain. Do not wash in water.
- Dehydrate rapidly in alcohol. Rapid dehydration is necessary since the alcohol removes the red components of the stain.
- Clear in xylol and mount.

Results

- *Nuclei, mitochondria, fibrin, alcoholic hyaline, and neuroglial fibrils*: Blue
- *Contractile portions of voluntary (striated) and heart muscle*: Blue
- *Bone, cartilage, and matrix*: Shades of yellow
- *Reticulum and elastin*: Orange to brownish red

Note

- Mallory bleach, i.e., steps 4–7 may be omitted for tissues other than nervous tissue.
- Mordanting is not necessary if mercurial fixative has been used. In that case, remove mercury with iodine and iodine with alcohol (hypo ruins the stain)
- Staining is progressive and microscopic examination of intervals of 1 hour is recommended. Heat accelerates staining and 1–2 hours at 60°C is often adequate.

Stain Components

Mallory's PTAH stain solution

- *Hematoxylin (or hematein)*: 0.1 g
- *Phosphotungstic acid*: 2.0 g
- *Distilled water*: 100 mL

Dissolve the hematoxylin in one-half of the water with the aid of gentle heat. Dissolve the phosphotungstic acid in the remainder of the water. When cool, combine the two solutions. The stain will ripen in several months or in 5–7 weeks if placed in warm sunshine. Add 17.7 mg of potassium permanganate for immediate ripening. When properly ripened the stain has a rich purple color and will be opaque.

STAINS FOR LIPIDS

Oil Red O Stain[7]

Introduction

Simple lipids are usually found in adipose tissues as energy stores. Fatty acids and their derivatives—both saturated and unsaturated, triglycerides such as neutral fats, waxes (fatty acids joined with long-chained alcohols), and phospholipids (fatty acids joined by phosphorous groups); stain with oil red O, Sudan Black B, and osmium tetroxide.

Indications

- The oil red O stain identifies lipids in tissue as well as smears.
- Helps in identifying fat globules in sebaceous carcinoma.
- Lipoblasts in liposarcoma contain lipid vacuoles. The importance of lipid stains has been overtaken by immunohistochemical markers, such as MDM2, CDK4, and S100.

Principle

Lipids are insoluble in water but soluble in fat solvents, such as ethyl alcohol, xylene, and chloroform. Therefore, routine processing dissolves fat. They are best demonstrated on frozen sections of tissues preserved in formal calcium acetate (2% calcium acetate + 10% formalin). They are leached out by prolonged exposure to buffered neutral formalin. Phospholipids and lipofuscin bind to tissue elements and may resist paraffin processing.

Technique

For about 8–10 μ frozen sections.

Procedure

- Rinse the slides with frozen sections in distilled water.
- Absolute propylene glycol for 2 minutes.
- Oil red O solution for 16 hours.
- Differentiate in 85% propylene glycol solution for 1 minute.
- Rinse in two changes of distilled water.
- Mayer's hematoxylin solution for 15–60 seconds.
- Rinse thoroughly in changes of distilled water.
- Mount in glycerine jelly.

Results

- *Lipids*: Red
- *Nuclei*: Blue

Stain Components

- 100% propylene glycol
- 0.5% oil red O solution
    - Oil red O: 0.5 g
    - Propylene glycol: 100 mL
    - At first add a small amount of propylene glycol to oil red O and mix them together by crushing large pieces. Keep stirring while adding the remaining propylene glycol. Heat gently to 95°C but not to reach 100°C. Filter through coarse filter paper and stand at room temperature. Filter till clear.
    - 85% propylene glycol solution
    - Propylene glycol 100%: 85L
    - Distilled water 15 mL

Mayer's Hematoxylin Solution (Appendix 3)

Glycerin jelly

- *Gelatin*: 10 g
- *Distilled water*: 60 mL
- Heat until gelatin is dissolved, then add, glycerine 70 mL and phenol 1 mL.

Other Silver Stains (Besides Reticulin)[2-4]

Introduction

Silver stains have varied applications in histopathology, they stain not only reticulin fibers but also neuroendocrine granules, microorganisms as well as have applications in renal biopsies. "Argentaffin reaction" is the ability of a silver complex solution to blacken a tissue element *without the need for a reducing bath.* It is most commonly used to describe the brown-black granularity observed in carcinoid tumors. The tumors arises from the Kulchitsky cells or neuroendocrine cells. The cells manufacture the 5-hydroxytryptamine (5-HT) from tryptophan and are responsible for the argentaffin reaction. Midgut carcinoids (appendix and small intestine) almost always react and are argentaffin-positive. Foregut and hindgut carcinoids are only argyrophilic, i.e., react only when a reducing substance is added, e.g., rectum, stomach, bronchus, more frequently fail to give argentaffin reaction but are argyrophilic. All argentaffin tumors are also argyrophilic but not vice versa.

Melanin also reduces solutions of ammoniacal silver nitrate to black metallic silver.

This depends on their unique ability to precipitate metallic silver which is subsequently reduced to give a black color. Fungi, for example, have polysaccharides in their cell walls which on oxidation release dialdehyde groups. These aldehyde groups, besides being stained by the Schiff's reagent, can also be demonstrated by their ability to reduce methenamine silver nitrate in an alkaline solution. The Grocott's alkaline methenamine silver nitrate solution represents a vehicle that, upon reduction, precipitates nascent silver ions, thus blackening the site. Similarly, spirochetes also have the capacity to bind to silver which can be reduced by other agents to black silver.

Indications

With the name of stains:

- Grimelius stain (argyrophilic) shows positive granules in carcinoid tumors of the foregut and hindgut (bronchial, stomach, first part of duodenum, esophagus, pancreas, transverse colon last third, descending colon, and rectum).
- Fontana Masson's silver staining technique (argentaffin)-midgut carcinoids (second part of duodenum onward to first two-thirds of the transverse colon). Also stains melanin.
- Gomori's methenamine silver stain for fungus and *Pneumocystis jirovecii*
- Gridley's silver stain for fungus and bacteria (*Chlamydia* and *Klebsiella granulomatis*)
- PAS-methenamine silver stain—basement membrane in glomeruli
- Levaditi's stain—spirochetes
- Warthin starry sky stain—*Helicobacter pylori*

Masson-Fontana Silver Staining Technique for Melanin and Argentaffin Granules

Indications

- To show the presence of argentaffin granules in tumors
- To detect traces of melanin in tumors.
- To demonstrate 5-hydroxytryptamine in certain endocrine cells of the epithelium of the stomach and small intestine, known as *enterochromaffin cells.*

Principle

The ability of a silver complex solution to blacken a tissue element *without the need for a reducing agent.*

Technique

For about 5 μm thick paraffin sections.

Fixation

Formalin is best; chromate and mercuric chloride fixatives are to be avoided.

Control

Skin

Procedure

- Bring sections to the water.
- Immerse slides in Fontana-silver solutions for 1 hour at 56–58°C in a Coplin jar covered with aluminum foil or overnight at room temperature. The sections appear light brown.
- Rinse well in distilled water.
- Tone in gold chloride for 2 minutes.
- Place in 5% aqueous sodium thiosulphate for 2 minutes.
- Wash thoroughly in tap water followed by distilled water.
- Counterstain with aqueous neutral red, 0.5%.
- Rinse in distilled water.
- Dehydrate, clear, and mount in DPX.

Results

- *Melanin pigment*: Black
- *Other elements*: According to the counter stain used.
- *Argentaffin granules*: Brown black in carcinoid tumors of the midgut **(Fig. 10)**

Stain Components

- Stock 10% silver nitrate solution
- *Silver nitrate AR grade*: 10g
- *Distilled water*: 100 mL

Take the solution in a glass flask. Use a finely pointed dropping pipette and add concentrated ammonia drop by drop, constantly agitating the flask until the formed precipitate dissolves—the endpoint is faint opalescence. To this add 20 mL of triple distilled water and then filter into a dark bottle.

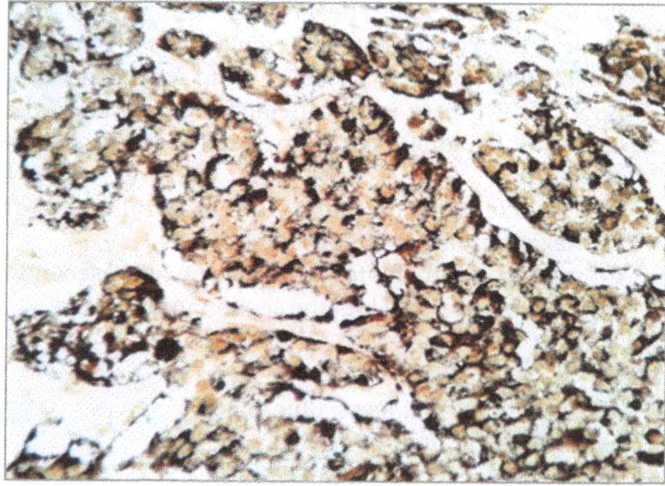

FIG. 10: Black granularity of neoplastic cells in carcinoid indicating the presence of neurosecretory granules. Masson's Fontana ×100.

Advantages

Neurosecretory granules are well demonstrated.

Disadvantage

Ammonical silver solutions are potentially explosive if stored incorrectly. (Store in a refrigerator and use within 4 weeks.) Thoroughly clean glassware used for silver solutions as explosive silver compounds might be formed with residues left on glassware.

Grimelius Staining Technique

Introduction

To demonstrate argyrophil substances, i.e., react only when a reducing substance is added.

Indications

Foregut and hindgut carcinoids are only argyrophilic, e.g., stomach, bronchus, and rectum more frequently fail to give argentaffin reaction but are argyrophilic. All argentaffin tumors are also argyrophilic but not vice versa.

Principle

The probable mechanism of argyrophil staining is the rapid absorption of silver salts in certain types of neurosecretory granules. The nonabsorbed granules are washed from the section. The absorbed silver is reduced by an external reducing agent (hydroquinone-sodium sulfite solution) to elemental silver.

Control

Pancreas (islets of Langerhans).

Procedure

- Deparaffinize using xylene for 5 minutes each × three changes.
- Take to alcohol 5 minutes each × two changes.
- Bring sections to water.
- Transfer to preheated silver solution at 60° for 3 hours.
- Drain the silver solution from the slide thoroughly.
- Place in freshly prepared reducing solution for 1 minute. The solution should be kept at 45°C for 4 hours before reducing.
- Rinse with distilled water.
- Counterstain if required (light green 0.5% aqueous is recommended)
- Dehydrate through graded alcohol, clear, and mount.

Result

- Argyrophilic substances (islet cells, argyrophil, and argentaffin tumors)—black
- Background—golden yellow

Notes:
- The most important or critical point to get a good result is the temperature of the solution at which the reaction takes place.
- The temperature of the reducing solution also is critical.
- The tail of the pancreas is most appropriate as control.

Stain Components

Silver Solution

- *0.2 M acetate buffer (pH 5.6)*: 10 mL
- *1% aqueous silver nitrate*: 3 mL
- *Double distilled water*: 87 mL

Reducing Solution

- *Hydroquinone*: 1 g
- *Sodium sulfite*: 5 g
- *Distilled water*: 100 mL

Acetate Buffer

- *Acetic acid*: 1.2 mL
  - Distilled water: 100 mL
- *Sodium acetate*: 2.7 g
  - Distilled water: 100 mL

Mix solution A: 9 mL + 91 mL B/adjust pH to 5.6

SPECIAL STAINS FOR MICROORGANISMS[3,4,7,8]

Stains for Bacteria: Gram Stain

Introduction

Microorganisms encountered in routine pathology specimens include bacteria, fungi, protozoa, and viruses. The most basic application is to classify bacteria into gram-positive and gram-negative bacteria. When the gram-positive bacteria die, they become gram-negative. Several histochemical stains help in identifying these organisms. The Gram stain was devised by Christian Gram (1884) to differentiate between gram-positive and gram-negative bacteria.

Indications

- The Gram stain is used to stain both bacillary and coccal forms of bacteria.
- It enables the identification of organisms causing lung abscesses, wounds, septicemic abscesses, or meningitis.
- It can be used on sections and smears.

Principle

All bacteria take up the primary stain. Bacteria that have large amounts of peptidoglycan in their walls retain the primary stain after decolorization with acetone/alcohol, i.e., they are gram-positive. Whereas, those who do not retain the color, have more lipids and lipopolysaccharides in their cell walls and are termed as gram-negative.

Indications

- Differentiation of gram-positive and gram-negative bacteria for classification.
- Screening of clinical samples.
- In the presumptive rapid diagnosis of gonococcal urethritis in men, acute purulent meningitis, pneumococcal pneumonia, aerobic infection, and selection of culture media.

Control

Gram-positive and gram-negative organisms on the tissues harvested from the microbiological plates.

Fixation

- Smears are fixed by passing on a flame
- Sections by routine fixatives, e.g., 10% neutral buffered formalin.

Technique

On fixed smears or 5 µm paraffin sections.

Procedure

- Make a thin smear of the clinical material/culture on a clean grease-free glass slide.
- Fix the dry film by passing it three times through a flame or placing it on a heat block.
- Stain in 1% crystal violet or methyl violet for 1 minute.
- Wash and stain with Gram's iodine for 30 seconds, pour off the excess, wash with tap water (enhances the crystal violet adherence to the walls of gram-positive bacteria)
- Decolorize with acetone—alcohol mixture for 2–3 seconds, until no stain comes out.
- Counterstain with dilute carbol fuchsin for 20 seconds.
- Wash with water and blot the section until it is dry.

Results (Fig. 11)

- *Gram-positive organisms*: Blue-black
- *Gram-negative organisms*: Red

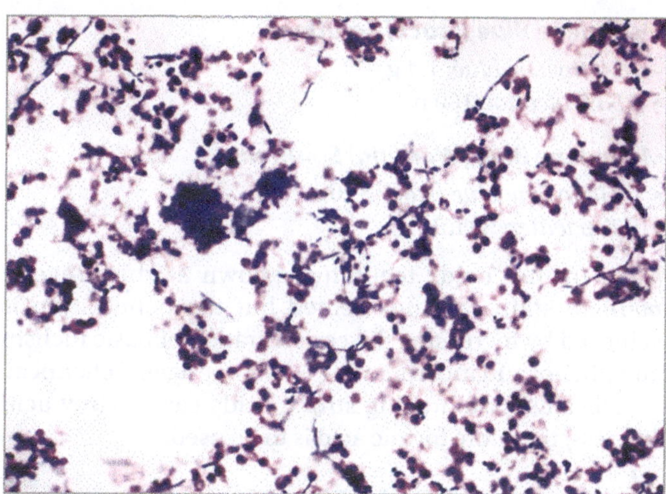

FIG. 11: Section shows gram-positive cocci seen as a group and pseudohyphae of *Candida* stained blue by the stain. Gram stain ×200.

Stain Components

- 1% crystal violet or methyl violet
- Gram's or Lugol's iodine is made up of iodine and potassium iodide.

Albert's Stain

Introduction

It is a metachromatic stain that stains granules of *Corynebacterium diphtheriae*.

Indications

Used mostly on smears; can be used on sections too. Identifies *Corynebacterium diphtheriae*.

Principle

The granules stain *purple black against the light green counterstained cytoplasm*. This helps to distinguish diphtheria from most of the short nonpathogenic diphtheroids which lack granules.

Procedure

- Prepare the smear from the sample and heat fix.
- Stain with Albert's A for 3–5 minutes; pour out the stain, do not wash with water.
- Stain with Albert's B for 1–2 minutes.
- Wash with water and blot dry.
- Observe under oil immersion.

Results

- *Bacilli*: Green
- *Granules*: Bluish black

Stain Components

- *Albert's A*: Toluidine blue, Malachite green, glacial acetic acid in 95% alcohol and deionized water.
- *Albert's B*: Iodine dissolved in potassium iodide and deionized water.

Stains for Mycobacteria Bacilli: Ziehl–Neelsen stain (Carbol Fuchsin Acid–Alcohol Stain)

Introduction

Gram stain is an aqueous stain that cannot penetrate the lipid-rich waxy mycobacterial cell walls and mycobacteria have large amounts of lipids called mycolic acid in their cell walls which stain by carbol fuchsin as well as resist decolorization by acid-alcohol. The latter property is responsible for the commonly used term "acid-fast bacilli." When these organisms die, they lose their fatty capsule and consequently their carbol fuchsin positivity.

Indications

- Extensively in the detection of *Mycobacterium tuberculosis*.
- Members of the *Actinomycetes*, genus *Nocardia* (*Nocardia brasiliensis* and *Nocardia asteroides* are opportunistic pathogens) are partially acid-fast.
- Oocysts of coccidian parasites, such as *Cryptosporidium* and *Isospora*, are also acid-fast.

Principle

The mycobacterial cell walls are stained by carbol fuchsin. The organisms stain pink with the basic fuchsin, a component of carbol fuchsin. Staining is followed by decolorization in acid-alcohol; mycobacteria retain the carbol fuchsin in their cell wall (acid-fast); whereas, other bacteria do not retain carbol fuchsin. Counterstaining is carried out by methylene blue. Care has to be taken not to over-counter stains as this may mask the acid-fast bacilli.

Control

Smear/section of known positive case with easily identifiable acid-fast organisms.

Fixation and Technique

- Smears fixed on flame or in cytological fixative.
- Paraffin processed 5 µm thick sections.

Procedure

- Deparaffinize and rehydrate through graded alcohols to distilled water.

- Cover the smear will carbol fuchsin stain.
- Heat the smear until the vapor just begins to rise (i.e., about 60°C). Do not overheat (boil or dry). Add additional stain if necessary. Allow the heated stain to remain on the slide for 5 minutes.
- Wash well in tap water.
- Differentiate in sulfuric acid solution or acid alcohol until solutions are pale pink (2–5 dips).
- Wash well in tap water for several minutes; rinse in distilled water.
- Counterstain with methylene blue solution until sections are pale blue.
- Rinse in tap water then with distilled water.
- Dehydrate, clear, and mount.

Results (Fig. 12)

- Mycobacterial, hair shafts, Russell bodies, mast cell granules, fungal organisms, and Splendore-Hoeppli zone around actinomyces—red
- Background—pale blue

Stain Components

Carbol Fuchsin

- *Basic fuchsin*: 0.5 g
- *Absolute alcohol*: 5.0 mL
- *5% aqueous phenol*: 100 mL
  (Mix well and filter before use with filter paper)

Decolorization Acid Solution

- 20% sulfuric acid, or
- 3% v/v acid alcohol

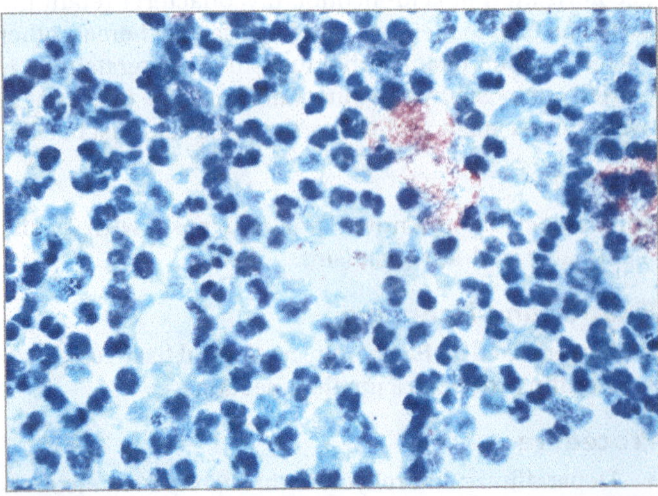

FIG. 12: Section shows a group of acid-fast bacilli (pink to red) against a pale blue background of inflammatory cells Z-N stain ×1,000.

Methylene Blue (Stock) Solutions

- *Methylene blue*: 1.4 g
- *95% alcohol*: 100 mL

Methylene Blue (Working) Solutions

- *Methylene blue (stock)*: 10 mL
- *Tap water*: 90 mL

Note: In the "cold" technique known as the *Kinyoun method*, stains are not heated but the penetration is achieved by increasing the concentration of basic fuchsin and phenol and incorporating a "wetting agent" chemical.

Decalcification using strong acids can destroy acid fastness, therefore formic acid is to be used.

Modified Fite (Wade-Fite) Method for *Mycobacterium leprae* and *Nocardia*

Introduction

The above stain is designed for detecting *Mycobacterium leprae*. *Nocardia* species of organisms that are weakly acid-fast positive also stain with this. These organisms are much less acid- and alcohol-fast and need a weaker concentration of acid in the staining procedure.

Indications

To detect the presence of *M. leprae* and *Nocardia*.

Principle

As compared to *M. tuberculosis*, *M. leprae* produces much less acid and alcohol quickly. The Wade-Fite stain is used for staining of *M. leprae* which has cell walls that are more susceptible to damage in the deparaffinization process. Solvents (fat-dissolving agents) such as alcohol and xylene when used directly damage the fragile fatty capsule of *M. leprae*. The inclusion of peanut oil in the deparaffinization solvents helps to protect the bacterial cell wall. (Xylene-peanut oil: 1 part oil: 2 part of xylene is used for deparaffinization.)

The acid used for decolorization in the Fite procedure is also weaker and generally 0.5% or 1% of aqueous sulfuric acid solution is used.

Control

Section from known cases of lepromatous leprosy.

Fixation

- Smears fixed on flame or in cytological fixative.
- Routine fixatives

Technique

Smears and paraffin processed 5 µm tissue sections.

Procedure

- Deparaffinize in two changes of xylene-peanut oil, 6 minutes each.
- Drain slides vertically on a paper towel and wash in warm running tap water for 3 minutes. (The residual oil preserves the sections and helps accentuate the acid fastness of the bacilli.)
- Pour carbol fuchsin solutions for 25 minutes (solvent may be reused).
- Wash well in tap water for 3 minutes.
- Drain excess water from slides on a paper towel.
- Differentiate with 0.5% or 1% sulfuric acid in 25% alcohol or water, two changes of 1.5 minutes each. (Do not allow the slides to dry between carbol fuchsin and acid alcohol. Sections should be pale pink.)
- Wash in tap water for 5 minutes.
- Counterstain in working methylene blue solutions, one quick dip. (Do not overstain the slide. Sections should be pale blue.)
- Blot sections and dry in 50–55°C oven for 5 minutes.
- Once dry, one quick dip in xylene.
- Mount with permanent mountant.

Results (Fig. 13)

- *Acid-fast bacilli including M. lepra*: Bright red
- *Nuclei and other tissue elements*: Pale blue

Stain Components

Carbol Fuchsin

- *Basic fuchsin*: 0.5 g
- *Absolute alcohol*: 5.0 mL
- *5% aqueous phenol*: 100 mL
  (Mix well and filter before use with filter paper)

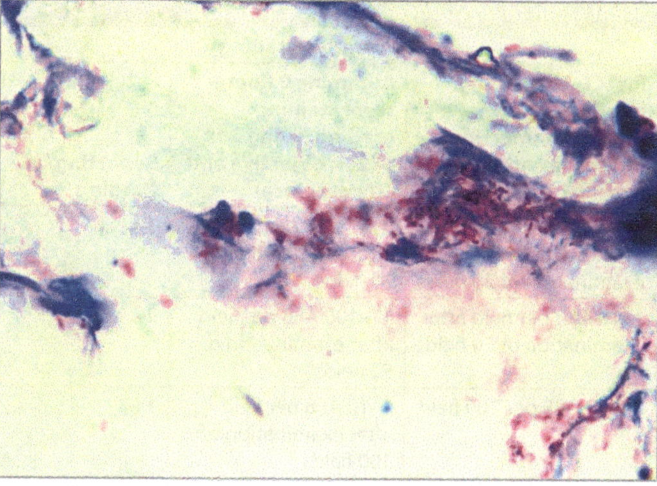

FIG. 13: Modified Fite–Faraco stain shows clusters of mycobacteria leprae in the macrophages in an aspirate of primary neuritic leprosy. Fite–Faraco ×1,000.

0.5% Sulfuric Acid in 25% Alcohol or Water (Aqueous Sulfuric Acid)

- *25% ethanol*: 95 mL
- *Sulfuric acid, concentrated*: 5 mL

Methylene Blue (Stock) Solutions

- *Methylene blue*: 1.4 g
- *95% alcohol*: 100 mL

Methylene Blue (Working) Solutions

- *Methylene blue (stock)*: 5 mL
- *Tap water*: 45 mL

Auramine–Rhodamine Fluorescence Method

Introduction

The unique cell wall character of mycobacteria prevents them from being stained by the standard Gram stain procedure. Due to this "acid-fastness," specific diagnostic tests are required, such as auramine-rhodamine and Ziehl–Neelsen staining. Fluorescence staining utilizes basically the same approach as Z-N staining but carbol fuchsin is replaced by a fluorescent dye (auramine O, rhodamine, auramine-rhodamine, acridine orange, etc.).

Indications

To detect the presence of *M. tuberculosis* or other acid-fast organism.

Principle

The exact mechanism of the stain is unknown. Both the dyes auramine-rhodamine used are basic dyes that fluoresce at short wavelengths for the mycolic acid in the cell walls. Both dyes are used in combination to yield better staining than either dye alone. Rhodamine alters the color from the yellow of auramine alone to a reddish or golden yellow. Both the sensitivity and specificity of fluorescence microscopy are comparable to the characteristics of Z-N staining.

Control

A section containing acid-fast bacilli must be used.

Fixative

For about 10% neutral buffered formalin is preferred. Slides should be scratch-free.

Technique

In the case of secretions, smears can be made directly. In the case of solid or semisolid material, an aqueous suspension of the material is made by taking a small amount of the material and suspending it in a drop of distilled water on a microscope slide, and making a smear that should not be too thick. The smear made by either method is air-dried and then "fixed" by passing rapidly through a Bunsen burner two to three times. The smear is allowed to cool before staining.

Procedure

- Place slides in Auramine O–Rhodamine B solution in a glass Coplin jar and stain for 10 minutes at 50°. In the case of sections, deparaffinized in two parts xylene + one part peanut oil, two changes each of 3 minutes duration. Drain and blot to opacity.
- Rinse smears/sections for 2 minutes in tap water.
- Differentiate in two changes of 0.5% acid alcohol for 1½ minutes each (for *M. leprae* use 0.5% aqueous HCl)
- Rinse smears/sections for 2 minutes in tap water.
- Differentiate for 2 minutes in 0.5% $KMnO_4$-quenches fluorescence of tissue cells.
- Wash in tap water for 2 minutes.
- Blot dry or stand slides on end and thoroughly air dry. (for *M. leprae* sections should be mounted in glycerol or liquid paraffin)
- In the case of *M. tuberculosis* smears/sections may be dehydrated in absolute alcohol (not >10 seconds) cleared quickly in xylene (for sections) and mounted with a synthetic resin (Harleco fluorescence mountant)
- Examine with a high-dry objective, a UG1 or UG2 exciter filter, and a colorless UV barrier filter.

Results (Fig. 14)

- *Acid-fast organisms*: Golden to yellow green
- *Background*: Black
- Slides can be screened on high power (400×) and verified under oil immersion. Staining times vary to suit one's preferences.

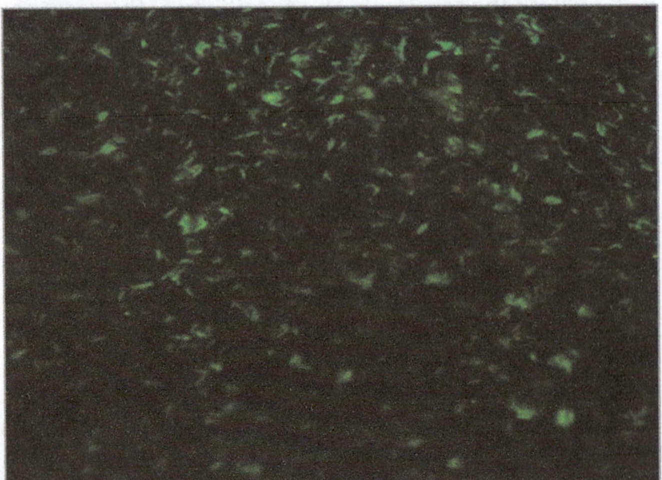

FIG. 14: Section shows several yellow-green, fluorescent bacilli by the rhodamine–auramine stain.

Stain Components

Formula: Auramine O–Rhodamine B Solution

- *Auramine O*: 1.5 g
- *Rhodamine B*: 0.75 g
- *Glycerol*: 75 mL
- *Phenol crystals*: 10 mL (liquified at 50°C and dissolved by shaking at room temperature in 50 mL distilled)

Advantages

The most important advantage of this technique is that the strain of examining slides under oil immersion to cover a large surface area is avoided as the examination is done with 10× and easily identifies the organisms.

Disadvantage

Expensive procedure.

Table 2 shows the Revised National Tuberculosis Control Programme (RNTCP) comparative grading in the ZN stain and fluorescent stain of *M. tuberculosis*.

Silver Stains (Warthin Starry Stain)

Introduction

Silver stains are very sensitive to the staining of bacteria and are reserved for visualizing spirochetes, *Legionella, Bartonella*, and *H. pylori*.

Treponema pallidum or spirochete causes syphilis. These organisms are infrequently seen in biopsies and a primary chancre is usually diagnosed clinically. The causative organism is seen using dark ground microscopy and is an 8–13 µm corkscrew microorganism, with

TABLE 2: Revised National Tuberculosis Control Programme (RNTCP) comparative grading in the Z-N stain and fluorescent stain of *Mycobacterium tuberculosis*.

Comparative grading		
RNTCF ZN staining grading (using 100× oil immersion objective and 10× eyepiece)	**Auramine 0 fluorescent staining grading (using 20× or 25× objective and 10× eyepiece)**	**Reporting/ Grading**
>10 acid-fast bacilli (AFB) per field after examination of 20 fields	>100 AFB per field after examination of 20 fields	3+
1–10 AFB per field after examination of 50 fields	11–100 AFB per field after examination of 50 fields	2+
10–99 ABF per 100 field	1–10 AFB per field after examination of 100 fields	1+
1–9 AFB per 100 field	1–3 ABF per 100 fields	Doubtful positive/repeat
No AFB per 100 fields	No ABF per 100 fields	Negative

a kink in the center. The modified Steiner method, Dieterle method, or Warthin Starry stains are used for staining spirochetes. *Leptospira interrogans* is also a spirochete (13 μm) with curled ends and causes Weil's disease. This can also be visualized by the above stains. *Legionella pneumophila* is a gram-positive organism causing pneumonia. *H. pylori* associated with chronic gastritis is also very well visualized by these silver stains. The gram-negative organisms (bacteria) *Afipia felis* and *Bartonella henselae* causing Cat scratch disease are also demonstrated by the silver stains.

Principle

Spirochetes and other bacteria can bind silver ions from solution but cannot reduce the bound silver. The slide is first incubated in a silver nitrate solution for half an hour and then "developed" with hydroquinone which reduces the bound silver to a visible metallic form.

Control

Known case with *Treponema pallidum* positivity or known case of *H. pylori* positivity of 3+ grade in Sydney system.

Fixation

Routine fixation.

Technique

Paraffin fixed 5 μm sections.

Procedure

- Deparaffinize and rehydrate through graded alcohols in distilled water.
- Celuloidinize in 0.5% celloidin, drain, and harden in distilled water for 1 minute.
- Impregnate in preheated 55–60°C silver solution for 90–105 minutes.
- Prepare and preheat the developer in a water bath.
- Treat with developer (solution) for 3½ minutes at 55°C. Sections should be golden brown at this point.
- Remove from the developer and rinse in tap water for several minutes at 55–60°C, then in buffer at room temperature.
- Tone in 0.2% gold chloride.
- Dehydrate, clear, and mount.

Results (Fig. 15)

- *Spirochetes, H. pylori, etc.*: Dark brown to black
- *Background*: Golden yellow

Stain Components

- Acetate buffer, pH 3.6
- *Sodium acetate*: 4.1 g

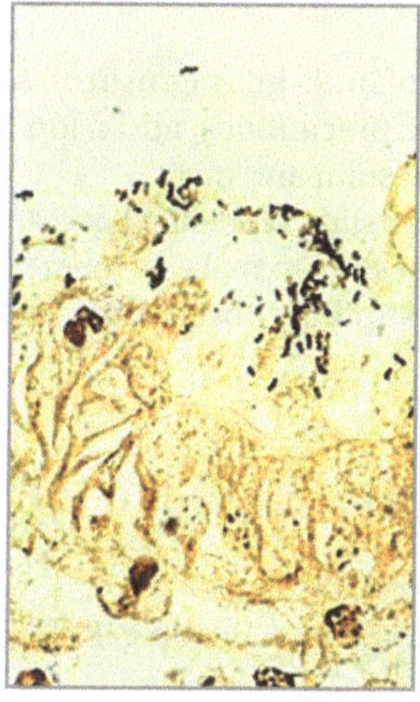

FIG. 15: Section demonstrates brown-black stained *Helicobacter pylori* in a gastric biopsy. Warthin–Starry stain ×1,000.

- *Acetic acid*: 6.25 mL
- *Distilled water*: 500 mL

1% silver acetate nitrate in pH 3.6 acetate buffer

Developer

Dissolve hydroquinone in 10 mL pH 3.6 buffer and mix 1 mL of this solution and 15 mL of warmed 5% scotch glue or gelatin; keep at 40°C. Take 3 mL of 1% silver nitrate in pH 3.6 buffer solutions and keep it at 55°C. Mix the two solutions immediately before use.

0.2 % gold chloride (optional).

Negative Staining with India Ink or Nigrosin[9]

Introduction

India ink or nigrosin can be used to demonstrate the capsule of microorganisms.

Indications

To demonstrate and identify capsulated organisms including *Cryptococcus*, *Klebsiella* species, and *Streptococcus pneumoniae*.

Principle

The stain is a suspension of carbon, formed in India ink or nigrosin. The carbon particles are negatively charged as in the cell membrane. As they repel the dye cells (capsules) remain clear and the background looks black or dark green.

Technique

Usually done on smears.

Procedure

- Place a drop of India ink/nigrosin on a clean glass slide.
- Using aseptic precautions, add a lop full of organisms to the drop of stain and mix.
- Using another slide (spreader) at a 45° angle spread it along the first slide to make a smear.
- Add a coverslip and observe under low/high power objective.

Results

Capsules do not take up the stain.

Stain Components

- *Nigrosin stain*: Nigrosin 100 g/L; formalin 5 mL/L in water
- *India ink stain*: Black Pelican drawing ink No. 17; deionized water
- Thimerosal (preservative)

STAINS FOR FUNGI

Introduction

Most fungi can be readily demonstrated with the common special stains, Gomori's methenamine silver, Gridley's fungus stain, and PAS; also referred to as "broad spectrum" fungal stains.

The fungal stains such as Alcian blue and Mayer's or Southgate's mucicarmine, that readily demonstrate the mucoid capsule of *Cryptococcus neoformans* are termed "narrow spectrum" stains for fungi. This staining reaction differentiates *Cryptococcus neoformans* from other fungi of similar morphology, such as *Coccidioides*, *Candida*, and *Histoplasma*.

Various Fungal Stains

Various fungal stains include:

- *H&E stain*: This is not a special stain but stains *Aspergillus* species and the *Zygomycetes* (mucormycosis and *Rhizopus*). It also demonstrates the reaction of tissues around fungi and is used as an accompaniment to silver stains.
- *Grocott's stain (GMS)*: GMS is preferred for routine use as it stains most fungi and even nonviable fungi that are sometimes refractory to H&E stain.
- *Gomori's stain*: This is an adaptation of the GMS stain.
- *Gridley's stain*: Stains most fungi
- *PAS stain*: Stains most fungi **(Fig. 16)**; mucin stains—Mayer's mucicarmine, Southgate's mucicarmine, and Alcian blue, stain the mucopolysaccharide capsule of *Cryptococcus neoformans*. *Blastomyces dermatitidis* and *Rhinosporidium seeberi* are also stained by it.

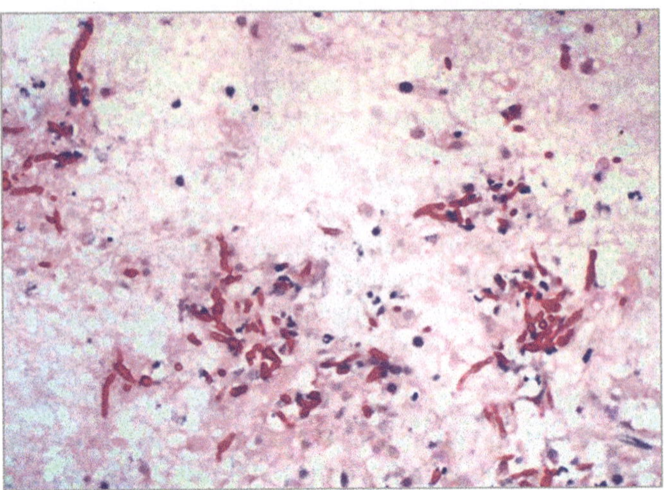

FIG. 16: Periodic Acid–Schiff (PAS) stain ×400 shows fungal filaments in tissue.

Grocott Methenamine Silver Stain for Fungi

Indications

Demonstrates most fungi; cysts of *Pneumocystis jirovecii* stain as cup-shaped structures; "also called cup and saucer appearance."

Principle

Most fungal cell walls are rich in polysaccharides which can be converted by oxidation to dialdehydes. The aldehyde groups reduce silver ions in the alkaline pH (alkaline methenamine silver nitrate solution) to metallic silver, which appears black.

Control

Any positive section with fungal elements, such as *Candida*.

Fixation

Routine fixatives.

Technique

For about 5 µm sections from paraffin-embedded tissue.

Procedure

- Bring sections to distilled water.
- Oxidize with 5% aqueous chromic acid for 1 hour
- Wash in water for a few seconds.
- Treat sections with 1% sodium metabisulfite for 1 minute.
- Wash in running tap water for 5 minutes
- Rinse thoroughly in distilled water.
- Place in preheated working silver solution in a water bath at 56°C for 30–40 minutes until the section turns yellowish-brown. (The incubation time is variable and

depends upon the type and duration of fixation—may also be 1-3 hours at 37-45°C.)

- Rinse well in distilled water. Check for adequate silver impregnation under the microscope after half an hour of incubation. The endpoint is when glycogen mucous, basement membrane, and fungi stain dark brown.
- Tone sections with 0.1% gold chloride for 4 minutes.
- Rinse in distilled water.
- Treat sections with 3% sodium thiosulphate for 5 minutes (to remove unreacted silver).
- Wash with running tap water for 5 minutes.
- Counterstain in working 1% light green for 15-30 seconds or H&E.
- Rinse excess light green off-slide with alcohol.
- Dehydrate, clear, and mount.

Advantages

- GMS is preferred for routine use as it stains viable and nonviable fungi.
- GMS also stains algae, intracytoplasmic granular inclusions of cytomegalovirus (CMV), *Actinomyces israelii*, *Nocardia*, *Mycobacterium*, *Klebsiella pneumoniae,* and *Streptococcus pneumoniae.*

Disadvantages

- The stain masks the natural color of pigmented fungi whether colorless, hyaline, or pigmented.
- GMS does not adequately demonstrate the inflammatory response to fungal invasion and a comparison of the same area has to be done with an H&E stain.

Results (Fig. 17)

- *Fungi, Pneumocystis carinii, and Histoplasma*: Black
- *Inner parts of mycelia and hyphae*: Old rose
- *Leishmania and Toxoplasma*: Negative
- *Mucin*: Dark gray
- *Red blood cells (RBCs)*: Yellow
- *Background*: Pale green

Stain Components

Stock Methenamine–Silver Nitrate Solution

- Silver nitrate, 5% solution—5 mL
- Methenamine, 3% solution—100 mL
- Add the silver nitrate to the methenamine solution, shaking until the precipitate which first forms, later dissolves. This mixture will keep for 1-2 months at 4°C.

Working Methenamine–Silver Nitrate Solution

- Borax 5% solution—5 mL
- Distilled water—25ml
- Mix and add methenamine-silver nitrate (stock solution)—25 mL

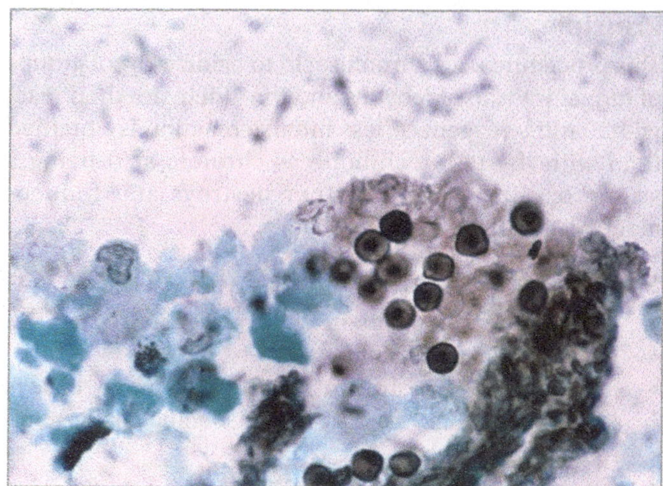

FIG. 17: Grocott's stain shows circular forms (cup and saucer appearance) of *Pneumocystis jirovecii* in bronchial lavage.

Stock Light Green Solution

- Light green, SF—0.2 g
- Distilled water—100 mL
- Glacial acetic acid—0.2 mL

Working Light Green Solution

- Light green (stock solution)—10 mL
- Distilled water—50 mL

Note:

- After treatment with the silver solution, fungi should be dark brown in color. It is advisable to check this with the microscope and a control section known to contain fungi should always be run at the same time.
- Reticulin fibrils and threads of fibrin will also be blackened by this method and must not be confused with fungi.
- The borax ensures an alkaline pH.
- When tissue details are important, some workers prefer a light H&E as a counterstain.

Gomori's Technique

This technique is similar to that of Grocott's; in fact, the latter is an adaptation of Gomori's technique with a difference in incubation times.

Gridley's Stain

Indications

Stains most fungi. Rickettsia is also stained: Rickettsial infection, causes Q fever, rocky mountain fever, or typhus, and rarely needs to be demonstrated on tissue sections as it can be diagnosed serologically.

Principle

This procedure uses chromic acid to oxidize glycol groups of fungal walls to aldehydes and the aldehydes then react with Schiff's reagent. A less intense reaction is obtained than with the PAS technique as chromic acid being a strong oxidizing agent further destroys and reduces aldehyde groups.

Stain Components

- 4% chromic acid solution
- Lillie's cold Schiff solution
- Sulfite rinsing solution (used to remove excess leucofuchsin, i.e., to remove nonspecific background reaction products)
- Gomori's aldehyde fuchsin solution
- 0.25% Metanil yellow/light green

Procedure

- Bring the sections to water.
- Oxidize with 4% chromic acid.
- Wash in running tap water.
- Treat sections with Schiff's reagent for 15–20 minutes.
- Give two sulfite rinses.
- Wash in water for 15 minutes.
- Treat the sections with Gomori's aldehyde-fuchsin solution for 15–20 minutes.
- Rinse in 95% alcohol.
- Wash in water for 5 minutes.
- Counterstain with 0.25% Metanil yellow/light green.

Results

- *Mycelia*: Deep blue
- *Conidia*: Deep rose to purple
- *Background*: Yellow
- *Elastic tissue and mucin*: Deep blue

IDENTIFICATION OF VIRUSES

Identification is difficult under a light microscope, but the outlines of the virus can be made out under an electron microscope. Some viruses aggregate within cells to produce viral inclusion bodies, which may be both intranuclear and extranuclear and can be stained with a Feulgen reaction. These intranuclear inclusion bodies (e.g., in CMV) are acidophilic and impart an owl-eye appearance to the nucleus. The extranuclear inclusion bodies can be basophilic and cytoplasmic and are PAS-positive. Special staining methods are Feulgen reaction; and modified trichomes using contrasting acid and basic dyes to exploit the differences in charges on the inclusion body and host cell. For example, Mann's methyl blue eosin stain for Negri bodies of rabies, a phloxine-tartrazine technique for viral inclusions, Shikata's orcein for hepatitis B surface antigen, Macchiavello stain for inclusion bodies (and rickettsiae).

PROTOZOAN ORGANISM

The identification can be made on morphological appearance using H&E and Giemsa stain. Wet mount preparations may be used particularly in flagellate organisms like *Entamoeba histolytica*. PAS stain is used to demonstrate cysts of *Entamoeba histolytica* and iron hematoxylin stain highlights the nuclear features. The availability of antisera against organisms such as *Entamoeba histolytica*, *Toxoplasma gondii*, and *Leishmania tropica* has made diagnosis much easier in difficult cases.

STAINS FOR PIGMENTS[3,4,8]

Fixation Artifacts

- *Formalin pigment* (artifactual pigment), also called *acid hematin*, is formed after several weeks in specimens by the interaction of acidic or alkaline formaldehyde solutions with blood. This dark brown pigment, a product of the degradation of hemoglobin, settles out as an insoluble product and can be identified by its presence extracellularly. This artifact is not formed in a neutral, buffered formaldehyde solution.
- *Mercury pigment*: These deposits occur in all tissues fixed in liquids containing mercuric chloride, including "B5," Heidenhain's solution, and Zenker's fluid. They occur as uniformly distributed brown black, extracellular crystals. The material is removed by brief treatment of sections with alcoholic iodine solution, followed by treatment with sodium thiosulfate which in turn removes the iodine.
- *Chromic oxide*: These are brownish-black granules that are the result of alcohol treatment following chrome fixation. Such pigment cannot be removed. Therefore, chrome-fixed tissue must be washed in running water for 12–18 hours immediately following fixation. This washing removes excess chromates and then the tissue can be safely dehydrated in alcohol.
- *Malarial pigment (hemozoin)*: It is formed within RBCs that contain the malarial parasite. They can be seen inside the macrophages if infected RBCs are ingested; seen in Kupffer's cells of the liver, sinus lining cells of the lymph node and spleen, and within phagocytic cells in the marrow. This can be removed with saturated alcoholic picric acid and requires 12–24 hours for complete treatment.

Formula

Picric acid (saturated in the alcohol) as up to 50 mL.

Procedure

- Bring sections to water.
- Place the sections in alcoholic picric acid.
- Rinse sections in 90% of alcohol.
- Rinse sections in 70% of alcohol.
- Place sections in tap water (alternatively, 10% ammonium hydroxide can be used).
- Stain with H&E or other routine stains.

Melanins

Introduction

Melanins are brown to black or yellowish polymeric pigments formed from the amino acid tyrosine by oxidation with tyrosinase [dihydroxyphenylalanine (DOPA) oxidase] in skin cells, hair, eyes (retina, iris, and choroid), and in the cell bodies of some neurons, notably in the substantia nigra and locus coeruleus of the brain stem. In skin, *melanocytes,* which are the branched cells at the junction of the epidermis with the dermis, synthesize the pigment and package it into protein-containing granules called melanosomes. Excess melanin production in the neoplasia of melanocytes obscures morphology, in such cases, bleaching of sections is done, and removing the pigment entails better study of cell nuclear detail.

Indications for Demonstration of Melanin

- In abnormal states melanin is found in the cells of malignant melanomas and various benign nevi derived from melanocytes.
- Histochemical staining of melanin is required when amelanotic melanomas are to be diagnosed or to differentiate minimal pigment from other pigments, such as hemosiderin.
- Special stains confirm its presence and therefore presence of neoplasms.

Removal of Melanin Pigments (Bleach)

Principle

Melanin can be bleached by strong oxidizing agents, such as potassium permanganate. A H&E stain is done after the bleaching procedure for each patient. Removal confirms that the pigment is melanin.

Control

Hematoxylin and eosin section from the same block without bleaching procedure.

Procedure

- Deparaffinize and hydrate to distilled water.
- Oxidize in permanganate solution for 30 minutes.
- Wash in water.
- Bleach in oxalic acid until white (oxalic acid removes potassium permanganate besides its bleaching action).
- Proceed as usual to H&E.

Stain Components

- 0.25% aqueous potassium permanganate
- 5% aqueous oxalic acid

Results

- Skin melanin is bleached within 30 minutes.
- Ocular melanin takes 2–4 hours.

Masson–Fontana Silver Staining Technique for Melanin

Refer to the stain described earlier.

Schmorl's Reaction

Principle

Melanin has the ability to reduce ferricyanide to ferrocyanide, which in the presence of ferric ions forms Prussian blue. This reaction is also seen with lipofuscins, bile, and neuroendocrine cell granules.

Control

Melanin pigment in skin biopsy.

Fixation

For about 10% buffered neutral formalin.

Procedure

- Deparaffinize and hydrate to distilled water (control and test).
- Treat with a working solution for 10 minutes.
- Wash in running water for several minutes to ensure that all the residual ferricyanide is completely removed from the section.
- Counterstain with 0.5% aqueous nuclear red for 5 minutes.
- Dehydrate rapidly in alcohols.
- Clear and mount.

Result

- Melanin, argentaffin cells, and chromaffin cells
- *Lipofuscins, bile, and colloid*: Dark blue
- *Nuclei*: Red

Stain Components

- 1% aqueous ferric chloride (freshly prepared)
- 0.4% aqueous potassium ferricyanide (freshly prepared)

Working Solution

To add 30 mL of 1% ferric chloride add 4 mL of 0.4% aqueous potassium ferricyanide, then add 6 mL of distilled water. Use within 30 minutes.

Enzyme Methods: Dihydroxyphenylalanine Oxidase (Tyrosinase) Method for Tissue Blocks

Introduction

The most specific method of all is an enzyme histochemical method called *DOPA-oxidase*. It requires frozen sections for the best results, but paraffin sections of well-fixed tissues may also be used. The procedure for the latter is given.

Indications

Dihydroxyphenylalanine reaction is used in diagnosing amelanotic melanoma. Amelanotic melanoma is a neoplasm that has no melanin but possesses the enzyme tyrosinase.

Principle

The stain works because the DOPA substrate used here is acted upon by the enzyme DOPA-oxidase in the melanin-producing cells to produce a brownish-black deposit. The enzyme catalyzes the oxidation of tyrosine to DOPA and its final oxidation to melanin pigment.

Primary Fixative

- For about 10% formalin in pH 7.4 buffer to which is added 0.44 sucrose. (tissue is fixed for 2–3 hours)
- *pH buffer 7.4*: Dissolve 42.8 g sodium cacodylate and 9.6 mL M hydrochloride acid in 1 L of distilled water. (Sodium cacodylate is a better buffer than phosphate buffer, which may also be used.)

Procedure

- Fix two pieces of the tissue for testing in the primary fixative for 3 hours at 4°C.
- Rinse in cold (4°C) pH 7.4 buffer for 5 minutes.
- Incubate one piece of tissue in the buffered DOPA solution for 16–20 minutes at 37°C. The other piece of tissue (negative control) is incubated in the buffer only, at 37°C for the same time as the test.
- Wash both tissues in distilled water for 5 minutes and then fix in a conventional 10% formalin solution for 1–2 days.
- Paraffin process in the usual way. Cut sections at 10 µm and, mount them on poly-L-lysine-coated slides.
- Lightly counterstain with Mayer's hemalum for 2 minutes. Wash and blue sections in tap.
- Dehydrate, clear, and mount.

Results

- *Cells with DOPA oxidase*: Brown
- *Nuclei*: Blue

Formaldehyde-induced Fluorescence

Introduction

Formalin-induced fluorescence can be used to highlight biogenic amines (chromaffin, dopamine, epinephrine, norepinephrine, and argentaffin) and melanin in tissues.

Indications

- Formalin fixation imparts a strong yellow autofluorescence to unstained tissues containing these substances—aromatic amines, such as 5-hydroxytryptamine (5HT), epinephrine, and histamine.
- An amelanotic melanoma is a tumor with no pigment but possesses the enzyme tyrosinase. It is diagnosed by autofluorescence of tyrosine or by the DOPA reaction.

Procedure

Frozen sections are fixed in 10% buffered formalin for 5 minutes dehydrated and placed in xylene; then mounted in the media that is fluorescent-free and examined using a fluorescent microscope with BG38, UG1, and a barrier filter.

The best results are seen using tissue that has been freeze-dried (snap-frozen) and then fixed using paraformaldehyde vapors.

Hematogenous Pigments

Hemosiderin is an aggregate of proteins (ferritin) containing ferric hydroxide. It is an intracellular granular yellow-to-brown pigment seen in the mitochondria (siderosomes) of histiocytes. Stainable ferric iron is normally found in the bone marrow and in the spleen. In pathological states, it is seen in sites of old hemorrhage, hematomas, and in hemochromatosis.

Commonly ferrous iron is of little interest and may be demonstrated by Tirmann's method where 20% potassium ferricyanide and 2% hydrochloric acid in equal parts are mixed and the sections exposed to this mixture for 1 minute. The results are similar to Perls' reaction.

Perl's Persian Blue Stain for Ferric Iron

This is also called the Prussian blue reaction; Turnbull's blue method.

Principle

Ferric iron combines with potassium ferro cyanide to form ferric-ferro cyanide, which gives a bright blue color (precipitate). This method demonstrates only ferric iron and not ferrous iron.

Historical Note

The characteristic blue-green color developed by this reaction is called Prussian blue after the uniform worn by the Prussian army. Prussia was a sovereign state established in the 13th century and became a kingdom in 1701 and is associated with Frederick the Great and Bismarck. At its height, it covered the area of North Germany and parts of Poland. It was formerly dissolved after World II (1939–1945). Berlin was the capital.

Control

Tissue with areas of old hemorrhage.

Indications

Some of the pathological conditions with hemosiderin deposits (ferric iron) are hemorrhages of any kind, hemolytic anemia, some liver diseases, the lungs in congestive heart failure, and in the liver, pancreas, and skin in hemochromatosis.

Procedure

- Bring sections to water.
- Rinse in distilled water.
- Transfer to Perl's solution.
- Rinse in distilled water.
- Counterstain with 1% nuclear fast red.
- Rinse in tap water.
- Bring to mountant.

Results (Fig. 18)

- *Hemosiderin*: Blue
- *Nuclei*: Red

Note:

- At stage 5, H&E stain may be used.
- Perl's stain should be fresh and filtered.
- Use only AR-grade chemicals. All glassware should be cleaned with distilled water to avoid extraneous ferric iron contamination.
- Use known control slides.
- Where excessive iron is present, the timing will need to be reduced.

Stain Components

Perl's Solution

- *2% aqueous potassium ferrocyanide*: 25 mL
- *2% aqueous hydrochloric acid*: 25 mL

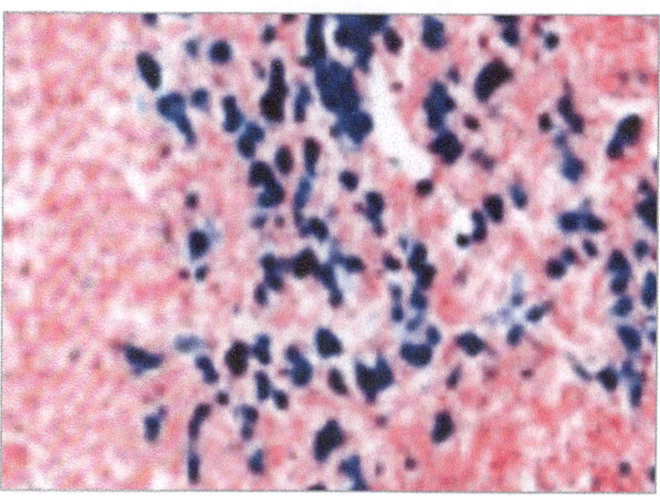

FIG. 18: Positive reaction for iron in a liver section in hemochromatosis. Perl's stain ×400.

Turnbull's Reaction

It can be performed on gross tissue specimens which are treated with an acidic solution of potassium ferricyanide, any ferrous iron present will *react* to form an insoluble bright blue pigment called *Turnbull's blue* (ferrous ferricyanide).

Modified Fouchet's Technique for Bile Pigments

Introduction and Indications

The pigments include both conjugated and unconjugated bilirubin, biliverdin, and hematoidin, all of which are chemically distinct and show different physical properties. They are seen elevated particularly in patients of obstructive jaundice due to blockage in the normal flow of bile from the liver into the gallbladder. In H&E staining, bile is stained as yellow-brown globules. It needs to be distinguished from lipofuscin which stains similarly. Lipofuchsin is autofluorescent while bile pigments are not. Hematoidin appears as a bright yellow pigment within the old hemorrhagic areas and in old splenic infarcts, where it contrasts well against the pale gray of the infarcted tissue.

The most commonly used routine method for bile pigments is the modified Fouchet's technique.

Principle

The pigment is converted to biliverdin which gives a green color and cholecyanin (blue) by the oxidative action of the ferric chloride in the presence of trichloroacetic acid.

Control

Liver section with bile stasis.

Procedure

- Take a test and control to distilled water.
- Treat with the freshly prepared Fouchet's solution for 10 minutes.
- Wash the well in running water for 1 minute.
- Rinse in distilled water.
- Counterstain with van Gieson's solution for 2 minutes.
- Dehydrate, clear, and mount in synthetic resin.

Results

- *Bile pigments*: Emerald to blue green
- *Muscle*: Yellow
- *Collagen*: Red

Stain Components

- Fouchet's solution
- *25% aqueous trichloroacetic acid*: 36 mL
- *10% aqueous ferric acid*: 4 mL
- Freshly prepared before use
- *van Gieson*: Dissolve 100 mL of acid fuchsin in 100 mL of saturated aqueous picric acid

MINERALS/ENDOGENOUS DEPOSITS[3,4]

Calcium

Calcium is present in hydroxyapatite, the insoluble mineral of bones and teeth. Abnormal deposits of calcium phosphate or carbonate can be associated with dystrophic calcification with lesions of atherosclerosis, infarction (Gandy-Gamna bodies), malakoplakia of the bladder (Michaelis-Gutman bodies), hyperparathyroidism, nephrocalcinosis, sarcoidosis, tuberculosis, and in some tumors. Calcium phosphate crystals can be seen in joints in chondrocalcinosis or pseudogout. Calcium salts are monorefringent but calcium oxalate is birefringent.

There are many ways to stain calcium, but only two methods are routinely used in histopathology. These are the von Kossa and Alizarin red S techniques.

Modified von Kossa's Method for Calcium

Introduction

The classic method for the demonstration of calcium and certain other salts in tissues is that of von Kossa (1901). Calcification in degenerative tissues, arteries, caseous foci of tuberculosis, malakoplakia, and Gamna-Gandy bodies is demonstrated.

Principle

This method demonstrates calcium in combination with phosphate and carbonate (cationic radicals), giving good results with both large and small deposits of calcium (anion). Silver compounds replace calcium and reduction to metallic silver is achieved by light or hydroquinone. This method is not specific, as melanin will also reduce silver to give black deposits.

Fixation

As a general rule, fixation of tissues containing calcium deposits is best done using nonacidic fixatives, such as buffered neutral formalin, formol alcohol, and alcohol.

Control

Calcium in tissue—Monckeberg's medial calcific sclerosis; calcified leiomyoma.

Procedure

- Deparaffinize sections and bring them to water. Rinse well in distilled water.
- Place in 1% silver nitrate solution under exposure to strong light (60–100 W bulb at a range of 4–5") for 60 minutes.
- Wash in three changes of distilled water.
- Treat with sodium thiosulphate for 5 minutes.
- Rinse well in distilled water.
- Counterstain with 1% neutral red for 3 minutes.
- Dehydrate in graded alcohol, clear, and mount.

Results

- *Mineralized bone*: Black
- *Osteoid*: Red

Stain Components

- 1% aqueous silver nitrate
- 2.5% sodium thiosulfate
- 1% neutral red

Note:

- This method is not specific for calcium ions but an indirect demonstration of it; melanin also reduces silver to give black deposits.
- As a general rule, fixation of tissues containing calcium deposits is best used using nonacidic fixatives, such as buffered neutral formalin, formol alcohol, and alcohol.

Alizarin Red S Method for Calcium

Alizarin red S gives more reliable results with small deposits and is said to be specific for calcium salts at pH 4.2.

Control

Calcium in tissue, as mentioned earlier.

Procedure

- Bring sections to 95% alcohol.
- Allow the slides to air dry thoroughly.
- Place sections in a Coplin jar filled with alizarin S solution for 5 minutes.
- Rinse quickly in distilled water.

- Counterstain with fast green for 1 minute.
- Rinse in three changes of distilled water.
- Dehydrate, clear, and mount in synthetic resin.

Results

- *Calcium deposits*: Orange red
- *Background*: Green

Stain Components

- 1% aqueous alizarin red S adjusted to pH 4.2 or 6.3–6.5 with 10% ammonium hydroxide.
- 0.05% fast green and 0.2% acetic acid.

Copper

Copper is an essential nutrient, contributing to blood vessels and bone stability. Excess deposition of copper is associated with Wilson's disease, primary biliary cirrhosis, and other liver disorders.

Two reagents are suitable for the histochemical demonstration of copper by virtue of reactions employing the oxidative catalyst properties of copper. Dithiooxamide (also known as rubeanic acid) gives a stable dark green polymeric product that can be mounted in a resinous medium.

Modified Rhodamine Method for Copper

Principle

Para-dimethylaminobenzylidene rhodamine (DMABR) gives a red product that dissolves in organic solvents and therefore requires an aqueous mounting medium.

Control

Liver with positive material.

Reagents

Rhodamine stock solution

- *5-p-dimethylaminobenzylidene-rhodamine*: 0.05
- *Absolute ethanol*: 25 mL
- Prepare fresh and filter before use

Working solution: Take 5 mL of the stock solution and add to 45 mL of 2% sodium acetate trihydrate

Borax solution

- *Disodium-tetraborate*: 0.5 g
- *Distilled water*: 100 mL

Procedure

- Take test and control sections to water.
- Incubate in the rhodamine working solution at 56°C for 3 hours or overnight in a 37°C.
- Rinse in several changes of distilled water for 3 minutes.
- Stain in acidified Lillie-Mayer or other alum hematoxylin for 10 seconds.
- Briefly rinse in distilled water and place immediately in borax solution for 15 seconds.
- Rinse in distilled water.
- Mount with Apathy's mounting media.

Results

- *Copper deposits*: Red to orange
- *Nuclei*: Blue
- *Bile*: Green

Rubeanic Acid Technique (Modified Okamoto and Utamura 1938)

Principle

Rubeanic acid (dithiooxamide) forms a colored copper rubeanate compound with copper.

Fixative

Mercury-containing fixatives are not recommended.

Control

Liver with positive material.

Procedure

- Bring sections to water.
- Place in a Coplin jar filled with rubeanic acetate solution for 8-16 hours at 37°C
- Wash briefly in distilled water and blot dry.
- Counterstain in 0.5% aqueous neutral red.
- Dehydrate, clear, and mount.

Result

- *Copper rubeanate*: Greenish black
- *Nuclei*: Red

Stain Components

- *Formula*: Stock solution
- *Rubeanic acid*: 100 mg
- *Ethanol*: 100 mL

Working Solution

- *Rubeanic acid stock solution*: 2.5 mL
- *10% aqueous sodium acetate*: 50 mL

Endogenous Deposits

Amyloid

Alkaline Congo red method for amyloid.

Principle of Stain

The tinctorial property of the amyloid is due to its fibrillar structure.

Fixation

Alcohol fixation gives the best results. Formalin fixation is also suitable, but prolonged fixation reduces the intensity of staining. Fixatives that contain dichromate or chromic acid are best avoided.

Technique

Use paraffin-embedded or frozen sections.

Procedure

- Bring sections down to water.
- Stain nuclei in alum hematoxylin
- Differentiate and blue.
- Treat with a working alkaline solution for 20 minutes.
- Stain in a working solution of Congo red for 20 minutes.
- Dehydrate with three brief rinses in absolute alcohol.
- Clear in xylene and mount in a synthetic resin medium.

Results (Fig. 19A)

- *Nuclei*: Blue
- *Amyloid*: Deep pink (salmon pink) to red
- *Background*: Light yellow
- Elastic fibers and some cytoplasmic granules may be stained pink to red.

Stain Components

- Alkaline solution
- *Stock solution*: 80% alcohol saturated with sodium chloride.
- *Working solution*: Add 0.5 mL of 1% aqueous sodium hydroxide to 50 mL of the stock solution.
- Filter and use within 15 minutes.

Congo Red Stain

- *Stock solution*: 80% alcohol saturated with Congo red and sodium chloride.
- *Working solution*: Add 0.5 mL of 1% aqueous sodium hydroxide to 50 mL of the stock solution. Filter and use within 15 minutes.

Note:

- Both stock solutions will keep for several months.
- Freshly prepared Congo red solution should be allowed to stand for 24 hours before use. It must be saturated with dye.
- The working solutions are not stable and should be used in 15 minutes.
- Examination of stained sections by polarized light should not be omitted as the green birefringence **(Fig. 19B)** is diagnostic of amyloid and that which is pink by congo red stain (elastic tissue) **(Fig. 20)** and negative for birefringence is not amyloid.
- Unstained paraffin sections of amyloid material often fail to stain if kept longer than 3–4 months.
- *Typing of amyloid*:[10] Amyloid proteins can be further distinguished by autoclaving. Autoclaving the tissues at 120°C for 30 minutes causes protein AA to lose its affinity for Congo red. Prolongation of autoclaving to 120 minutes abolishes the congophilia of protein AL.
- Treatment of the tissue with potassium permanganate causes protein AA and B2-microglobulin amyloid to lose their affinity to Congo red stain. Also, protein AA fails to stain with Congo red after treatment with alkaline guanidine for 1 minute, and protein AL and systemic senile amyloid (SSA) protein after treatment for 2 hours.
- Other methods of detection of amyloid include fluorescent stains, e.g., thioflavin T or S.

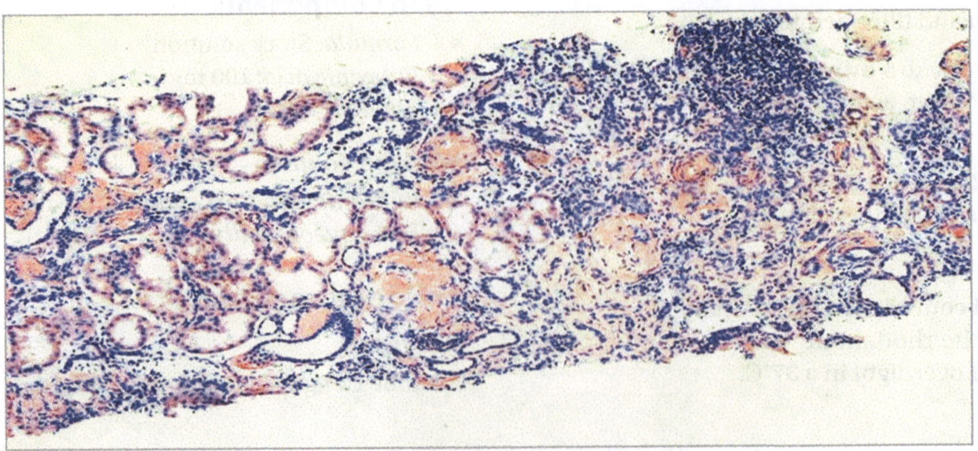

FIG. 19A: Amyloid stains pink to red (salmon pink) in glomeruli and blood vessels (amyloidosis of the kidney). Congo red stain ×100.

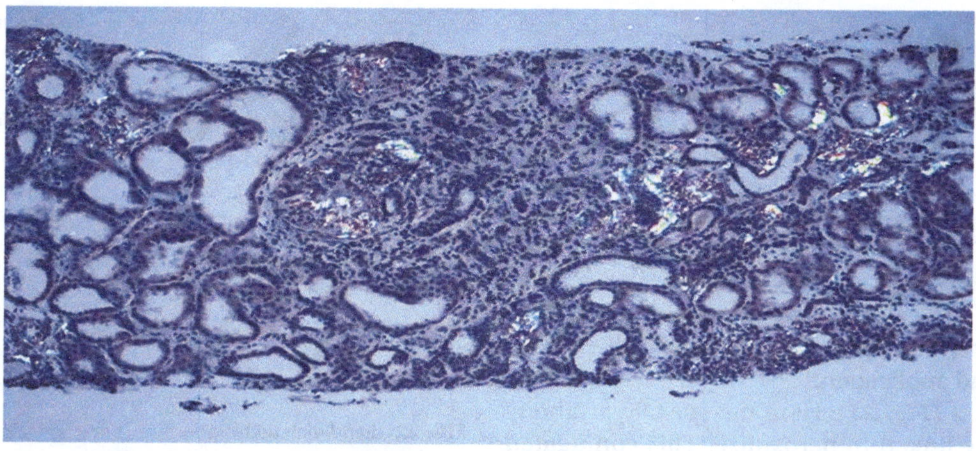

FIG. 19B: Apple green birefringence with the polarized light. This is diagnostic of amyloid. Congo red stain under polarized light ×100.

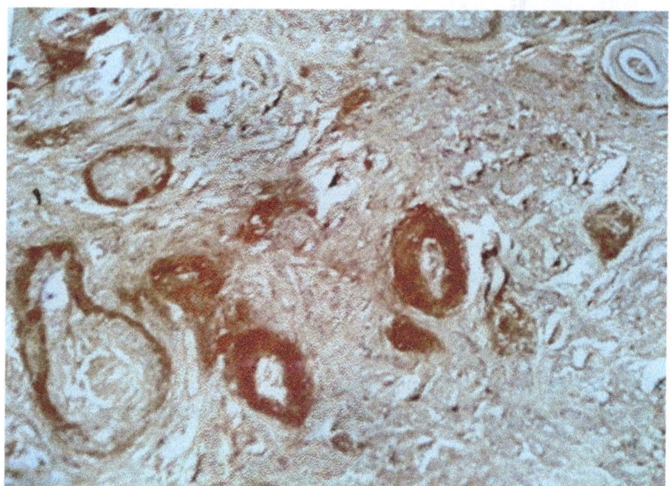

FIG. 20: Section shows periductal elastic tissue of breast staining salmon pink by the amyloid stain; but fails to show apple green birefringence by polarized light (not shown), ruling out the presence of amyloid.

- Metachromatic stains, such as crystal violet and methyl violet. van Gieson stain colors amyloid khaki brown and immunoperoxidase staining can be specific for the P component, proteins AA and AL, and familial amyloid protein (FAP).

IMMUNOHISTOCHEMISTRY[2,7,8]

Immunohistochemistry (IHC) is a staining technique that deals with the study of tissue sections stained with labeled antibodies, an antibody induced by a specific antigenic determinant on the tissues. Thus, specific antibodies are used as probes to detect the morphological position of antigens within cells and tissue sections. In order to visualize this antigen-antibody complex these complexes are either "colored" by dyes or "tagged" by some method that permits their visualization, e.g., immunohistochemical/immunofluorescent methods.

Immunoperoxidase (Immunoenzyme) Methods

These methods are based upon the attachment of an active enzyme, e.g., horseradish peroxidase (HRP), to a specific antibody. This antibody may be the one detecting an antigen in the tissue (as in the direct method) or one that combines with other specific antibodies acting as probes to detect antigens in tissues (as in other methods). This enzyme (HRP) also has the ability to produce a visible color change in a 'substrate system' thus enabling visualization of the 'antibody-enzyme complex' or indirectly the antigen-antibody reaction.

The "substrate system" refers to consists of hydrogen peroxide and a chromogen such as 3,3 diaminobenzidine tetrahydrochloride (DAB) or 3-amino-9-ethyl carbazole (AEC). The enzyme HPR reacts with this "substrate system" to produce a colored molecule and water.

Although other enzymes such as alkaline phosphatase and glucose oxidase may also be used, peroxidize is commonly preferred because:

- It is available in a highly purified form so that the chance of contamination with other enzymes is minimized.
- It is very stable and relatively inexpensive.
- Only small amounts are present in tissue specimens and the endogenous peroxidase activity is easily quenched.
- Several coloring chromogens are available which can be acted upon by peroxidizing to form a colored end product that will precipitate at the morphological site of the antigen to be localized.

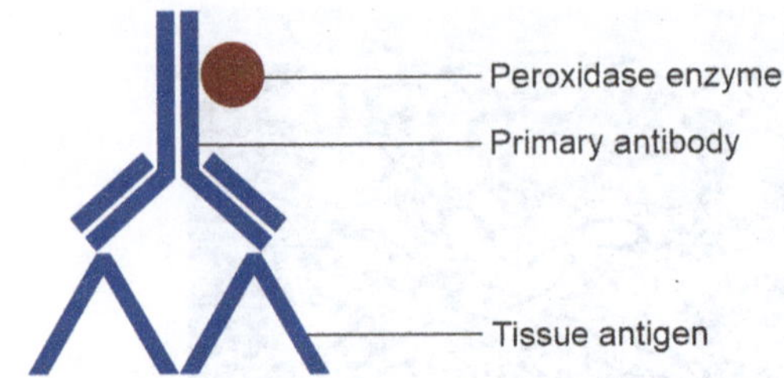

FIG. 21: Direct method.

The following are the important techniques which have found widespread application:

- *Direct method* ***(Fig. 21)***: Here the specific antibody is chemically linked to peroxidize. This conjugated antibody reacts with the antigen. "A substrate system" applies a colored end product precipitating at the site of antigen-antibody interaction.

  The most common application of the direct immunoperoxidase method is for the detection of immunoglobulin, complement, and immune complex deposits in kidney biopsies from patients with various types of renal disease, in skin biopsies from cases of systemic lupus erythematosus and other connective tissue disorders.
- *Indirect method (sandwich technique)* ***(Fig. 22)***: An unconjugated antibody reacts with the antigen. A conjugated antibody is then applied which binds to the first antibody, now acting as an antigen. A substrate system is added to localize the reaction.

  The advantage of this technique over the former one is the fact that a variety of primary antibodies made in the same animal species can be used with one conjugated secondary antibody.

  The method gains popularity in the identification of antibodies in the serum of patients with various autoantibodies as well as bacterial and parasitic diseases - thyroidal, nuclear, mitochondrial, smooth muscle antigen, treponemal palladium, herpes simplex virus, and CMV virus.
- *Peroxidase-antiperoxidase (PAP) method* ***(Fig. 23)***: Three reagents are utilized there. The primary antibody reacts specifically with the antigen. The secondary antibody or link antibody binds to the primary antibody and the PAP complex. The PAP complex comprises the enzyme peroxidize and an antibody against peroxidize. The peroxidize enzyme is then visualized via a substrate chromogen reaction.

  The primary antibody and PAP complex are both produced in the same animal species and the link antibody (produced in another species) is; therefore, capable of binding to both.

  This system has greater sensitivity as compared to the above procedures and can detect small traces of antigen in paraffin-embedded tissue when much of it is lost by fixation and processing. The direct and indirect techniques on the other hand are usually performed on cryostat sections.

  One of the most important applications of the PAP method is in determining the origin of a neoplasm in undifferentiated tumors by identifying specific antigenic components of a tumor, e.g., prostate-specific antigen (PSA); K and λ light chains, immunoglobulin G (IgG), immunoglobulin A (Ig)A, immunoglobulin M (IgM), GFAP (glial fibrillary acidic protein), etc.
- *Alkaline phosphatase-antialkaline phosphatase method (APAAP)*: The principles of the APAAP method are the same as that of PAP except that the PAP complex is replaced with the APAAP complex.
  - Major applications:
    - Staining of tissues with high levels of endogenous peroxidize (e.g., bone marrow).
    - Double immunostaining in conjunction with peroxidize.
    - Specific cell types stand out due to the bright red color of alkaline phosphatase.

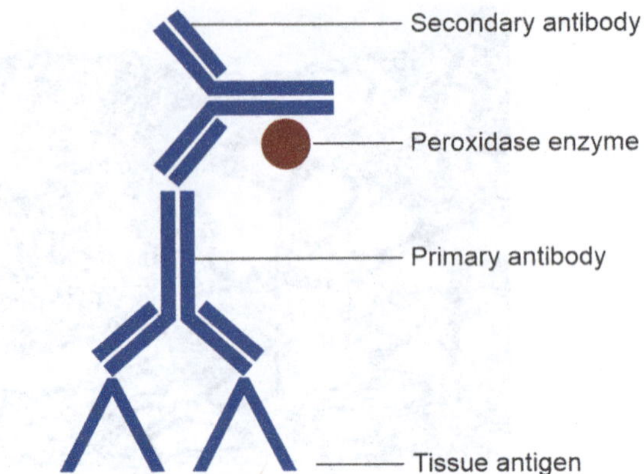

FIG. 22: Sandwich technique.

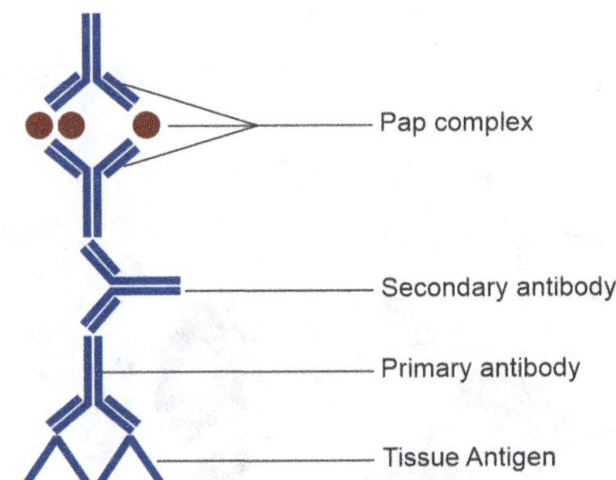

FIG. 23: Peroxidase-antiperoxidase (PAP) complex attached to a secondary antibody which in turn is bound to the primary antibody.

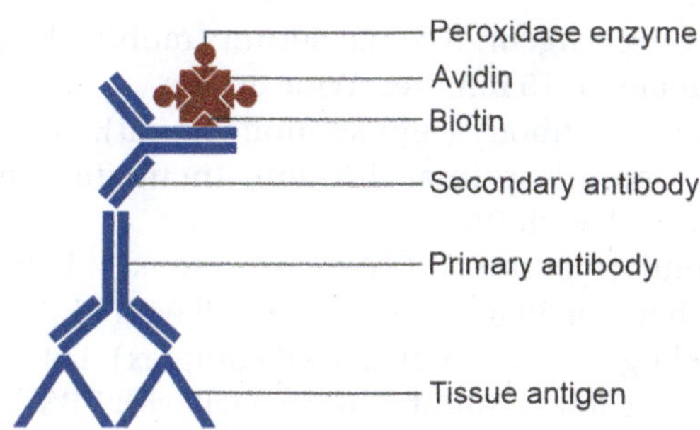

FIG. 24: Avidin biotin method.

- *Avidin-biotin method* **(*Fig. 24*)**: The avidin-biotin method utilizes conjugated antibodies. Avidin is an egg white glycoprotein and binds nonimmunologically to four molecules of the vitamin biotin.

  The primary antibody is specific for the antigen to be localized. A secondary antibody capable of binding to the primary antibody is conjugated to biotin. The third reagent is a complex of peroxidize, avidin, and conjugated biotin (the free sites on the avidin molecule are bound to the biotin on the secondary antibody). Visualization is done by using an appropriate chromogen.

  The strong affinity of avidin for biotin gives this method greater sensitivity, and excellent results can be achieved on fixed paraffin-embedded specimens. The technique lends itself to the localization of numerous antigens in a variety of specimens—identification of hormones, cell markers in neoplasia, lectin binding sites, viral proteins, and intermediate filaments.
- *Polymeric labeling-two step methods* **(*Fig. 25*)**: These methods utilize a unique technology based on a polymer backbone to which multiple antibodies and enzyme molecules are conjugated. This polymer system contains a dextran backbone to which enzyme molecules (HRP or AP) are attached along with secondary antibodies with antimouse Ig and antirabbit Ig specificity. This universal reagent can detect any tissue-bound primary antibody of mouse or rabbit origin.

Advantages

- Increased sensitivity
- Minimized nonspecific background staining due to the absence of the endogenous biotin.
- Associated nonspecific staining.
- A reduction in the total number of assay steps as compared to conventional techniques.

Interpretation

Deposits of the colored chromogen indicate the presence of antigen and represent specific positive staining.

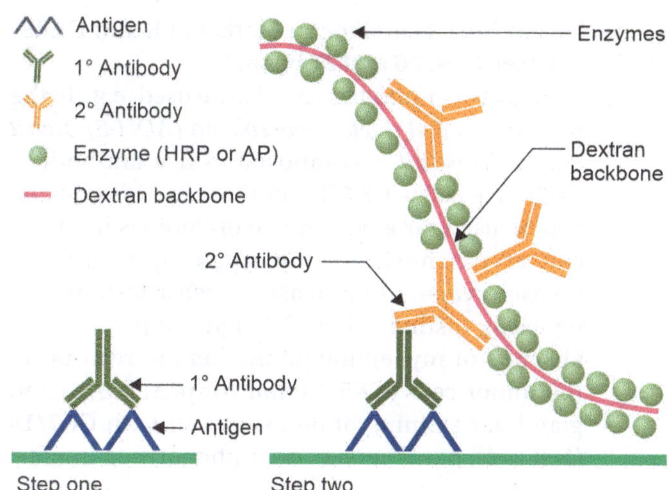

FIG. 25: Two-step polymer method.

Besides frozen sections and paraffin-embedded sections, these procedures can be carried out on smears. The most common fixative for smears is acetone in 10% buffered saline in which smears can be fixed for 15 minutes.

The practical applications of immunohistochemical stains lie in the following:

- *Histogenesis and typing of neoplasia where* IHC has gained widespread popularity. A variety of markers are available for use in the market which include epithelial and nonepithelial antibodies, hormones- and related proteins, intermediate filament proteins, leukocyte markers, hormone receptors in breast, and other carcinomas **(Appendix 4)**.
- *IHC markers*: The positivity of either a single marker or a group of markers used simultaneously can prove useful. For example:
  - In a round cell tumor the first line of markers would be leukocyte common antigen (LCA), cytokeratin (CK), and neuron-specific enolase (NSE) and positivity of any of these would signify lymphoma, small cell carcinoma, and neuroendocrine carcinoma respectively.
  - In infectious disease, in the detection of tissue antigens of herpes simplex virus, measles, CMV and human papillomavirus, Hantavirus, and Rocky Mountain spotty virus.
  - IHC in Hirschspring disease: This demonstrates nerve fiber hypertrophy and ganglion, markers include NSE, S-100, Synaptophysin
  - IHC in Alzheimer's disease: Identifies major protein amyloid fibril.
  - IHC in Barrett's esophagus: MUC5AC and MUC3 in superficial columnar epithelium, MUC2 in the goblet cells, and MUC6 in the glands.

- IHC in breast carcinoma: Markers ER/PR, HER2-neu (see **Figs. 26 and 27** below)
- Cocktails of antibodies can also be used, e.g., in the breast; *atypical ductal hyperplasia (ADH-5) breast marker cocktail* is composed of five antibodies: CK5/14 + p63 + CK7/18 antibodies. This cocktail can be used for a wide range of findings in breast cancer diagnosis in one single application—invasive versus noninvasive breast lesions can be easily distinguished through the presence or absence of myoepithelial markers in relation to the tumor cells (CK5/14 and /or p63) (DAB) and glandular staining of breast cancer with CK7/18 (fast red); basal versus other phenotypes in most breast cancers.
- Luminal (7/18) positivity signifies a glandular differentiation with a good prognosis, both 7/18 or cytoplasmic staining (CK5/14) signifies a bimodal cell pattern (not such a good prognosis). In certain cases, only CK 5/14 luminal staining is observed, representing a basal phenotype classification of breast cancer that has a poor prognosis.

IHC Staining Procedure

- Deparaffinize the 4 μm fixed section.
- Treat with different grades of alcohol and finally bring to PBS buffer, i.e., 100% alcohol two changes 3 minutes each. 95% alcohol two changes 3 minutes each. PBS buffer for 5 minutes.
- Blocking reagent 3% hydrogen peroxide. Incubate for 10 minutes. Rinse well with PBS. Incubate for 10 minutes.
- *Blocking reagent*: Normal serum (rabbit). Dilute 1:5. Incubate for 15 minutes. Wipe excess.
- Primary antibody (mouse monoclonal). Dre-diluted or prepared optimal dilution. Incubate overnight. Rinse well with PBS.
- Secondary antibody (rabbit antimouse). Dilute 1:50. Incubate for 30 minutes. Rinse well with PBS.
- Labeling reagent (mouse PAP complex). Dilute 1:100. Incubate for 30 minutes. Rinse well with PBS.
- Acetyl ethyl carbazole solution. Incubate for 30 minutes. Rinse in distilled water.
- Flood distilled water. Incubate for 2 minutes.
- Counterstain with hematoxylin.
- Wash in tap water.
- Mount while wet with glycerin jelly.

The incubation is carried out at 37°C. All stains should be carried out with a known positive control slide and a negative control slide. Slides may be coated with polylysine before sections are taken onto them. This ensures better fixation of sections onto the slides through all steps of staining.

- Never allow sections to dry at any step of staining.
- All reagents should be stored in the refrigerator. They should be allowed to reach room temperature before use.
- Fresh dilution of antibodies should be made prior to use.

Results

The brown to red color of nuclei, or cytoplasm as per the marker indicates positivity (**Figs. 26A and B** below for ER positivity and **Fig. 27** showing distinct membranous positivity for Her2neu)

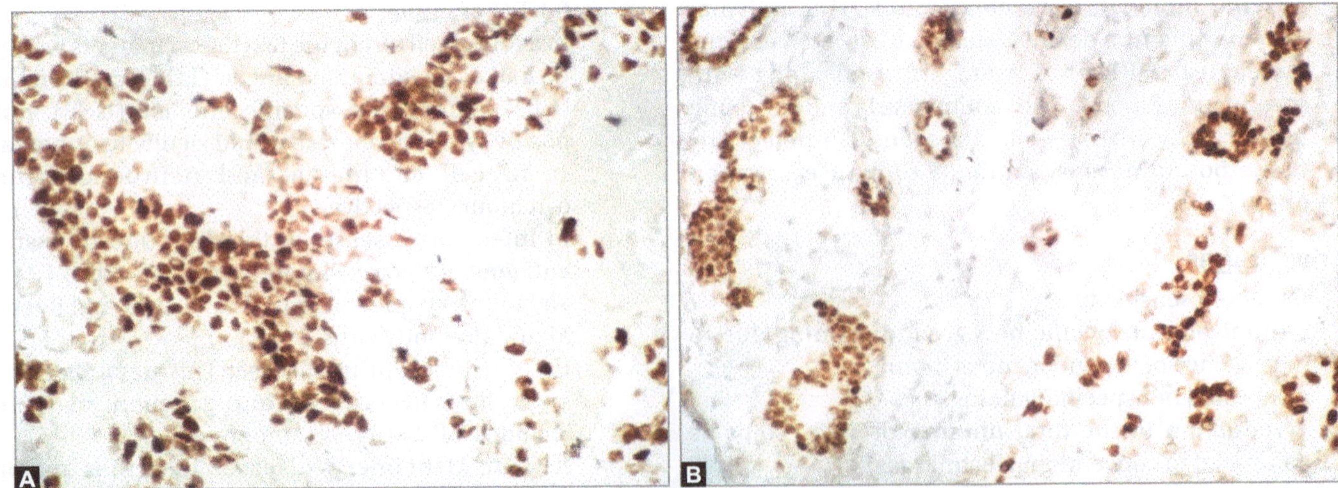

FIGS. 26A AND B: Estrogen receptor (ER) positivity in breast carcinoma. (A) Strong nuclear positivity ×400 and (B) In-built control of ER showing positivity in nuclei of ductal cells ×400.

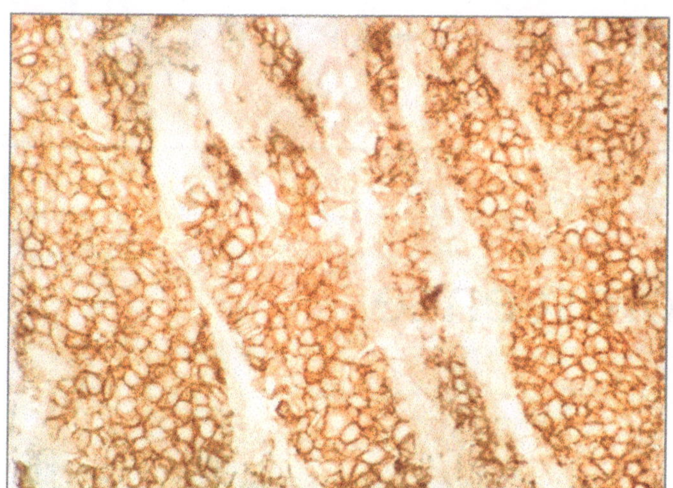

FIG. 27: Her2neu positivity (3+) in carcinoma breast.

CONCLUSION

Special stains unveil substances that would normally escape the eye, they are additive to morphology and though it is the era of immunohistochemistry, all special stains including marker positivity should be read keeping in mind the morphology at histology and not in exclusion.

REFERENCES

1. Myers R. Special stain techniques for the evaluation of mucins. [online] Available from https://www.leicabiosystems.com/en-in/knowledge-pathway/special-stain-techniques-for-the-evaluation-of-mucins/ [Last accessed March, 2024].
2. Shariff S. Laboratory Techniques in Surgical Pathology. India: Prisms Pvt Ltd; 1996.
3. Raphael SS. Lynch's Medical Technology, 3rd edition. London: WB Saunders Company; 1976.
4. Bancroft JD. Theory and practice of Histological techniques, 5th edition. Philadelphia, USA: Churchill Livingstone; 2005.
5. Winsor L. In: Woods AE, Ellis RC (Eds). Tissue processing in Laboratory Histopathology: A complete Reference. Philadelphia, USA: Churchill Livingstone; 2000.
6. In: Kumar GL, Kiernan JA (Eds). Educational guide, special stains and H & E, 2nd edition. Carpinteria, California: Dako North America; 2010.
7. Laboratory manual of the armed forces. In: Prophet EB, Bob Mills, Arrington JB, Sobin LH (Eds). Armed Forces Institute of Pathology. Washington DC: American Registry of Pathology; 1994.
8. Shariff S, Kaler AM. Principles and Interpretation of laboratory practices in Surgical Pathology, 1st edition. New Delhi: Jaypee Brothers Medical Publishers (P) Ltd; 2010.
9. Nigrosin Tulips Diagnostics, http://www.tulipgroup.com>PackInsert>Stains>2. https://www.microxpress.in/product.php?type=C&c_id=5&id=714
10. Elghetany MT, Saleem A. Methods for staining amyloid in tissues: a review. Stain Technol. 1988;63(4):201-12.

CHAPTER 21

Immunofluorescence

INTRODUCTION

Immunofluorescence is a very sensitive and special method, used for topographical detection of antigens by antibodies, labeled with fluorochromes. Immunofluorescent methods have the potential to define antigen-antibody interactions at the cellular level, e.g., mitochondria and microsomes, and identify small cell surface structures, such as receptors. Also, these highly specific reactions can be seen in the background of general histological topography of the tissue sections.

TYPES OF IMMUNOFLUORESCENCES[1-4]

- Direct immunofluorescence (DIF)
- Indirect immunofluorescence
- Microimmunofluorescence

Direct Immunofluorescence[1-4]

This technique was introduced by Coons in 1941.

Principle

It is used to detect antigens using specific fluorochrome-labeled antibodies. The steps involved are fixation of smear/section on the slide, treatment with the labeled antibody, incubation, washing to remove unbound excess labeled antibody, and visualization under a fluorescent microscope. When viewed under a fluorescent microscope, the field is dark, and areas with bound antibodies are fluorescent green.

Advantages

This technique has several advantages as the steps involved are few; therefore, it is fast and therefore is no question of nonspecificity as the site of reaction alone fluoresces and is visualized.

The disadvantages include limitations due to the unavailability of commercially available direct conjugates against antigens, the signal is weak.

Disadvantages

It include lower signal, generally higher cost, less flexibility, and difficulties with the labeling procedure when commercially available direct conjugates are unavailable.

Applications

The best application of direct immunofluorescence is in the evaluation of renal glomerular disease and bullous diseases of the skin.

Procedure: Immunofluorescence on Frozen Sections

Tissue Preparation

- The tissue is snap-frozen in isopentane in liquid nitrogen; alternatively, can be frozen in a cryostat at –28 to –30° whatever the protocol in the laboratory.
- Cut sections 5 µm thick and mount onto poly-L-lysine-coated glass slides or readymade adhesive slides
- Air-dry sections under a fan for a few hours.
- If poly-L-lysine solution is prepared in the lab it should be coated on absolutely clean detergent washed (to remove grease) and distilled water washed slides. Slides are then dried and stored at room temperature in a closed dust-free wooden box.

Direct Immunofluorescence Staining Method (Fig. 1)

- Sections are thawed at room temperature and dried for 30 minutes.
- Wash sections in 0.1 m phosphate-buffered saline (PBS) with three changes over a period of 30 minutes.

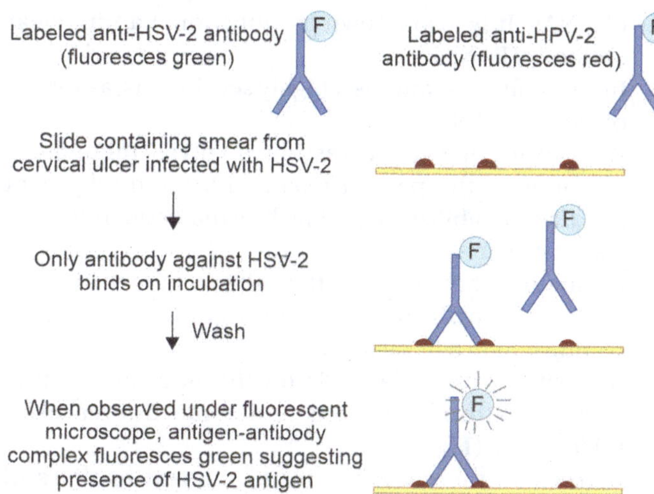

FIG. 1: Direct immunofluorescence.
(F: fluorescence; HPV: human papillomavirus; HSV: herpes simplex virus)

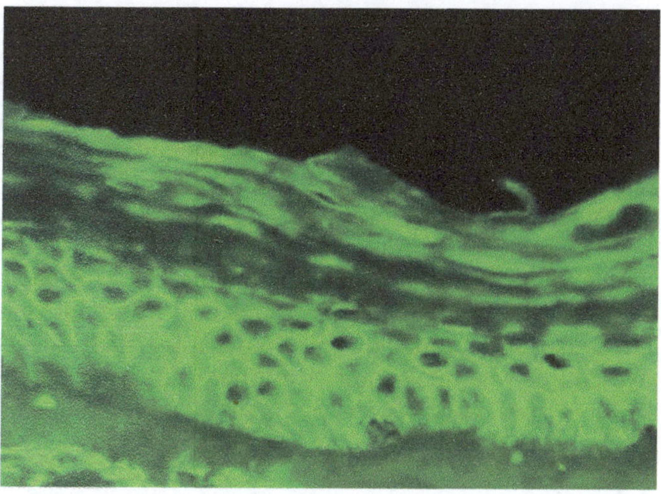

FIG. 2: Section shows basket weave positivity of immunoglobulin G (IgG) antibody in pemphigus vulgaris.

- Drain off the excess PBS and wipe sections with cellulose tissue. Cover the section with diluted conjugate and allow it to react with for at least 30 minutes at room temperature.
- Drain off the conjugate and wash off three changes of PBS over a period of 30 minutes.
- Drain off the excess PBS; sections are dried with cellulose tissue. The sections are mounted with fluorescence mounting medium (Dako, Code S3023)/ glycerol/DABCO solution.
- The edges of the coverslip are sealed with nail varnish.
- Preparations are read on a fluorescent microscope and stored at 4°C.

Immunofluorescence on frozen sections is considered the gold standard for the evaluation of renal biopsy specimens. The antibodies routinely used are immunoglobulin G (IgG), immunoglobulin A (IgA), immunoglobulin M (IgM), and component complements C3 and C1q. Results are always superior by the immunofluorescence technique as compared to immunohistochemistry.

Immunofluorescence is also of immense importance in the diagnosis of bullous lesions of the skin. **Figure 2** shows its application in pemphigus vulgaris.

Salt split immunofluorescence technique in the diagnosis of skin biopsies: The patient's skin sample is incubated in 1 mol/L normal saline which results in the split of the epidermis at the level of lamina lucida. Then the skin is subjected to direct immunofluorescence. Pemphigoid antibodies bind to the blister roof (basal keratinocytes) in 80% of cases and to the roof and floor of the blister in 20% of cases. In epidermolysis bullosa acquisita the antibodies bind only to the floor of the blister.

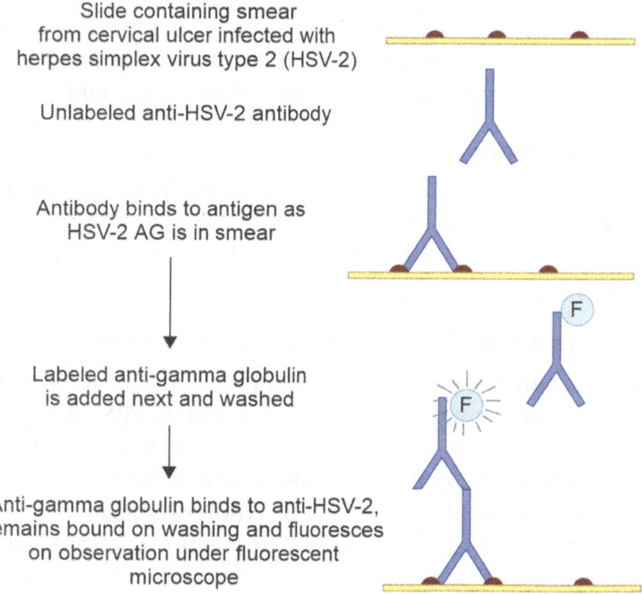

FIG. 3: Indirect immunofluorescence.

In the indirect immunofluorescence test, normal skin is used as the substrate with the patient's serum.

Indirect Immunofluorescence[1-4] (Fig. 3)

Indirect immunofluorescence was introduced by Weller and Coons in 1954.

Principle

Indirect immunofluorescence uses two antibodies; the first (the primary antibody) recognizes the target molecule and binds to it, and the second (the secondary antibody), which carries the fluorophore, recognizes the primary antibody and binds to it. The second antibody is labeled antigamma globulin antibody. This antibody binds to the Fc portion (constant) of the first antibody and persists despite washing. The presence of the second antibody is detected by observing under a fluorescent microscope.

Different primary antibodies with different constant regions are typically generated by raising the antibody in different species as compared to the secondary antibody, e.g., primary antibodies can be created in a goat that recognizes several antigens, and then employ (fluorescent) dye-coupled rabbit secondary antibodies that recognize the goat antibody constant (Fc) region ("rabbit antigoat" antibodies).

Advantages

Though this protocol is more complex than the direct protocol above and takes more time it allows more flexibility. It has a greater sensitivity than direct immunofluorescence as several secondary antibodies (each with a fluorophore) can attach to a single primary antibody resulting in a strong signal. Commercially produced secondary antibodies are cheap and easily available.

Applications

It is often used to detect autoantibodies, e.g., in the detection of antinuclear antibodies (ANAs) found in the serum of patients with systemic lupus erythematosus (SLE) and other autoimmune disorders.

Method of Indirect Immunofluorescence

- Prepare the patient's serum dilution in PBS in the ratio of 1:10. (Conventionally, 50 uL + 450 uL PBS are used.)
- Expose sections to serum dilution of primary antibody for at least 30 minutes at room temperature.
- Wash over 30 minutes in PBS (three changes).
- Drain off the excess PBS and wipe sections with cellulose tissue.
- Cover sections with appropriately diluted antihuman Ig/fluorescein isothiocyanate (FITC) conjugate for 30 minutes.
- Drain off the excess conjugate and wash with three changes of PBS.
- Mount coverslip as outlined under "direct technique" and view under the microscope.

Antinuclear Antibody Test[5,6]

- ANA test is an indirect immunofluorescence test and one of the primary tests in helping to diagnose a clinically suspected autoimmune disorder, in particular, SLE.
- An ANA test is based on immunofluorescence and remains the gold standard technique for the detection of ANAs. It is also known as "functional antinuclear antibody (FANA)."
- Immunofluorescence is a highly sensitive assay for the presence of ANAs.
- Immunofluorescence testing involves incubating dilutions of the patient's sera with a monolayer of fixed, permeabilized cells (such as the frequently used Hep-2 cell line)
- Antibodies that attach to the cell layer are visualized with an antihuman immunoglobulin reagent conjugated to a fluorescent dye.
- A positive result depends on the nuclear staining and its pattern observed under the fluorescence microscope **(Fig. 4)**.
- Increasing the cut-off point of the test to titers of 1:320 or greater leaves only 3% of normal people with positive values, indicating a specificity of ANA testing of 97%.

Enzyme-linked Immunosorbent Assay

The other common method for ANA testing currently in use is the enzyme-linked immunosorbent assay (ELISA).

- In this technique, multiwell plates are coated with a homogenate of antigens. Preparations of these are derived from cell nuclei and nuclear proteins.
- Patient's sera in dilutions is incubated in antigen-coated wells.
- Followed by incubation with an antihuman immunoglobulin reagent linked to a tagged enzyme.
- Antibody binding is quantitated by colorimetry, adding a substrate to the wells; this substrate changes color in the presence of the enzyme tag.

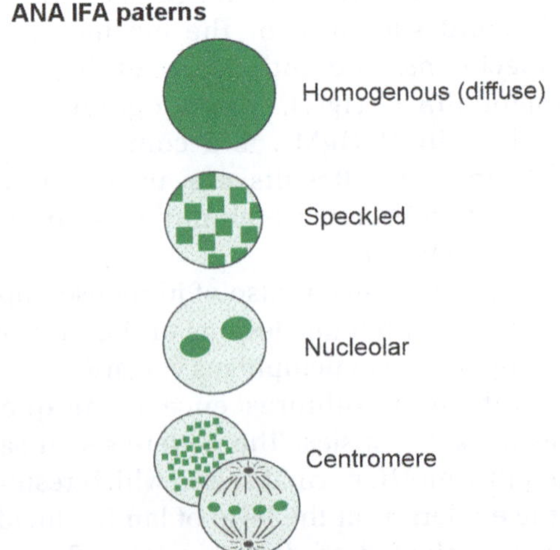

FIG. 4: The four major patterns of antinuclear antibody seen when using indirect immunofluorescence. The centromere pattern can be distinguished from other "speckled" patterns by seeing the fluorescent dots along the chromosomes in cells that are dividing.
Courtesy: James Faix, MD.

The main advantage of ELISA testing is that it is easy to perform and the speed of its performance. ELISA assays give results close to immunofluorescence in their sensitivity and specificity for the identification of ANAs.

Antineutrophil Cytoplasmic Antibody Test[7]

Antineutrophil cytoplasmic antibody (ANCA) detects autoantibodies [perinuclear antineutrophil cytoplasmic antibodies (p-ANCA) or cytoplasmic antineutrophil cytoplasmic antibodies (c-ANCA)] in the bloodstream of a patient in conditions like necrotizing vasculitis such as granulomatosis with polyangiitis (GPA), microscopic polyangiitis (MPA), and to a lesser extent, eosinophilic granulomatosis with polyangiitis (EGPA). There are two main kinds of autoantibodies that can be detected by ANCA testing. One is called *p-ANCA*. This p-ANCA type of autoantibody usually targets and attaches to myeloperoxidase (MPO), in neutrophils. The other one is called c-*ANCA*. This c-ANCA autoantibody usually targets and attaches to proteinase 3 (PR3), in neutrophils. Cytoplasmic ANCA (c-ANCA) with specificity for PR3 is found in patients with GPA; whereas, perinuclear ANCA (p-ANCA) in patients with MPA and EGPA.

Principle of ANCA Test

Most often, ANCA tests are performed using the indirect immunofluorescence technique. The patient's serum sample is mixed with neutrophils and in the presence of autoantibodies these react with the neutrophils. The sample is then smeared on a slide and treated with a fluorescent stain and the fluorescence is detected by a fluorescent microscope.

Alternately, neutrophils can be fixed onto a slide. Serum from the blood sample is mixed with the neutrophils on the slide and any ANCAs in the sample attach to the neutrophil proteins. Detection is done by the fluorescent stain.

Results

A positive test on the indirect immunofluorescence microscopy method shows different ANCA patterns:

- p-ANCA—most of the fluorescence occurs around the nucleus; about 90% of samples with a p-ANCA pattern will have MPO antibodies.
- c-ANCA—the fluorescence occurs throughout the cytoplasm of the cell; about 85% of samples with a c-ANCA pattern will have PR3 antibodies.
- Negative ANCA—no fluorescence.

According to the current recommendations, indirect immunofluorescence if positive is followed by proteinase 3 (PR3) and MPO antigen-specific immunometric assays for proper diagnostic specificity.

Advanced automated image analysis of immunofluorescence patterns, so-called third-generation PR3-ANCA and MPO-ANCA ELISA, and multiplex technology are also presently available.

Microimmunofluorescence

Works on the same principle as that of indirect immunofluorescence and has applications in the detection of IgG, IgA, and IgM antibodies to infections, such as chlamydia, toxoplasmosis, epidemic typhus, and Q fever. It makes use of Teflon-coated slides with many wells dotted with different antigens.

APPLICATIONS OF IMMUNOFLUORESCENCE IN DIAGNOSTIC PATHOLOGY[1,5,6]

- Detection of microorganisms, e.g., *Mycobacterium tuberculosis*
- Detection of antigens in fresh frozen and fixed tissues
- Testing of bacterial and parasitic infections
- Detection and localization of specific deoxyribonucleic acid (DNA) sequences on chromosomes
- Detection of antibodies in autoimmune disorders

LIMITATIONS OF IMMUNOFLUORESCENCE[4]

Photobleaching

Photobleaching is the photochemical destruction of a fluorochrome due to the reductive of reactive oxygen species as a result of fluorochrome excitation. Loss of activity can be controlled by reducing the intensity or timespan of light exposure and by increasing concentration.

Fluorescence Overlap

When multicolor fluorescence is used the emission signals may overlap and these may give a false level of more than one color.

This overlap of excitation and emission intensities and wavelengths must be eliminated, using the appropriate selection of an excitation filter, and barrier or emission filter.

For a given fluorochrome, the manufacturers indicate the wavelength for the peak of the illumination excitation intensity and the wavelength for the peak of fluorescence emission intensity.

CONCLUSION

In summary, immunofluorescence is the visualization of antigens within the cells using antibodies as fluorescent probes. Indirect immunofluorescence deals with the detection of antibodies. The benefits of the immunofluorescence technique have proved to be a powerful tool for determining the distribution of antigens in frozen sections and in the localization of specific DNA sequences.

REFERENCES

1. Bancroft JD. Bancroft's Theory and Practice of Histological techniques, 5th edition. Philadelphia, USA: Churchill Livingstone; 2005.
2. www.imperial.ac.uk. Beta Cell Genome Regulation Laboratory. [online] Available from https://www.imperial.ac.uk/medicine/beta-cell-genome-regulation-laboratory/ [Last accessed March, 2024].
3. Taylor CR, Rudbeck L. (2013). Immunohistochemical Staining Methods. [online] Available from https://www.agilent.com/cs/library/technicaloverviews/ public/08002_ihc_staining_methods.pdf. [Last accessed March, 2024].
4. Wikipedia. (2019). Immunofluorescence. [online] Available form https:// en.wikipedia.org/wiki/Immunofluorescence [Last accessed March, 2024].
5. Greidinger EL, Hoffman RW. Antinuclear antibody testing: Methods, indications, and interpretation. Lab Med. 2003;34(2): 113-7.
6. Association for Diagnostics & Laboratory Medicine. (2019). A basic guide to ANA testing. [online] Available from https://www.myadlm.org/cln/articles/2019/april/a-basic-guide-to-antinuclear-antibody-ana-testing [Last accessed March, 2024].
7. Csernok E, Moosig F. Current and emerging techniques for ANCA detection in vasculitis. Nat Rev Rheumatol. 2014;10(8):494-501.

CHAPTER 22

Automation in Histopathology

INTRODUCTION

Like all fields in health care, the histopathology laboratory is turning to automation and advanced technology in order to meet the increasing demands of work and quality services. Automation and procedures have become the core of anatomic pathology reporting. The automated testing laboratory (ATL), without which no hospital (or even a small private medical group!) can function, is the emerging result. This chapter will review the various types of automation and technology available to histopathology laboratories and the possible impact it can have on histology workflow.

DEFINITION OF AUTOMATION

- Automation is the independent accomplishment of a function by a device or system that was formerly carried out manually.
- There are many machines that are used at different stages of tissue treatment till a thin section is obtained to be viewed under the microscope, e.g., tissue processors and microtomes.

NEED FOR AUTOMATION

- Increased workload
- Saves technician's time and labor
- Gives reliable quality control
- Fast reporting in surgical pathology where treatment decisions must be taken

AUTOMATED INSTRUMENTS[1-3]

- *Tissue processing*:
  - Automated tissue processor: Two types are available—(1) open (tissue basket mobile) and (2) closed (tissues static) types
    - Vacuum histoprocessor
    - Microwave histoprocessor
- *Tissue embedding*: Automated tissue embedding
- Section cutting machine
- Manual
- Semiautomatic
- Automatic
- *Automated slide stainer*:
  - Two types are available: (1) Circular and (2) linear
- Automated coverslipping machine

Tissue Processing

Principle

The principle are treated with various fluids using a series of solutions for a predetermined length of time in a controlled environment. Tissue thus processed is embedded in a medium such as paraffin which is firm and supports it thus making it easy for sectioning.

Automation in tissue processing has two principles:

1. Tissue is mobile and moves through a series of chambers containing fluids arranged in the order desired. The tissue is housed in cassettes which are placed in a perforated metal cylinder. This cylinder is automatically transported through a series of reagents

in the chambers (in the form of glass jars that are stationary) the basket of tissues travels from jar to jar.

2. Tissue is static and housed in a closed chamber and the series of fluids moves in and out of these chambers at predetermined regular intervals.

In such an automated tissue processor:

- The length of time the tissues are exposed to each reagent container is electronically programmed.
- Vertical oscillations or the mechanical raising and lowering of the tissue basket/agitation (closed type) in the reagent container provide the impetus needed for processing the tissue
- About 12 containers (or more) containing different solutions are used for processing in the order as per the schedule of the lab, for example:
    - 10% formalin—container numbers 1 and 2
    - 50% alcohol or 60% alcohol—container number 3
    - 70% alcohol—container number 4
    - 90% alcohol—container number 5
    - Absolute alcohol—container numbers 6 and 7
    - Acetone/toluene—container numbers 8 and 9
    - Xylene—container number 10
    - Paraffin wax—container numbers 11 and 12
- For overnight processing, the schedule can be programmed

Tissue Processor (Open Type) (Fig. 1)

- The tissue is mobile and moves automatically through a series of solutions.
- Comes with programmable 24-hour clock
- Thermostatically controlled wax bath
- Uses vacuum function to accelerate the speed of tissue processing

Advantages

- The progress of tissue processing is visible
- Easy to troubleshoot as compared to the closed system

Tissue Processor (Closed Type)

- Tissue is static and the fluid moves through a series of chambers containing fluids.
- This is called continuous input, rapid tissue processor.
- This uses vacuum infiltration.
- Agitation—accelerates the rate of diffusion of solvents into the tissues

Advantages of this Automatic System

- Acceptance of tissues into the system at timed intervals
- Improving turnaround time
- Morphology and quality of the specimen is consistent with that of traditional tissue processing
- Enclosed system
- Vacuum facility
- Capacity of up to 360 cassettes
- 12 reagent containers with three paraffin stations
- Fixation to paraffin infiltration
- Has a unique linear design
- Reliable technique in a small space in the laboratory
- Tissues are loaded in a static container where they remain throughout the process.
- Reagents and melted paraffin are moved in and out of the chamber one after the other as per the programming using vacuum/pressure.
- By reducing the pressure during wax impregnation—air bubbles and clearing agents are rapidly removed from the tissues resulting in more rapid impregnation

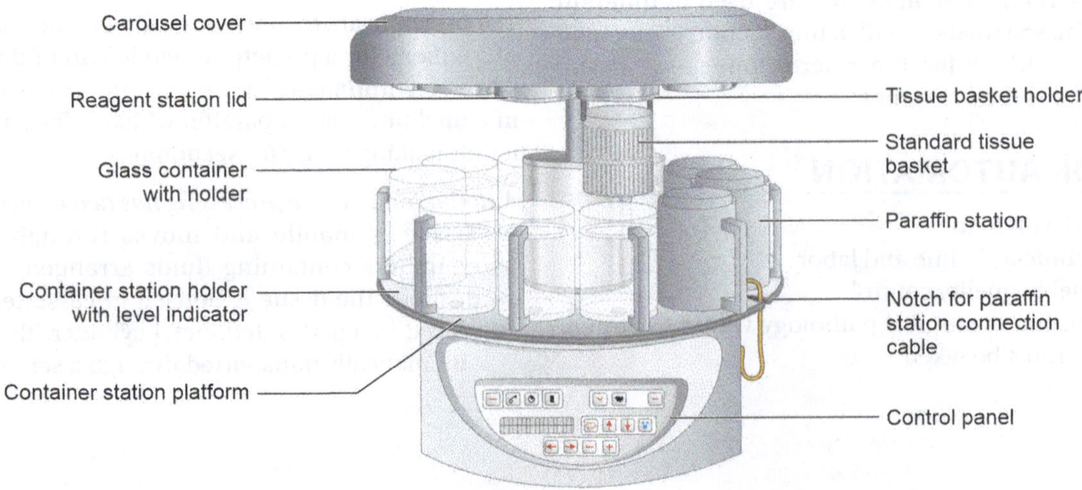

FIG. 1: Tissue processor open type.

Vacuum Tissue Processor

Vacuum tissue processor is commonly used in closed type.

Factors Influencing the Rate of Infiltration and Impregnation

- Specimen size
- Agitation
- Heat
- Viscosity

Microwave Histoprocessor

- Ethanol/isopropanol/polyethylene glycol
- Proprietary mixtures of alcohol and paraffin.
- Graded concentration of alcohol is not required
- Marked Reduction in processing time
- 110 biopsies every 45 minutes can be processed.
- Processing with single dehydration/clearing reagent
- Clearing agents are not required (the temperature of the final paraffin step facilitates the evaporation of alcohol from the tissue).
- Xylene and formalin are not used (eliminates toxic fumes)
- Properly controlled processing provides uncompromised morphology and antigenicity of the specimen
- Increased efficiency through improved turnaround times.

Advantages

- The embedding time is half that of the routine wax embedding
- Any air in the tissue is extracted
- Shortens the processing time from hours to minutes
- Stimulates the diffusion of solutes into the tissue by increasing the internal heat of the specimen.
- Accelerating the reaction time
- They have precise temperature controls, timers, and a fume extraction system.
- Time for processing is dependent on the thickness and density of the specimen.

Disadvantages

- The process is cumbersome as everything is performed manually.
- The use of the microwave should be monitored and calibrated regularly.

Maintenance of Microwave Histoprocessor

- All automatic tissue processing should adhere to a standard program with regard to the changing of solutions and the duration of tissues in each, this should be placed near the machine in a written format.
- The above will in turn depend on the surgical load, the size and types of tissue processed, and the reagents used.
- Solutions should be carefully monitored and frequently change depending on tissue load to ensure quality.
- The manufacturer's handbook outlining preventive maintenance should be followed.
- The temperature of paraffin in the infiltration containers should be set 2–3°C above the melting point of the paraffin.
- Spillage and hardening of wax on any surface should be cleaned and removed from time to time.
- Timing should be checked each time before placing tissue cassettes in the processor.

Tissue Embedding Machine

- The machine is convenient for quick and meticulous paraffin embedding of a large number of tissue specimens carried out simultaneously.
- All functions should be checked separately, in particular, the heat regulation function should be controlled by an accurate digital thermostat mechanism, not to exceed 70°C.

Components

- Magnifying lens
- Prewarming chamber
- Warming chamber
- Electrically heated forceps
- Programmable timer
- Flexible magnifier
- Sealed surface

Advantages of Automated Tissue Embedder

- Marble working platform is easy to clean up
- Separate temperature control

Section Cutting: Microtomy

- Microtomy is sectioning of tissue from paraffin blocks at 5–6 μm thickness in a machine called the microtome and mounting of these onto glass slides to enable staining.
- The basic instrument used in microtomy is the microtome.
    - Manual: Completely manipulated by the operator
    - Semiautomatic: One motor to advance either the fine coarse hand wheel
    - Automatic: Two motors that drive both the fine and coarse advanced hand wheel

Semiautomatic

Features

- Section and trimming mode have control systems
- The LCD screen provided gives information on section thickness, section trimming thickness range, number of sections, etc.
- Hand wheel can be locked at any position to ensure user safety
- Has a large waste tray, easy to unload
- Universal cassette clamp and standard specimen clamp; alarm system and emergency stop systems

Rotary Microtome (Automated)

- The rigid base provides stability to the machine
- A protective hood is attached to the base and swings back to expose the parts for easy handling while cleaning and lubrication.
- Automatic feed release, safety device, and wheel lock
- LCD slice counting device
- Easy to clean sealed box cover
- Easy adjustment of sample slice angle

Advantages

- Improved section quality
- Increased productivity
- Improved occupational safety for the technologist
- Eliminates manual hand-wheel operation; reduces the incidence of repetitive motion disorders.

Slide Stainer (Circular Type)

- Up to 70 slides can be stained
- Continuous loading
- Automated water flow system
- Simultaneous staining of H&E, Pap, and special stains
- Integrated oven for optimal slide drying
- Fume extraction system
- Continuous loading and unloading

Slide Stainer (Linear Type)

- Enables concurrent staining of routine H&E and special stains
- It has a provision to stain up to 60 slides at each run; and up to 500 slides in 1 hour
- It can be programmed for cytology staining as well as histopathology.

Cover Slipping Machine

- About 150 slides can be coverslipped in 1 hour.
- All steps of mounting are done automatically—the mounting media is placed on the slide, the slide is placed horizontally on a rack for coverslipping, air bubbles are removed as the cover slip gets laid over the section, and the positioning is done automatically.
- The mounted slide is moved mechanically to a storage rack by a metal fork.
- The cycle is repeated for every slide and the time taken for each slide is 22.5 seconds.

CRYOSTAT

- The automatic cryostat has a facility for taking temperatures down to −35°C for rapid freezing of specimens; this temperature is electronically controlled.
- It also has an electronically controlled advance and retraction of the block.
- It has a specimen orientation facility with digital visualization of chuck and cabinet temperature.
- Section thickness can be adjusted, sections are spread through a vacutome attachment, and the speed of cutting can be controlled.
- The machine has an automatic defrost system as well as automated decontamination and sterilization.

IMMUNOSTAINER

- There are instruments available offering various levels of automation in immunohistochemical techniques.
- *Two types of reagent delivery systems are there*:
  i. Capillary action used by Shandon Sequenza, Shandon Cadenza and Ventana-Techmate
  ii. Spray delivery: Dako Autostainer
- The latest innovation in immunostaining is the development of automated systems capable of carrying out both antigen retrieval and immunostaining, e.g., Bond-Max autostainer—polymer-labeled antibodies.

Inbuilt Characteristics of Immunostainer

- *Power failure safeguard*: If any power failure occurs in operation, the external UPS will provide a power supply to keep the procedures running.
- It has a programming capacity to stain paraffin sections, frozen sections, and smears; can stain 50 slides in each batch.
- The inside environment is moist and suitable to prevent sections from drying during the procedure.
- The equipment can estimate automatically whether the amount of static reagent in the machine is enough or not for the current procedure and gives an automatic warning of reagent shortage.
- The system automatically cleans burettes each time after dropping the reagent in order to avoid cross-contamination.

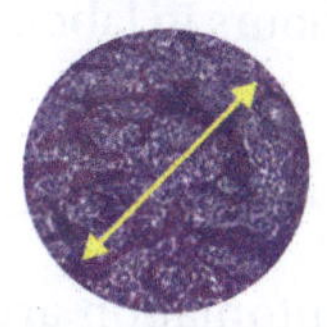

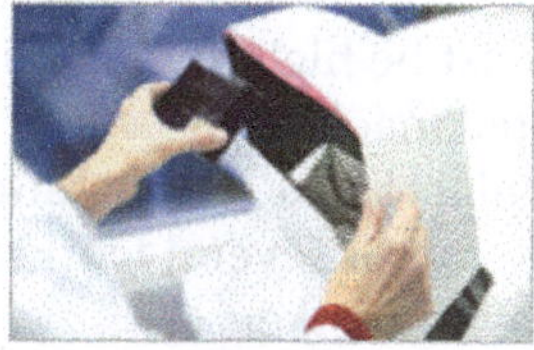
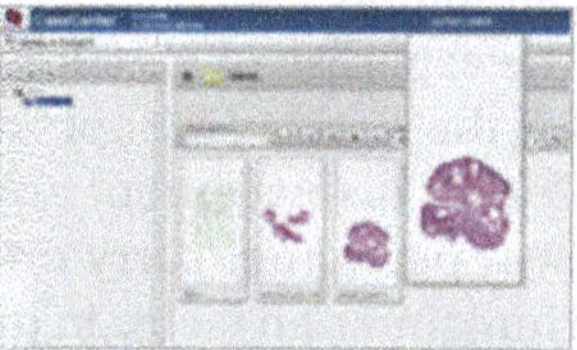

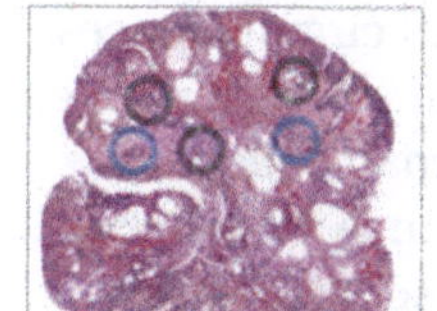
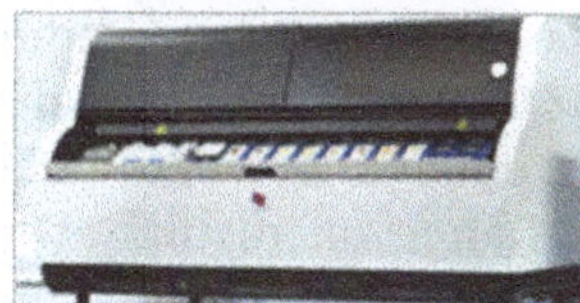

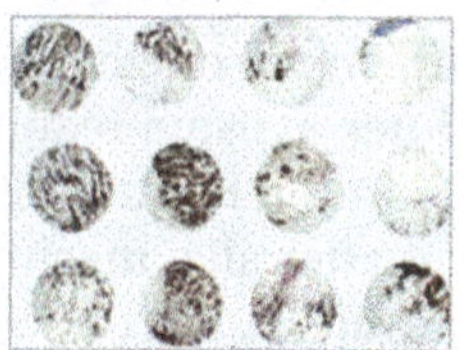

FIG. 2: Diagrammatic representation of automated tissue microarray plan with a digital selection of images and tissue microarraying.

- It is ideal for increased load and automation ensures standardization of technique
- A single computer can control several immunohistostainers simultaneously.
- The machine is easy to operate and has a facility for adding or removal of slides during the procedure.

TISSUE MICROARRAY[4-6]

- Automated machines can place 100 or more samples in a single block depending on the size of the core.
    - There are two types of TMA techniques that are (1) automated and (2) manual. Automated method is depicted in **Figure 2.**
- It can perform visual selection in a section for punching, using a magnifying glass or a stereomicroscope as a guide.
- It marks, edits, and saves punched tissue with the help of coordinates on an on-screen display with software tools.
- Punch speed and the block capacity are much faster (7 times more) than the manual method.
- A video merge unit displays premarked slide images side-by-side with the donor block image, in the automated method.
- The operative level begins with slide scanning and the use of a digital platform.
- Histological expertise is necessary to perform precise annotations.

Advantages

- Easy to use; has a specimen tracking software system
- About 120–80 cores can be punched per hour

DISTANCE LEARNING[7]

Slides can be digitally scanned (Aperio scanner, Leica Biosystems, Nussloch, Germany) and stored on the virtual pathology website, and the links to the slides can be made available for university trainees and consultant pathologists as part of continuing medical education programs and for discussions and lectures.

DIGITAL PATHOLOGY AND TELEPATHOLOGY FOR CONSULTATIONS[8,9]

Digital pathology is a branch of pathology that deals with the analysis of pathology material based on information generated from digitized slides on a particular case or specimen. With the aid of computer-based technology, digital pathology uses virtual microscopy for data analyses. It employs static images, live streaming of images, and whole-slide imaging (WSI). WSI permits digitization of the entire glass slides, thereby eliminating the need for pathology practices to be limited by conventional microscopes or transfer of fixed images taken by an inbuilt camera. A digital slide image is generated which allows for high-resolution viewing, interpretation, and image analysis of digital pathology slides. Glass slides are converted into digital slides that can be viewed, marked on the areas of interest, and analyzed on a computer monitor with as many consultants as possible using magnification of various dimensions on these images.

With the practice of WSI, the field of digital pathology is growing and has applications in diagnostic medicine, and the prediction of disease prognosis due to its success and on-par efficiency as compared to real-time microscopy.

Recent challenges in technical requirements (scanner, storage, and network) still pose limitations for the dissemination of digital pathology data. Over the last 5 years this has changed as new and powerful and affordable scanner technology as well as mass/cloud storage technologies have emerged in the field.

Digital pathology enables pathologists to view, evaluate, and collaborate images and data rapidly and remotely, with consistency, thus improving efficiency and productivity.

Digital images lend themselves to many clinical and nonclinical applications, such as research. Clinical uses include making primary pathology diagnoses directly from digital images, telepathology, archiving, and image analysis. Nonclinical uses include research and education. Digital pathology is nevertheless deemed to become increasingly vital for the future practice of pathology.

Digital pathology has been approved by the United States Food and Drug Administration (FDA) for a primary diagnosis. The approval is based on studies in which WSI is shown to be not inferior to microscopy across a wide range of surgical pathology specimens.

ADVANTAGES AND LIMITATIONS OF AUTOMATION

Advantages

- Higher production rates and increased and quick turnover of work
- More effective and economic use of raw material, better, standardized, and neat product turnover
- No human bias
- Improved safety measures for personnel, less occupational hazards, and shorter working hours in labor.
- Manpower can be used for other jobs

Disadvantages and Limitations

The disadvantages and limitations of automation are as follows:

- High cost of machines and maintenance; frequent calibration.
- The expertise of personnel must be high in maintaining the working of sophisticated machines.
- Person displacement and replacement by machines. Less personnel carry out the job of several workers. Humanitarian factor in displaying workers.
- Less flexibility in carrying out procedures. Less scope for maneuvering procedures to suit circumstances.
- In the long run personal skills will suffer dependence on automation will supersede human abilities.
- Reliance on results at the expense of mechanical performance versus common sense.

CONCLUSION

Automation is a double-edged sword, on the one hand, it hastens sample analysis, and computer-assisted reading is of immense help; on the other hand, all equipment should be supervised constantly, it is after all a machine unlike the human brain and elicits results based on what is fed! It lacks analysis and therefore cannot replace the comprehension of a human brain.

REFERENCES

1. Lynch MJ, Raphael SS. Medical Laboratory Technology, 3rd edition. Philadelphia: WB Saunders Company; 1976.
2. Bancroft JD. Bancroft's Theory and Practice of Histological techniques, 5th edition. Philadelphia, USA: Churchill Livingstone; 2005.
3. Prophet EB, Mills B, Arrington JB, Sobin LH. Armed Forces Institute of Pathology: Laboratory Methods in Histotechnology. Washington DC: American Registry of Pathology; 1994.
4. Aktas S. Tissue microarray: Current perspectives in pathology. Aegean Pathol J. 2004;1:27-324.
5. Zlobec I, Koelzer VH, Dawson H, Perren A, Lugli A. Next-generation tissue microarray (ngTMA) increases the quality of biomarker studies: an example using CD3, CD8, and CD45RO in the tumor microenvironment of six different solid tumor types. J Transl Med. 2013;11:104.
6. Fejzo MS, Slamon DJ. Frozen tumor tissue microarray technology for analysis of tumor RNA, DNA, and proteins. Am J Pathol. 2001;159(5):1640-50.
7. Rotimi O, Orah N, Shaaban A, Daramola AO, Abdulkareem FB. Remote Teaching of Histopathology Using Scanned Slides via Skype between the United Kingdom and Nigeria. Arch Pathol Lab Med. 2017;141(2):298-300.
8. Leong JWM, Graham AK, Gahm T, McGee J. Telepathology : Clinical utility and methodology. In: Lowe D, Underwood J (Eds). Recent advances in histopathology 18. Edinburgh: Churchill Livingstone; 1999. pp. 217-39.
9. Winstein RS, Graham AR, Richter LC, Barker GP, Krupinski EA, Lopez AM, et al. Overview of telepathology, virtual microscopy, and whole slide imaging: prospects for the future. Hum Pathol. 2009;40(8):1057-69.

CHAPTER 23

Systematized Nomenclature of Pathology

INTRODUCTION

As the subject of pathology assumes growing importance in the field of medicine, there is a need to collate data with regard to the prevalent diseases and lesions in various organ systems across geographic regions. In order to achieve uniformity in communication and for ease of compilation it became necessary to code lesions and neoplasia so that an indexing system could be maintained in every institution and center of reporting.

The chief reasons for indexing are:

- To study the pattern of diseases at the geographical and socioeconomic levels.
- To provide statistics with regard to a particular disease process.
- To make a follow-up of individual patients possible.
- To provide feedback to the pathologist/cytologist on the accuracy of a particular diagnosis.

Various indexing systems have been used to advantage in histopathology.

HISTORICAL ASPECTS[1]

- In the 1950 and 1960s, the principal system for classifying diseases was the International Code of Diseases (ICD); a series published by the World Health Organization (WHO). ICD was used to code and tabulate the diagnoses on all patient medical records to be stored.
- The first "code manual" for the morphology of neoplasms was published by the American Cancer Society (ACS) in 1951 as the Manual of Tumor Nomenclature and Coding (MOTNAC).
- The Second Edition of the International Classification of Diseases for Oncology was published by WHO in 1990 (first edition in 1976) for use in cancer registries and in pathology and other departments specializing in cancer.
- The Third Edition of the International Classification of Diseases for Oncology (ICD-O) was published in 2000 and is intended to be used for cancer cases diagnosed from January 2001 onward.

SYSTEMATIZED NOMENCLATURE OF PATHOLOGY

The systematized nomenclature of pathology (SNOP),[2-4] a coded vocabulary of diseases was published by the College of American Pathologists (CAP) in 1965 and provided a morphology code as well as a topography code to cover every part of the human body; it was revised in the 1990s.

In the mid-1970s, SNOP was expanded beyond pathology to develop a terminology that would encompass the entire medical record. This was known as Systematized Nomenclature of Medicine (SNOMED)[5] and was designed to provide the terminology needed to code the entire medical record. The terminology is validated with careful quality assurance procedures in place to ensure that it is structurally sound, biomedically accurate, and consistent with current practice. Therefore, SNOMED is an offshoot of the work of the CAP, and supervision of the "content" is done by a multidisciplinary editorial board with broad representation from clinical practice.

This work was refined with another release, in 1993, of SNOMED International, which was updated annually through 1998. Work continued with the release of SNOMED Referral Terminology (RT) version 1.0 in January 2001 and SNOMED RT 1.1 in July 2001.

Systematized Medical Nomenclature for Medicine Clinical Terms

This is a systematically organized computer processable collection of medical terms providing codes, terms, synonyms, and definitions used in clinical documentation and reporting.

One of SNOMED CT's precursors focuses mainly on pathology, today's SNOMED CT has a broad scope that encompasses all of healthcare. SNOMED CT is the merger of SNOMED RT and the United Kingdom's CTV 3 terminology (connected TV 3), formerly known as the Read Codes. (Connected TV is video content on a TV screen, delivered via an internet connection.)

Systematized Medical Nomenclature for Medicine–Clinical Terminology

Mapping is designed to be integrated into a computerized patient record so that developers of software or systems might use it.

With regard to pathology, SNOP originally designed by Arnold Pratte (1966), is the scheme of classification for the filing and retrieval of case material in the four categories of topography (anatomic sites), morphology (tissue reactions, specific lesions, and diseases), etiology (organisms and chemicals), and function (including metabolic and endocrine states). It can be used both as a manual system and a computer-assisted system.

These codes of SNOP can be used for an indexing system for histopathology reports, slides, and museum specimens, both as card files and computer-based systems. In the latter, the rapidity of computer searches will allow the review of previous diagnoses in patients with the current material under examination. Several centers in most countries are establishing computer-based indexing systems for surgical pathology diagnoses.

By getting software done to incorporate SNOP phrases and diagnoses in the final typed report, a system of automatic encoding of surgical pathology and cytology data can be developed in all departments.

This SNOP[2-4] nomenclature is based on four areas:

1. *Topography*—where the portion of the body affected plays a part in the diagnosis, the code letter being "T," e.g., breast, liver, or abdomen. A two-digit form may be used, e.g., T43 which is designated for coronary artery. If a more anatomical detailed version is needed, then a four-digit system may be used, e.g., T4311 designating the anterior descending branch of the coronary artery. Some examples for topography T (topography) along with anatomic terms are as follows:
   i. (T-28000) Lung
   ii. (T-32000) Heart
   iii. (T-51000) Mouth
   iv. (T-D2500) Hip
   v. (T-D9600) Heel
2. *Morphology*—where structural changes are essential to the diagnosis, the code letter being "M," e.g., adenocarcinoma and papilloma.
   Examples of morphology are as follows:
   i. (M-40000) Inflammation
   ii. (M-44000) Granuloma
   iii. (M-54700) Infarcted
   iv. (M-54701) Microscopic infarct
   For example, thus suppose a patient has had a fibroadenoma of the breast diagnosed, the indexing card would read as:
   T-0400 M-9010
   Breast Fibroadenoma (**Appendix 5**, for more examples on SNOP dictionary)

   In certain instances, the term topography may be used to not only indicate anatomical organs in the strict sense but *an area too*. In such instances, a two-digit code is used. It was realized when this two-digit code was introduced for topography, that expansions on this coding system would be required and so the letters "X" and "Y" have been placed after the letter "T."

   Examples:
   a. T-Y 4 is abdomen and includes retroperitoneum.
   b. T-Y 5 is abdominal viscera in general.
3. *Etiology*—where the etiological agent is known, the code letter being "E," e.g., herpes simplex virus infection.
4. *Function*—where body functional manifestations are essential to the diagnosis, the morphology plays only an ancillary role, e.g., thyrotoxicosis.

In the utilization of this nomenclature, topography is always used in conjunction with any one of 2, 3, or 4.

INDEXING IN CYTOLOGY

Whereas the above system suffices for histopathology, the SNOP system can be modified for cytology. Three four-digit codes put forth by the SNOP are as follows:

1. *6971*: Cytological alteration, suspicious
2. *6972*: Cytological alteration, positive
3. *6973*: Cytological alteration, deferred classification

These can be combined with the topography and morphology to convey to the clinician the cytological alteration whether positive, suspicious, or deferred. For example, in **Table 1**, breast aspirate No. FNA-1240 for the year 2021 is diagnosed as fibroadenoma as a definite diagnosis; FNA-1241 for the year 2021 is diagnosed cytologically as suspicious for diagnosis.

FNA-1242 for the year 2021 is diagnosed as cytologic alteration classification deferred for fibroadenoma.

TABLE 1: Cytological indexing modified from SNOP indexing.

Organ code no.: T-0400	Diagnosis code no.: M-9010	Cytology code no.: 6972
Breast FNA-1240/2021	Fibroadenoma	Cytological alteration positive
Organ code no.: T-0400	Diagnosis code no.: M-9010	Cytology code no.: 6971
Breast FNA-1241/2021	Fibroadenoma	Cytological alteration Suspicious
Organ code no.: T-0400	Diagnosis code no.: M-9010	Cytology code no.: 6973
Breast FNA-1242/2021	Fibroadenoma	Cytological alteration deferred classified

It should be noted also that the intrinsic to this indexing system is the maintenance of a report copy and relevant requisition form on file. Once any cytological number is located on the index card the name, age, sex, and other details can automatically be derived by tracing the report copy and relevant requisition form.

CONCLUSION

As medical treatment advances due to technology, it becomes mandatory that maintenance of medical records is an essential requirement not only for patient care but also for interinstitutional comparative studies and epidemiology of disease.

REFERENCES

1. National Cancer Institute. Cancer Registration & Surveillance Modules. [online] Available from https://training.seer.cancer.gov/modules_reg_surv.html [Last accessed March, 2024].
2. ACI Open Thieme-Connect. Methods of Information in Medicine. Thieme. 2023;62(05/06):151-205.
3. Sommers SC. Systematized nomenclature of pathology. Path Microbiol. 1967;30(5):826-7.
4. Coles EC, Slavin G. An evaluation of automatic coding of surgical pathology reports. J Clin Pathol. 1976;29(7):621-5.
5. Imel M, Campbell JR. Mapping from a clinical terminology to a classification. [online] Available from https://www.coursesidekick.com/medicine/1739914 [Last accessed March, 2024].

CHAPTER 24

Quality Systems in Histopathology

INTRODUCTION

Quality control[1] is defined as a system for verifying and maintaining a desired level of quality in individual tests or processes in any laboratory. Quality control activities apply to all processes that are involved from the arrival of the specimen in the laboratory to its exit on completion of the test with the report.

Quality assurance (QA)[2] is defined by the College of American Pathologists as systematic monitoring of quality control results and quality practice parameters to assure that all systems are functioning in a manner appropriate to excellence in health care delivery. QA is a coordinated system designed to detect, control, and prevent the occurrence of errors. Quality control is an important part of the systematic approach to QA.

QUALITY CONTROL[1,3,4]

In histopathology, the laboratory requires basic minimum standards of acceptability for good laboratory practices. It means delivery of accurate, timely, and complete reports comparable to a referral standard. This results in efficient services and cost-effectiveness. For efficient services, the laboratory should outline objectives that should be met on a continuous basis. These objectives should outline the requirements of the clinician and patient and attempts should be made to meet these. Every stage that a specimen goes through after entry into the laboratory should be foolproof with guidelines to deal with a probable situation that the receipt of that specimen would face during the phase of preanalysis, analysis, and postanalysis.

Preanalysis

- Clear outlines and guidelines to receive specimens should be outlined with regard to checking for fixative; giving the correct accession number; entry into respective register or computer system; the date of receipt; information on the request form, requesting doctor's name, unit's previous biopsy accession number.
- The specimen should be duly "cut up" on the scheduled time as per laboratory norms; adequate description; mention of the person doing the cut-up and the technician receiving the bits. A complete description of the specimen which would enable any reader to visualize the features described.
- Any gross photographs to be taken should promptly be done and delay for cut up should be avoided due to this.
- Processing and staining of tissue should be as per standard protocol; timings should be adhered to. Technicians on duty should be alerted to receive any urgent samples as in transplant biopsies if that service is available.
- The infrastructure of the laboratory should be ideal with the workspace being bright and lit up with adequate light for work. Backup for electricity should be available so that tissue in automated machines does not get held up or dried. Protocols of action for stoppage of tissue in processing units due to electricity failure should be laid down.
- Fixation, processing, and staining procedures, standard operating procedures (SOPs) should be available at all times as hard copies.

- Staining of surgical biopsies should be checked by the technical supervisor on a daily basis before being handed to the reporting pathologist.
- A separate register should trace the journey of a specimen with regard to regross, special stains, and delays if justifiable.

Phase of Analysis

- Turnaround times should be adhered to and the workload of technicians and surgical pathologists should conform to international norms.
- Completed reports should be typed, checked by a junior pathologist, and given for signatures to the reporting pathologist who in turn checks it before signing.
- SOPs for specimen analysis should be typed and made available at all times.
- All problem cases should be brought to a table for consultation and adequate decisions should be taken.
- All reporting staff should be qualified with post-graduation and experience.
- Regular intradepartment discussions should occur with regard to interesting cases before the dispatch of the report.
- The department should have policies laid down as regards system-wise reporting of biopsies by consultants or general rotation of all specimens where all the consultants get to see all systems. The duty rota should be clear, and schedules put up on the notice board much in advance so as to let everyone be aware of them.
- Clinicopathological discussions should occur before reporting any out-of-the-ordinary case. Any interesting biopsy should be discussed at the departmental clinicopathological meetings which should be held at regular intervals in turn with all surgical departments, depending on the workload and free time.
- Indexing of all lesions should be done on a daily basis; the systematized nomenclature of pathology (SNOP) system may be used which has a facility for abridging or expanding the same.

Postanalysis Period

- A systematic dispatch of all completed reports should be done daily.
- The system streamlined and agreed upon for dispatching of reports in consultation with the hospital superintendent should be adhered to. Any deviation from the norm should be brought to the notice of the head of the department. Signatures should be taken from the nursing staff or the personnel in charge of receiving the reports and a record maintained.
- If urgent reports are orally conveyed, these should be followed by a written report. The name of the person receiving the oral report and the text of the report should be documented with time and date.
- Acceptable norms of turnaround time for small biopsies like endometrial curettage is 24–48 hours and for medium-sized biopsies is 3–4 days and for large specimen resections is about a week to 10 days. Any delay should be conveyed to the clinician with the reason for the same.
- The facility for archiving material and retaining it for a specified period of time as per international norms should be maintained.

QUALITY ASSURANCE[2,5]

The programs should encompass all of the aforementioned factors and ensure that an integrated system of operation exists for the smooth running of the laboratory.

- *Laboratory infrastructure*: The laboratory must be designed to have enough working, bright light in the area of work; space to accommodate all equipment, storage space for raw materials, block storage, and place for archives. Specimen preparation areas should be separate from the reporting side. Continuous water supply, electric connections for automated services, and backup for instruments.
- The hierarchy of the staff should be known to all employees and each employee should know who they can approach in times of troubleshooting.
- Regular meetings should be held in order to assess the working conditions of the laboratory with regard to equipment maintenance, calibration, and workload of personnel. Problems should be reviewed from time to time and solutions sought. All levels of staff should attend these meetings.
- *Intradepartmental, interdepartmental,* and *interinstitutional quality* assessment programs should be organized at every level so that staff is updated from time to time. Credit points for performance should be encouraged. Attendance for continuing medical education and conferences should be encouraged and made compulsory on an annual basis.
- The laboratory should be registered by national and international academic bodies and associations to ensure participation in External Quality Assurance (EQAs) programs.[5,6]
- *External quality assurance or assessment (EQA)* is carried out under Clinical Pathology Accreditation (CPA) and National Accreditation (NABL). Other schemes are those of the Indian College of Pathologists/ Indian Association of Pathologists and Microbiologists/

National Accreditation Board Laboratories/Quality Control Laboratories)

- *Accreditation* is the assessment or evaluation by an external agency of an individual or organization against defined criteria. It is the mechanism by which an agency or an organization, service, or program of study meets specific predetermined standards. It is also a professional recognition reserved for those who intend to provide high-quality health care. Accreditation is similar to licensing or registration but is voluntary and carried out by a recognized external agency like ISO 9001:2015 Quality Management System.
- *Audit* is defined as an assessment of the efficiency of the laboratories and allows the histopathologists to analyze their own work. It is a systematic activity, with a peer view of medical care, comparing actual practice with explicit standards of practice. The primary objective of medical audit and QA is to improve the outcome of medical care in community health care.
- Audit[5] conducted at the departmental level is a necessary component of laboratory management and examines many aspects of the reporting process. In most local histopathology audit schemes, overall staining quality, assessment of laboratory speed, and turnaround time are measured. The audit also assesses the workload both for the laboratory and for individual pathologists. The audit also plays a role in defining diagnostic criteria in histopathology—analyzing and evaluating patterns of diagnosis derived from matching the histological impression with other factors, such as age, sex, anatomical site, clinical history, and incidence ratio.
- A pathology service must audit its operations as part of the quality system in order to determine compliance of the service with current regulatory and accreditation requirements. Laboratories must be continuously enrolled, participate, and perform to an acceptable standard in external proficiency testing programs that cover all test methods performed in the laboratory where such programs are available.

CONCLUSION

There is a growing awareness that laboratory services are an inbuilt component of the medical care system. The total evaluation of laboratory services is judged as to how well the patient is served; therefore, both the pathologists and clinicians as well as administrators should be motivated to work while keeping in mind the welfare of the patient.

REFERENCES

1. Penner DW. Quality control and Quality evaluation in histopathology and cytology. Pathol Annu. 1973;8:1-19.
2. Batsakis JG, Lawson NS, Gilbert RK. Introduction to the report on quality assurance Programs of the College of American Pathologists, American Society of Clinical Pathologists; 1982.
3. Dorsey DB. Evolving concepts of Quality in Laboratory Practice. A Historical overview of Quality assurance in Clinical Laboratories. Arch Patholl Lab Med. 1989;113(12):1329-34.
4. Ramsay AD. Errors in histopathology reporting: detection and avoidance. Histopathology. 1999;34(6):481-90.
5. Morson BC. Quality assurance and medical audit in Histopathology. J Clin Pathol. 1983;36(10):1202.
6. Sherwood A J. An external quality assessment scheme in histopathology. J Clin Pathol. 1984;37(4):409-14.

CHAPTER 25

Laboratory Management and Laboratory Safety

INTRODUCTION

Laboratory management is an art; an amalgamation of experience, expertise, optimal utilization of financial resources, good interpersonal relationships, and the ability to troubleshoot so that the organization runs on oiled wheels. Though it is the norm to believe that experience is the most vital card for a well-organized laboratory adherence to planned objectives, review of goals laid down from time to time, and replan with change for the better enable a smooth running of any laboratory.

OBJECTIVES AND EXECUTION

The objectives and execution[1,2] *of these toward a well-functioning laboratory could be summarized as*:

- Plan for the future 5–10 years.
- Lay down the financial budget for each year with an expectation of a 20% increase in what one has estimated.
- Plan from where these finances will be raised. If any laboratory can pay off financial loans/commitments in a couple of years then it is extremely creditable, do not expect gains in the first few years.
- Set clear standards for laboratory procedures, quality control, and laboratory accreditation.
- Plan the staff and laboratory personnel as per workload, and sample expectation, do not compromise on quality and credibility. Focus on smooth running and quality maintenance.
- Personnel in charge should undertake courses for management skills. Optimize management skills for each section in a laboratory.
- Strive for good interpersonal relationships and aim toward keeping all members of staff under a "family umbrella."
- *Laboratory director*: They are responsible for the overall operation and administration of a laboratory and, the employment of competent personnel in each section for assuring compliance with the applicable regulations. If he is a medical person, he may be called a medical director.
- *Laboratory managers*: They ensure that laboratories run smoothly with regard to procedures, equipment, calibration of equipment, supplies, maintenance of records (equipment and client reports), and safety. A good laboratory manager knows every nook and corner of his laboratory, walks around his laboratory on a daily routine knows how to extract the best from each individual, and ignores the faults in the same. He takes responsibility for all aspects of the laboratory including equipment, employees, supplies, software, and documentation. Ensures the safety of all laboratory procedures and personnel.
- *Laboratory supervisor*: The laboratory supervisor oversees the operations of a laboratory—supervising personnel and procedures and facilitating collection of samples, procedures, and interpretation of results as per schedule for each procedure, maintaining the turnaround time.
- *Laboratory technicians*: They are responsible for the sample, its analysis, procedure, sticking to standard norms, and quality control procedures. Anything out of the ordinary is to be reported to the supervisor.
- A qualified and competent medical doctor should be responsible for signing out reports—these being pathologists, cytologists, microbiologists, biochemists, etc., in the respective sections and should be responsible for the results. Internal and external quality control programs should be a routine in the laboratory and the laboratory should aim to excel in its results.

- All the laboratories should be accredited to regulatory bodies[3] for their maintenance.
- The international standard of good laboratory practice (GLP) or standard laboratory practice (SLP). Until recently these practices were not consistently adopted or enforced upon, but the present era demands guidelines aimed at providing standard services from every laboratory and organization to meet the challenges of evidence-based medicine.
- A *laboratory management system (LMS)*, or as it is otherwise termed *laboratory information management system (LIMS)*[4] is basically a software designed to manage samples. It is a dynamic process and has to keep pace with laboratory demands and technological progress. Despite the dynamism the components of a LIMS include the following laboratory processing phases, supported by numerous software functions:
    - Reception and log-in of a particular *sample* and its associated details including clinical data, concerned referring physician/center, record of previous investigations, treatment, etc. The registration process may involve accessioning the sample and producing barcodes to affix to the sample container.
    - The assignment, scheduling, time taken tag for tracking of the sample, and methodology of analysis.
    - Equipment and inventory needed for processing of the sample.
    - Quality control measures for procedures associated with the sample. Internal quality audits for various Quality Management Systems (QMS) and methods of validation and quality assurance.
    - The inspection, approval, and compilation of the sample data for reporting and further investigations.
    - Provision for sample storage for further analysis—location tracking involves assigning the sample to a particular freezer location, often down to the detail of the level of the shelf, rack, box, row, etc. Event tracking such as freeze and thaw cycles that a sample undergoes in the laboratory may also be included.
    - The record of turnover time taken; storage of data associated with the sample analysis for future reference.
    - LIMS are unique to each laboratory and should be designed to match the capability, feasibility, and financial support of each organization. Modern LIMS have implemented extensive configurability for each laboratory's needs; for tracking additional data points can vary widely.
    - A key attribute of any technically advanced laboratory information management system is:
        - Avoidance of particular company and brand dependencies
        - Reduced costs and improved efficiency
        - Improved transparency of work in laboratories
        - Flexibility to accommodate new requirements
        - Improved quality and compliance
        - Easily available record of standard operating procedures (SOPs)
        - Access to the instrument data can sometimes be required based on circumstances and other security reasons.
        - Easily accessibility and inspection of a testing facility

GOOD LABORATORY PRACTICE

In order to meet the above, every modern laboratory should incorporate steps toward *GLP*, a managerial quality control system covering organizational processes and criteria for planning, performance, and monitoring the functioning of a laboratory by improving knowledge and understanding of GLP principles and its regulation; Understanding the requirements of a standard laboratory; comprehensive information about the documentation of all data, such as SOPs and protocols, data for quality measures and integrity, auditing, and accreditation.

- The key areas through scientific programs such as workshops, continuing medical educations (CMEs), and other educational processes that integrate theory and practice. Facility for application of this knowledge for all personnel particularly the junior staff.
- Knowledge of ongoing research and association with research organizations.
- Recent development in procedures and validation.
- Rewards and incentives to laboratory personnel as motivation modes.

LABORATORY SAFETY

All healthcare system workers should feel a sense of security in the environment in which they work in. For this, it becomes mandatory for all the laboratories to follow strict measures that would ensure the safety of the staff.[5,6]

Safety Manuals

Every laboratory should have a safety manual based upon guidelines laid down by the National/State Occupational Guidelines for Health Systems. The manual should contain SOPs to include all phases of safety. Safety training should be a part of the orientation program that all workers should undertake upon joining. All employees should be made aware of the hazards of working with chemicals and how to avoid them. These hazards that workers in pathology laboratories face usually include specific risks from (1) toxic chemicals that are used in routine processing procedures, (2) pathogenic microorganisms that patient's samples and tissues may harbor (e.g., tuberculous bacilli in resected lung specimens), and (3) general risks from mechanical, electrical, and fire hazards.

The danger can be aggravated by ignorance of the hazards, lack of knowledge on how to deal with them, and what safety measures are to be implemented to counter these. All the laboratories should have a well-outlined safety program which should begin with the recognition and understanding of laboratory dangers, followed by a policy for implementing safety rules and regulations outlined in the manual. Risk management pertains both to personal health and safety as well as environmental health.

TOXIC CHEMICALS

A wide range of chemicals that are potentially dangerous are used routinely in all laboratories. The risks associated with these chemicals may be controlled by having an adequate knowledge of the properties of these substances; their storage in protective containers, the quantities being timely monitored and issued, and protective equipment and gear while handling them.

Nearly all the chemicals are irritants to the eyes, skin, and respiratory passages on constant exposure. Strong acids, dehydrating, and oxidizing agents are particularly corrosive and can cause damage while handling. Chemicals cause allergic reactions, formaldehyde being the most common irritant causing skin allergies, dryness, and irritation to the nasal mucosa, etc. Chemicals such as chloroform, chromic acid, dioxane, and potassium dichromate and dyes such as auramine O, basic fuchsin, and Congo red are all proven carcinogens.

Cyanides and heavy metal salts cause acute or chronic poisoning. Mercury, lead, arsenic, and a number of organic substances are cumulative poisons and are injurious to health on long exposure. Chromic acid, osmium tetroxide, and uranyl nitrate are highly toxic. The effects may not be immediately evident but are cumulative and frequently irreversible. While dealing with these it should be realized:

- Use them using protective gear such as gloves and masks while weighing out powders. Monitor their usage by identifying the quantities needed.
- Frequently rotate staff dealing with these substances so as to avoid cumulative effects; make all of them aware of the hazards of mishandling them.
- Sleeves are disposable garments worn to protect the arms from contact with biohazards. The permissible exposure limits (PELs) of the Occupational Safety and Health Administration (OSHA) should be strictly observed.
- Containers of chemicals should be labeled with basic information such as "chemical name," manufacturer's name and address, storing and handling instructions, date of receipt and opening, date purchased, expiry date, hazard warnings, and safety precautions. Stored chemicals should be examined periodically for replacement, deterioration, and container integrity.
- Chemicals should be categorized for disposal. Identify those that can be disposed of safely in normal trash or sewage systems and other chemicals that must be placed in appropriate containers to be picked up by safety services.

FLAMMABLE AND EXPLOSIVE AGENTS

- Many of the commonly used organic solvents such as ethyl alcohol, methyl alcohol, and acetones are highly flammable. Some have low ignition temperatures and can be ignited on contact with heated surfaces.
- In the preparation of the commonly used silver impregnation solutions various chemical reactions occur. With aging or exposure of ammoniacal silver solutions to air or light, shiny black crystals of explosive silver compounds, e.g., "fulminating silver," silver nitride (Ag_3N) and silver azide (AgN_3) are formed. Oxidizers, e.g., sodium iodate, and mercuric oxide can initiate or promote combustion in other materials and may present a serious fire risk when in contact with other substances. A silver flask or a silver-paper coating of containers for silver solutions may be used to avoid oxidation. These solutions should be colorless and not black or brown at the time of usage.

Violent explosions may occur while removing a stopper, throwing a solution down a sink, or even when holding it up to light. In order to avoid this:

- All ammoniacal silver solutions should be prepared fresh just before use and not restored but discarded.
- Any used solutions should be inactivated by adding an excess of sodium chloride solution or dilute hydrochloric acid.
- Storage of flammables should be done in minimal quantities. Their area of storage should be separate and away from electric points. Safety inspections of these

storage areas should be undertaken from time to time both by intramural and extramural bodies conforming to health safety rules.

- Personal protective gear such as gloves, aprons, rubber shoes face shields, and safety glasses should be made available at all times for the handling of hazardous chemicals.
- Food or beverages, and drinking water should never be kept in storage areas, refrigerators, glassware, or utensils that are used for laboratory purposes.

Safety Showers/Eyewash Stations

Safety showers/eyewash stations should be provided in every laboratory so that measures can be taken by washing off any toxic substances.

Work Area

The work area should be adequately ventilated, and airy, with open windows. Where the area for use of chemicals is situated adequate exhaust fans should be provided for the exit of toxic fumes.

Pathogens

Fresh tissue and body fluids are the most common source of infection by microorganisms. Fixed tissue is less hazardous.

- All infective tissue sent to the laboratory should have a "biohazard" label on it.
- Disinfect the area routinely after the use of fresh infective tissue while grossing out specimens on the same day of surgery. All personnel handling the tissues should be masked and adequately gloved.
- Any cut/injury while cut up, on an acquired immunodeficiency syndrome (AIDS) patient or those having hepatitis should be reported to the physicians, and proper treatment measures taken. In accidental needle stick injuries.
- Fine needle aspiration (FNA); samples of blood for testing of the patient as well as attending doctor for the suspected infection should be collected for analysis.

Fire/Electric Hazards

Proper training for all staff should be given to combat unfortunate episodes of accidental fires. A fire extinguisher should be available and accessible at all times. Exits for emergency exit should be provided in case of any such accidents.

Electrical shock can be minimized by properly polarizing and grounding all the outlets. An electrician should be available on the premises. Refrigerators and freezers must never be used to store highly flammable chemicals.

Broken glass particles, needles used for fine needle aspiration cytology (FNAC), and disposable microtome blades should be disposed of in special "sharp" containers. Microtomes and cryostats must be cleaned after the removal of blades.

CONCLUSION

Laboratory access should be regulated by the supervisor of the laboratory area and permitted after working hours only to personnel on duty. For safety reasons, working alone in laboratories before or after hours should be strictly monitored.

REFERENCES

1. Harmening DM. Laboratory Management: Principles and Processes, 2nd edition. Pennsylvania: FA Davis Company; 2000.
2. Skobelev DO, Zaytseva TM, Kozlov AD, Perepelitsa VL, Makarova AS. Laboratory information management systems in the work of the analytic laboratory. Measurement Techniques. 2011;53(10):1182-9.
3. Iyengar JN. Quality control in the histopathology laboratory: an overview with stress on the need for a structured national external quality assessment scheme. Indian J Pathol Microbiol. 2009;52(1):1-5.
4. Gibbon GA. A brief history of LIMS. Laboratory Automation and Information Management. 1996;32(1):1-5.
5. Adyanthaya S, Jose M. Quality and safety aspects in histopathology laboratory. J Oral Maxillofac Pathol. 2013;17(3):402-7.
6. Prophet EB. Laboratory Safety. Laboratory Methods in Histotechnology. Armed Forces Institute Of Pathology; 1992.

CHAPTER 26

Advanced Techniques in Pathology

INTRODUCTION

The application of molecular techniques[1-3] has a substantial impact on diagnostic pathology. It has transformed the world of morphological pathology into precision diagnosis with insight into molecular targets that define disease more accurately toward a better therapeutic approach.

Molecular techniques give insight into genetic aberrations, mutations, prognostic markers, tumor gene signatures, etc. However, the analysis has to be interpreted in the light of clinical settings.

This chapter will focus on the applications of molecular techniques in diagnostic pathology.

KARYOTYPING

The basic principle and study of cytogenetic analysis is karyotyping, or the study of chromosomes. In this technique, metaphase chromosomes are obtained for analysis and the spread is photomicrographed. Individual chromosomes are then cut and arranged according to standard classification. This is called an ideogram or karyotype **(Fig. 1)**.

This can be performed on any cell. In many instances, the analysis is performed on circulating lymphocytes which can easily be stimulated to undergo mitosis. Such mitosing cells are treated with "colchicine" to arrest them in metaphase after they are spread on glass slides to disperse the chromosomes.

They are stained by standard techniques (e.g., Giemsa stain), which help in the more precise identification of chromosomes on the basis of distinct bands (G banding).

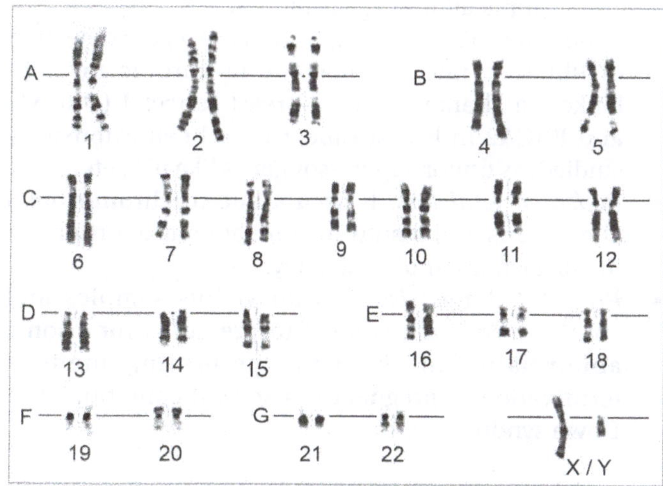

FIG. 1: Karyotyping.

Chromosome Classification[4]

The chromosomal study can be classified according to their length and positioning of their constriction or "centromere." The centromere is the point at which two identical sister chromatids attach to each other during mitosis. Based on their position the chromosomes may be metacentric (the centromere is exactly in the middle) in chromosomes 1, 3, 19, and 20. In such metacentric chromosome, the centromere divides the chromosome into a short arm (p, from the French and "petit" which means small) and a long arm (q, the next letter in the alphabet).

Chromosomes of many animal species have terminally located centromeres, and are called *telocentric chromosomes*, they are not found in humans.

Hematological stains like Giemsa bring out chromosomal characters which are used to classify chromosomes into seven groups concurrently labeled with letters from A to G and in their grouping, group A contains two large metacentric and one large subcentric chromosomes; group B contains two distinct large submetacentric chromosomes and group C contains six submetacentric chromosomes, etc.

Applications of Karyotyping

Genetic Disorders

It helps in detecting genetic diseases and arriving at a clinical diagnosis in patients with congenital abnormalities, delayed milestones, and mental retardation.

- *Gene analysis*: Chromosome analysis has great applications in human gene mapping, genetic mutations, and in applications of gene therapy.
- *In oncology*: Extensive applications, e.g., the detection of Philadelphia chromosome in chronic myeloid leukemia alters prognosis. Breast cancer 1 (BRCA1) and BRCA2 in breast cancer have been extensively studied, as tumor suppressor genes like p53, etc.
- *Repeated fetal loss*: It occurs due to chromosomal aberrations and results in spontaneous abortions in the first trimester of pregnancy.
- *Prenatal diagnosis*: Chorion villous samples and amniotic cells are studied to predict chromosome abnormality in the fetus permitting medical termination of pregnancy in several conditions like Down syndrome, etc.

IN SITU HYBRIDIZATION

In situ hybridization (ISH) is an established procedure for the detection and visualization of specific nucleic acid sequences whether deoxyribonucleic acid (DNA) or ribonucleic acid (RNA) in tissue sections, cytological preparations, and whole organisms. It is the study of genetic sequences. The technique has a history of applications going back over several decades and is routinely employed in laboratories where visualization of gene expression directly within the tissue of interest is necessary. Over the years modifications and refinements in visualization methods such as radioactive probes, fluorescent techniques, and multicolor fluorescence have evolved. It involves the application of a labeled probe to the tissue section and in detecting the label as a means of identifying where hybridization between probe and tissue has occurred.

Principle of the Technique

A nuclei acid probe (a string of nucleotides) is generated and detects complementary sequences on specific chromosomal sites where hybridization between probe and tissue has occurred. This is performed on a wide variety of tissue samples such as fixed tissues, frozen tissue, cells from touch preparations, and exfoliated, aspirated, or cultured cells by labeling the probe.

This allows DNA or RNA target molecules to be localized to specific cells and sites in the sections. The genetic target in the molecular analysis is a nucleic acid sequence—either DNA or RNA. The probe after hybridization can be detected by radioactive labeling or other method.

The tissue to be tested has to be treated before hybridization in order to open up the target nucleic acids to increase their accessibility. Subsequent to this is the process of hybridization of labeled probes to the pretreated tissue samples. The excess nonhybridized probe is washed off.

Detection of the labeled probe, revealing the location of the target cellular nucleic acid on the sample.

Types of Probes

A probe refers to a stretch of nucleotides that is used to detect a specific region of DNA or RNA, as a function complementary to the target sequence. Various probes are: DNA probes/RNA probes; single-stranded DNA probes (can be prepared by primer extension on single-stranded templates); oligonucleotides (short probes), typically 20–40 bases in length; radiolabeled probes, e.g., phosphorus 32, sulfur 35, and tritium have high sensitivity; nonradioactive labels, e.g., biotinylated probes, enzyme-conjugated probes, hapten conjugated probes (digoxigenin probes) and fluorescent probes.

Precautions for an Optimal Result

- *Coating of slides*: Slides are coated with poly L-lysine or aminopropyltriethoxysilane so that cells or tissues adhere on to the slides and are retained for the entire procedure.
- *Pretreatment of tissue*: Before hybridization, the tissues are subjected to a series of pretreatment that increases the efficiency of hybridization.
- Whole tissues or sections are usually treated with organic solvents (ethanol or methanol) to permeabilize the cells by removing lipid membranes.
- In order to increase the accessibility of the target RNA, the tissue is treated with protease (proteinase K)
- Nonspecific binding of the probe to positively charged amino groups can be prevented by acetylation of these residues with acetic anhydride.
- For whole-mount hybridization, tissues are prehybridized by incubation in a hybridization solution lacking a probe in order to block nonspecific binding.

- For double-stranded DNA targets, a heat denaturation step is carried out. This can be achieved either by chemical means or by heating the double-stranded DNA to above its melting temperature, either in an oven or using a microwave. For DNA detection using DNA probes, both probe and target molecules must be denatured.
- Denaturation is not necessary for RNA detection. Once the probe and target molecules have been rendered single-stranded, all that is required for annealing to take place is for the probe and target molecules to be brought together. For this, the incubation temperature is to be reduced to below the melting temperature of the required hybrids.
- Washing of the hybridized sections is carried out to remove excess probe that has bound to any sequences related to, but distinct from the integral target or nonspecifically to other cellular components.
- *Visualization of signal*: The method for this depends upon the type of label that has been incorporated into the probe.
- *Digoxigenin probes (hapten-related probes)*: The location of hapten-related probes can be visualized by fluorescence microscopy, directly if the probe is fluorescently labeled or indirectly with a conjugated antibody using high affinity anti-digoxigenin antibodies, coupled either to alkaline phosphatase (AP), horseradish peroxidase (HRP), fluorescein or rhodamine for colorimetric, and chemiluminescent or fluorescent detection.

Applications

- *Detection of infectious agents*: Gene probes are available for the identification of the genetic material of numerous bacteria, mycobacteria, and viruses.
    - Specific localization of the organism with a specific cell type or histologic lesion, thus providing an essential pathological link between the presence of an organism's genetic material and the presence of disease.
    - Valuable in viral infections, in which probes have the ability to detect the molecular mechanisms of viral-induced injury and detect viral oncogenesis.
    - ISH has the advantage over immunohistochemistry (IHC) in that it can detect latent infections as well as active infections.
    - ISH has the potential to elucidate the mechanism of the spread of viruses in tissues and to define their life cycles.
- *Cytogenetic:* ISH is the method of choice for localization of a gene at a specific locus. Nucleic acid probes are commercially available for large portions of every chromosome as well as specific gene arrangements associated with certain forms of neoplasia.
    - For chromosomal mapping of single and multiple genes in the haploid genome, for delineation and classification of many genetic diseases.
    - Prenatal and postnatal detection of several genetic diseases.
    - Used in genetic counseling.
- *Neoplasia:* ISH is used in the assessment of gene expression in tumors at the cellular level. It is superior to IHC in tumor studies as the latter detects proteins and protein products and ISH detects specific messenger ribonucleic acid (mRNA) encoding such products.
    - Can be used to study neoplasia at different levels of tumor differentiation.
    - Proven to be effective for the analysis of oncogene overexpression in a variety of different tumor types, e.g., lymphoma
    - The demonstration of mRNA of encoding cytoskeletal proteins including intermediate filaments, actin, and tubulin.
    - Considerable application for tumor typing when IHC techniques prove negative.
- *Neuroendocrinology*: ISH has proved to be of upgraded value in experimental and clinical neuroendocrinology.
    - mRNAs encoding a large series of regulatory peptides have been demonstrated in both the central and peripheral neuroendocrine systems. In some instances, positive hybridization signals for certain regulatory peptide mRNAs such as somatostatin have been observed in the presence of negative immunohistochemical reactions for the peptide.
    - The demonstration of a particular mRNA by ISH is a reflection of the rate of gene transcription and mRNA turnover. These methods have proven to be of particular value for the analysis of certain neuroendocrine tumors.
    - In instances of ectopic hormone production, e.g., ISH can resolve the question of whether cells are simply concentrating their product from circulation or whether they are actively transcribing the specific mRNA for peptide synthesis.

FLUORESCENCE IN SITU HYBRIDIZATION[5-8]

Principle

The procedure allows the ability of DNA probes to specifically hybridize to a DNA target sequence in tissue, cells, or isolated chromosomes by making a probe complementary to the known sequence. The probes are labeled with a fluorescent marker, e.g., fluorescein. In 1986 Pinkel and coworkers were the ones to apply the fluorescence in situ hybridization (FISH) technique in hybridization. Between 1986 and 1992 multicolor FISH experiments have been routinely performed for cytogenetic analysis.

Procedure

- The tissue is placed on a microscopic slide and the DNA is denatured.
- The probe is also denatured and added to the tissue on the microscope slide, letting the probe hybridize to its complementary site.
- The excess probe is washed off and the hybridization site is read in a fluorescent microscope. The probe will show as one or more fluorescent signals in a microscope, depending on how many sites it can hybridize to.

Types of Probes

Chromosome sequence probes (chromosome painting):

- The whole chromosome fluorescences.
- *Repeat sequence probes*: They are isolated from telomerase/centromere regions and used in chromosome enumeration.
- *Unique sequence probe*: Isolate from a clone disease-causing gene, used to identify the presence or absence of that gene.
- A marked increase in sensitivity can be achieved by enzyme-mediated signal amplification in FISH. Tyramide signal amplification (TSA)-FISH, also known as catalyzed reporter deposition (CARD)-FISH is based on the deposition of fluorescently labeled tyramide by peroxidase activity.

Clinical Applications in Cytogenetics

- By using a marked probe, various chromosomes can be identified. FISH allows rapid screening in cases of chromosomal mosaicism, and polymorphisms. Chromosomal aneuploidy (e.g., Down syndrome) in prenatal samples, monitoring bone marrow engraftment after transplantation.
- *For cancer diagnosis and prognosis*:
    - *Gains and losses*: The identification of abnormal chromosome numbers in cancer, e.g., trisomy 8 in many hematological tumors, trisomy 12 in CLL, a gain of chromosome 3, 7, and 17 in cancer of the urinary bladder.
        - *Gene deletions*: Inactivation of tumor suppressor genes, such as p53 and RB, is a commonly observed genetic event in cancer. FISH deletional analysis performed on urine cytology showed deletions of 9p21 deletions in transitional cell carcinoma.
    - *Chromosome rearrangements*: Identification of chromosomal translocation, e.g., the detection of the t(9;22) in >90–95% of chronic myeloid leukemia (CML) and resultant fusion of the *BCR* to the *ABL* gene; 8–14 translocation in Burkitt's lymphoma, the site of the *Myc* gene; in small round cell tumor, t(11;22) favors Ewing's sarcoma/primitive neuroectodermal tumor (PNET); and t(X;18) is characteristic of synovial sarcoma. The use of two differently labeled probes (dual color in FISH) for the two loci, e.g., BCR and ABL loci will show the presence of a fusion signal which strongly suggests the presence of BCR-ABL fusion, diagnostic of CML.
    - Gene amplification is an oncogene mechanism observed in most cancers, e.g., detection of multiple gene copies of Her2 neu in breast adenocarcinoma, c-MYC in carcinomas, and leukemias and n-MYC in neuroblastomas.
    - FISH detects breakpoint regions in chromosomes to a few hundred KB or even less, as compared to a level of 5–10 Mb in chromosome banding alone.

POLYMERASE CHAIN REACTION[9-11]

Polymerase chain reaction (PCR) is an invaluable technique that amplifies specific DNA fragments from minute quantities (from a few hundred base pairs of source DNA material) up to 40 megabases. PCR has rapidly become one of the most widely used techniques in molecular biology as it is quick and inexpensive.

Polymerase chain reaction copies DNA in repeated cycles, each consisting of three steps **(Fig. 2)**:

1. The reaction solution containing DNA molecules that need copying; polymerase (which copies the DNA), primers (which serve as starting DNA), and nucleotides (which are attached to the primers) is heated to 95°C.
    - The heating causes the two complementary strands of DNA molecules (to be copied); to separate, a process known as denaturation or melting. DNA polymerase known as Taq polymerase is an enzyme that can withstand high temperatures needed for DNA strand separation.
2. Lowering the temperature to 55°C causes the primers to bind to the DNA, a process known as hybridization or annealing. The resulting bonds are stable only if the primer and DNA segment are complementary, i.e., if the base pairs or DNA segments match.

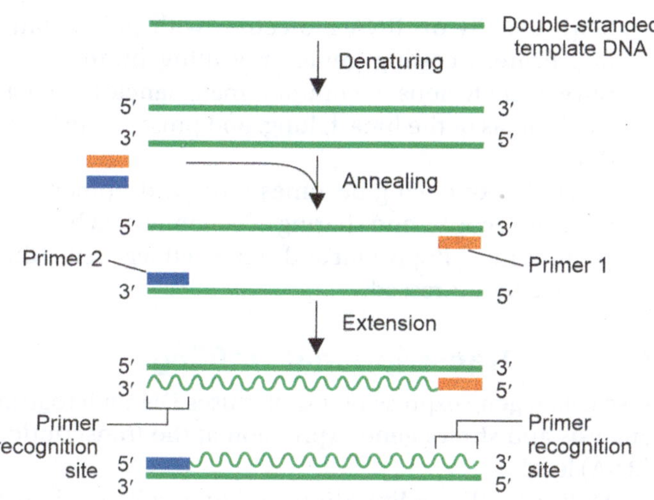

FIG. 2: Amplification of target sequence.

3. The polymerases then begin to attach additional complementary nucleotides at these sites, thus strengthening the bonding between the primers and the DNA.

Extension

The temperature is again increased, to 72°C which is the ideal working temperature for the polymerases to act. Further nucleotides are added to the developing DNA strand. At the same time, any loose bonds that have formed between the primers and DNA segments that are not fully complementary are broken.

- Each time these steps are repeated, the number of copied DNA doubles. After 20 copies a million copies are cloned from a single segment of double-stranded DNA.
- The reaction products are separated by gel electrophoresis. The reaction products are visualized by staining with ethidium bromide or a silver staining protocol, or by means of radioisotopes and autoradiography.

Reverse transcription polymerase chain reaction (RT-PCR), a variant of PCR, is a technique commonly used in molecular biology to detect RNA expression. RT-PCR is different from real-time PCR. RT-PCR is used to qualitatively detect gene expression through the creation of complementary DNA transcripts from RNA. This complementary deoxyribonucleic acid (cDNA) is amplified by the traditional PCR methods.

Quantitative real-time polymerase chain reaction (qPCR) on the other hand is used to quantitatively measure the amplification of DNA using fluorescent dyes.

Applications of Polymerase Chain Reaction

- Applications of small amounts of DNA for further analysis by DNA fingerprinting.
- Mapping the human and other species genome.
- The isolation of a particular gene of interest from a tissue sample. RT-PCR is extensively used in studying gene expression.
- *Generation of probes*: A large amount of probes can be synthesized by this technique.
- *Production of DNA for sequencing*: Target DNA is cloned using appropriate primers and then its sequence is determined.
- *Analysis of mutation*: Deletion and insertion in a gene can be determined by differences in the size of the amplified product.
- PCR is used to amplify DNA from fetal cells obtained from amniotic fluid. Fetal diseases and carrier testing can be diagnosed.
- In forensic medicine to amplify evidence, for example, from scanty human hair, single cell, body fluid stains (blood, saliva, and semen), etc.
- Study of microorganisms, viruses, etc.
- *Future prospects of PCR*: PCR-based recently developed methods search for unknown mutations by denaturing gradient electrophoresis, chemical mismatch cleavage, single-stranded conformation polymorphisms, and direct genomic sequencing. Known mutations in a particular gene can be detected by the allele-specific hybridization, the amplification refractory mutation system, the competitive oligonucleotide priming reaction, or the oligonucleotide ligation assay.

Limitations of Polymerase Chain Reaction

Polymerase chain reaction is an extremely sensitive technique and is prone to contamination from extraneous DNA, leading to false positive results.

- Cross contamination between samples can occur and should be avoided at all lost.
- Expensive and cannot be afforded by small laboratories.

DEOXYRIBONUCLEIC ACID SEQUENCING

- DNA sequencing is the process of determining the nucleic acid sequence, i.e., the order of nucleotides in DNA.[12,13] It includes any type of technology that is used to determine the order of the four bases: (1) Adenine, (2) guanine, (3) cytosine, and (4) thymine.

- DNA sequencing may be used to determine the sequence of individual genes, larger genetic regions, i.e., clusters of genes, full chromosomes, or entire genomes of any organism. It can indirectly sequence RNA also.
- Chromosomal rearrangements resulting in the fusion or exchange of regulatory sequences are present in approximately 20% of carcinomas. A strong association between the type of gene fusion and tumor type makes them highly useful diagnostic markers, particularly in tumors with similar morphology.
- Until recently, the vast majority of gene fusions were identified through changes in banding analysis, followed by use of the RT–PCR and Sanger sequencing (first-generation sequencing). The Sanger method (chain termination method) is the technology that produced the first human genome in 2001, ushering in the age of genomics, i.e., the study of the entire genome of an individual.
- In the late 1990s newer methods of DNA sequencing called "next generation sequencing (NGS)" technologies, came into existence, and detection of new gene fusions as well as mosaic variants increased dramatically. NGS technology is rapid, enabling information on the complete genome with DNA and RNA on just a few cells alone. RNA-seq can provide information on the entire transcriptome of a microorganism in a single analysis.
- "Shotgun sequencing" is a sequencing method designed for analysis of DNA sequences longer than 1,000 base pairs, up to and including entire chromosomes.
- High-throughput sequencing, which includes next-generation "short-read" and third-generation "long-read" sequencing methods, applies to exome sequencing, genome sequencing, genome resequencing, transcriptome profiling (RNA-Seq), DNA-protein interactions (ChIP-sequencing), and epigenome characterization.
- NGS (also known as second-generation sequencing, deep sequencing, massively parallel sequencing, etc.). is an umbrella term to obtain simultaneously both width (i.e., multiple nucleotide sequences analyzed at the same time) and depth (i.e., each target nucleotide sequence is analyzed several times, allowing for the detection of rare, mosaic variants) in the analysis of genetic material.
- It is currently possible to obtain information within a few days on the entire genome or transcriptome of any type of cell or organism, using as little starting material as the DNA or RNA of a few cells.
- NGS studies employing different variants of transcriptome sequencing (also known as RNA-Seq), usually on RNA molecules with poly-A tails, i.e., protein-coding genes, revealing hundreds of novel gene fusions in common malignancies, such as carcinomas of the breast, lung, and prostate are being done.
- As DNA sequencing becomes more widespread, the storage, security, and sharing of genomic data has also become more important and creates ethical issues that need to be addressed.

Genomic Transcriptional Profiling

Also called gene expression profiles uses DNA microarray analysis and shows gene expression at the transcription (RNA) level.

- Defines cell proliferation activity; cell regulatory mechanisms; and biochemical pathways and confers distinct gene signatures in neoplasia **(Fig. 3)**.

Applications

- In *classification of tumors* (widely used in breast and also in endometrial carcinoma)
- *Breast carcinoma*:[14-16] (1) Gene expression profiling shows four molecular subtypes of breast carcinoma, i.e., (i) luminal A, (ii) luminal B, (iii) human epidermal growth factor receptor 2 (HER2)-enriched, and (iv) basal-like. These have significant behavioral differences in incidence, response to treatment, disease progression, survival, and imaging morphology. Type A and B are the most common (60–70%) of breast carcinomas:
    - Luminal A tumors have the best prognosis of all subtypes, whereas patients with luminal B tumors have significantly shorter overall and disease-free survival. Distinguishing between these tumors is important because luminal B tumors require more aggressive treatment. Luminal B tumors are associated with axillary lymph node metastasis at presentation. Both A and B-type tumors present as large masses.
    - HER2+ disease carries a poor prognosis, but patients do well with anti-HER2 therapy. HER2+ tumors most commonly present as spiculated masses with pleomorphic calcifications.
    - Basal-like cancers (15% of all invasive breast cancers) are the most common "triple negative" cancers, which lack ER, progesterone receptor (PR), and HER2 expression.
- Combining histologic grade, ER/PR/HER2 status, multigene assay, and TNM staging can better dictate the clinical management of this carcinoma.
- *Identifies distinct subtypes of breast cancer*: Poor prognosis gene signature

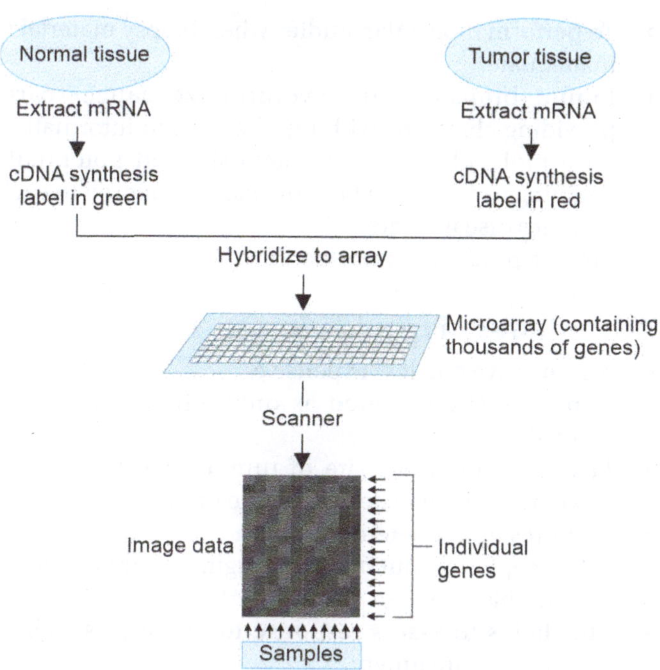

FIG. 3: Gene transcription profiling.
(cDNA: complementary deoxyribonucleic acid; mRNA: messenger ribonucleic acid)

- Gene-expression signatures, such as the 70-gene signature (MammaPrint[R]), were first:
  - Developed to assess the risk of distant recurrence in the first 5 years after diagnosis to predict outcome of breast cancer patients; but is able to accurately differentiate between patients at a low and a high risk of distant metastases up to 25 years after diagnosis. The low-risk tumors as shown by this gene signature have an excellent 20-year, long-term survival prognosis. Tumors of these patients are referred to as "indolent breast cancer."
- *Endometrial carcinoma*: In 2013, The Cancer Genome Atlas (TCGA) Research Network published an integrated genomic characterization of *endometrial carcinoma* into four groups based on genomic data from array and sequencing-based technologies. They are as follows:
  1. *Copy number*: High (frequently involving mutations of *TP53*); the majority of serous carcinomas and 25% of high-grade endometrioid tumors
  2. *Copy number*: Low (frequently involving mutations of *PTEN, PIK3CA, ARID1A,* and *KRAS*); this group is mostly composed of low-grade endometrioid carcinomas
  3. Microsatellite instability hypermutated (frequently involving alterations of mismatch repair protein genes)
  4. *Polymerase* ε (*POLE*) ultramutated; this group is mostly composed of endometrioid cancers; and appears to have a better prognosis and favorable outcome than others

LIQUID BIOPSY

Cancer diagnosis is no longer dependent on only biopsy specimens, the diagnosis is supported and contributed by assessments of DNA and mRNA as well as the proteomics of neoplastic cells.[17-19]

Liquid biopsy is a noninvasive procedure for the detection, diagnosis, and monitoring of cancer. The principle lies in the detection of circulating biomarkers in blood. Such biomarkers are the somatic mutations and epigenetic changes found in exfoliated cells and cell fragments in circulation in neoplastic conditions. To date, biopsies, exfoliated cells from body fluids, and aspirated material from tumors have been used to morphologically detect disease/neoplastic processes, supplemented by histochemistry and immunohistochemistry using the visualization of protein antigen-antibody complexes. In comparison Liquid biopsy is a unique noninvasive blood test that picks up circulating tumor cells and circulating DNA fragments that may be shed into the blood by primary or metastatic tumors leading to the study of genomic mutations in these cells and fragments. Cells, cell-free neoplastic nucleic acids (DNA fragments and RNA fragments), and exosomes (membrane-bound vesicles containing mRNA) may be subjected to study and give valuable and accurate information about the presence of cancer-specific genes (mutations).

Circulating Cancer Cells

The best example of this is in breast carcinoma where shed cancer cells were detected in circulation. Recent studies have also shown that blood-based testing can pick up HER2 mutations that emerge, or proliferate, in later-stage refractory breast cancer and might confer sensitivity to new anti-HER2 drugs.

Similarly, several solid tumors may shed cells into blood though in small numbers (<10 cells/mL of blood); that can be detected to monitor the presence of cancer/metastasis. Various methods for the detection and multiplication of these shed cells are used, including immunostaining; cell cultures, FISH, RT-PCR, etc.

Strategies to reprofile the molecular landscape of the tumor to identify new treatment targets for patients who are developing resistance to their current therapy are becoming more frequent.

Circulating Deoxyribonucleic Acid Fragments

These depend on the tumor burden in the body. The existence of cell-free deoxyribonucleic acid (cfDNA) molecules circulating in human blood was described as early as 1948 but it was much later that awareness of a higher quantum of cfDNA in cancer patients than in normal controls was reported. The circulating tumor deoxyribonucleic acid (ctDNA) load belongs to the pool of the total cfDNA in blood, but the main source being tumors. In individuals without cancer, fragments of DNA are also released into the blood due to apoptosis, but the concentration of cfDNA is low as a result of the clearance of dead cells by phagocytosis. Therefore, patients with neoplasms have significantly higher levels of cfDNA because of the high turnover of cancer cells. It has been observed that ctDNA has been confirmed to contain DNA mutations of both primary and metastatic lesions, such as point mutations, copy number variations, and insertions/deletions.

Presently, the most commonly used protocols to obtain cfDNA require approximately 1 mL of serum or plasma (3 mL of blood) and preparation should not exceed 4–5 hours following the blood draw as these have a short life span and are stable in the plasma at –80°. In order to isolate, this blood is collected in ethylenediaminetetraacetic acid (EDTA) tubes but the separated plasma/serum has to be stored at –8°. The DNA fragments are used for pyrosequencing, next-generation sequencing, and quantitative and digital PCR.

Exosomes

Exosomes are vesicles carrying DNA, RNA, and protein components that can be studied. In fact, the information obtained from the ctDNA can be further complemented through the analysis of mRNA contained within vesicles (exosomes) or sequestered in "tumor-educated platelets."

Besides tumor cells, normal cells around the vicinity of neoplasm are also released in circulation and give information as regards the tumor, the best studies among these have been on platelets these are called "tumor-educated platelets." This results in the study of altered tumor genes as well as mRNA reflected on the platelets.

Indications of Liquid Biopsy

- Monitor residual tumors in patients in cases of known tumor mutations.
- To monitor disease progression and detect tumor resistance and thereby find alternative treatment protocols.
- Try to detect the site of the unknown primary.
- To perform molecular studies when biopsy material is inadequate.
- Liquid biopsies can revolutionize cancer care, providing clinicians with rapid access to information on a molecular level at diagnosis, and potentially enabling treatment to be more closely tailored to each patient's disease state.
- Provide prognostic information.

Advantages of Liquid Biopsy

- Noninvasive and less expensive
- Can be easily repeated as only a blood sample is needed.
- Less dependent on site of tumor—can be used in unknown primary site/metastatic disease.
- Captures tumor heterogeneity.
- A few copies of mutant DNA fragments are adequate for amplification.
- This helps to assess response to therapy as well as resistance to treatment.
- Able to obtain serial samples during treatment to assess for drug resistance and tumor progression. This is not picked up with a tumor biopsy given that tumor biopsies are generally only done before treatment, therefore mutations indicating resistance would not be picked up as these generally arise after starting therapy.
- Evaluation of prognosis.

Disadvantages

- New tools and validity have to be tested.
- Results have to be authenticated against standard procedures and concordance between the somatic mutations of the "Gold standard" of biopsy should be well established.
- The potential role of liquid biopsies in detecting mutations, for targeted therapy, and prognosis of various cancers cannot be overemphasized.
- Lack of consensus in technical approaches of choice.

Though the advantages of liquid biopsy are appreciated as a noninvasive procedure (in comparison to tissue biopsies) and studies are encouraging as regards to somatic mutations being detected close to or equal to tissue biopsy findings, a liquid biopsy cannot replace the conventional tissue biopsies at this stage. Though promising, it is yet to be seen what the future holds for this technique in the routine treatment of cancer.

Liquid biopsy is a relatively new procedure. As such, present understanding restricts its use to certain forms of cancer, including breast cancer, prostate cancer, colon cancer, and nonsmall cell lung cancer.

New biomarkers can be detected by liquid biopsy as ongoing research. It has long been known that cell-free deoxyribonucleic acid (CF-DNA) could be a promising diagnostic and prognostic marker in different tumor types. Studies have been attempted to evaluate the prognostic role of CF-DNA quantity and integrity of *HER2*, *MYC*, *BCAS1*, and *PI3KCA*, markers frequently altered in breast carcinoma. CF-DNA, as a liquid biopsy for identifying patients at risk of relapse, is a prognostic biomarker for all breast carcinoma subtypes.

Mass arrays of DNA can be carried out on a few or multiple samples enabling clear decision-making for treatment.

TISSUE MICROARRAY[20]

Tissue microarray is a unique molecular technology that permits the assessment of many small representative tissue samples from hundreds of different cases gathered together on a single microscope slide for the study of genes and gene products. The format for the technique was conceived by Wan and colleagues in 1987 and meant for researchers in the molecular field. Large-scale analysis of hundreds of tissues can be done using the FISH/ISH technique on a single slide. It differs from DNA microarrays where each spot represents a cloned cDNA (complementary DNA) or oligonucleotide. In tissue microarrays, the spots are larger and represent small histological sections from varied tumors.

Technique

The principle is the arrangement of minute amounts of tissue samples on one platform. These are nothing but cylinders of paraffin with tissue (core biopsies) extracted from regular paraffin blocks. These cylinders taken from various donor blocks are reembedded into a single recipient block (microarray) at well-defined and planned distances **(Fig. 4)**.

- Standard hematoxylin and eosin (H&E) sections are studied from regular paraffin blocks to identify the area of interest in the tumor.
- A special tissue microarray instrument (e.g., Beecher instrument, Wisconsin, USA) is made use of to acquire a tissue core (from the area of interest) from the donor block. The core is then placed in an empty paraffin block—the recipient block.
- The currently available Beecher instruments arraying device is designed to produce sample circular spots that are 0.6 mm in diameter and placed at a spacing of 0.7–0.8 mm. The surface area of each sample is about the size of 2–3 high power fields (0.282 mm^2).
- The recipient block receives cores from hundreds or even thousands of blocks depending on the array design.
- Currently about 600 spots can be made with ease on one slide with a needle core of 0.6 mm

Advantages and Applications of Tissue Microarray

- *Amplification of material for analysis*: On average, each archived block yields material for a maximum of 50–100 assays. If the same block is processed for optimum micro assay construction, it would routinely yield 200–300 times or even more depending upon the size of the tumor in the original block. Thus, the technique amplifies (up to 10,000-fold) the limited source.

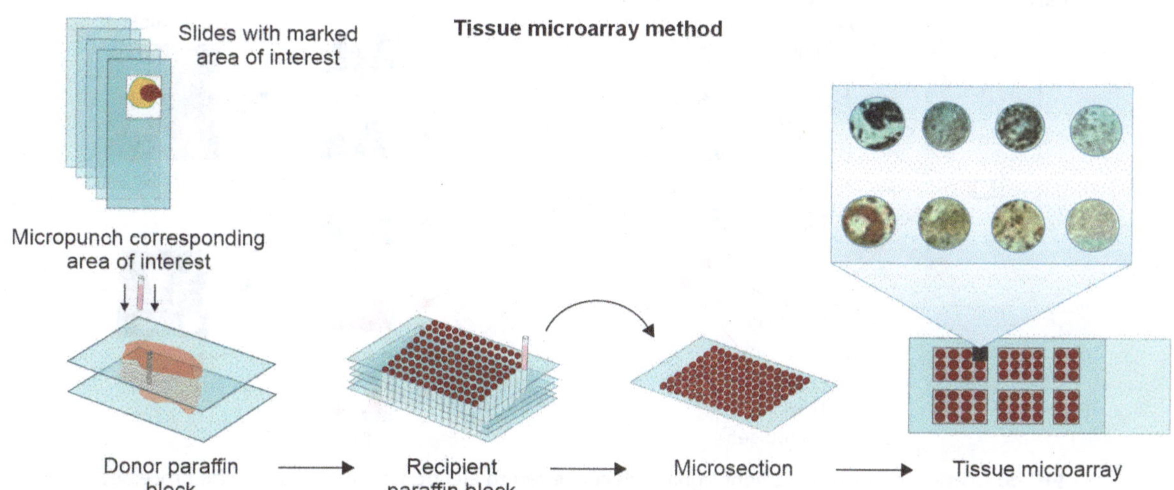

FIG. 4: Diagrammatic representation of tissue microarray system.

- Simultaneous analysis of very large numbers of different specimens. It enables pathologists to perform large-scale analysis using immunohistochemistry, FISH, or RNA ISH at substantially faster and at markedly lower costs compared with conventional approaches.
- *Uniformity in performance*: Each tissue sample is treated in an identical manner and microarrays are amenable to a wide range of techniques, including histochemical and immunologic stains with either chromogenic or fluorescent visualization, ISH (including both mRNA, ISH, and FISH) and even microdissection techniques.
- *Cost-effective*: Only a small amount of reagent is required to analyze an entire cohort. This method has proven to be very efficient, of shorter duration, and cost-effective, especially with expensive reagents.
- *Conserves valuable tissue*: There are occasions where the original tissue block must be returned to the patient or donating institution. In these cases, the block may be cored a few times without destroying the original.

Disadvantages

The main disadvantage is that the small cores sampled may not be representative of the whole tumor, particularly in heterogenous cancers, such as germ cell tumors and Hodgkin lymphoma.

This technology should not be confused with DNA microarrays where each tiny spot represents a unique cloned cDNA or oligonucleotide. In tissue microarrays, the spots are larger and contain small histological sections from unique tissue or tumors.

FLOW CYTOMETRY[21]

Flow cytometry is a technology based on the principle that when single particles (cells) flow through a fluid medium through a beam of light, their properties with regard to size, granularity, and relative fluorescence make them scatter incident light and emit fluorescence in varying proportions **(Fig. 5)**. An optical and electronic coupling system records this scatter. Measurement of light scattered by the cell in a forward direction is proportional to cell size, whereas light scatter at 90° is related to cell granularity. By using these two physical parameters it is possible to differentiate lymphocytes, monocytes, and granulocytes.

The images are stored in a computer and can be analyzed later.

Flow cytometry has applications in the categorization of normal and neoplastic hemopoietic cells, of great value in lymphomas and leukemias. Immunophenotyping of these is based on the use of fluorescein-tagged specific monoclonal antibodies to cell surface antigens and intracellular components of the cells in the flow.

Any suspended particle or cell from 0.2 to 150 μm in size is suitable for analysis. Cells from solid particles (as in freshly removed lymph nodes) are disaggregated before analysis.

Although flow cytometry technology offers the advantage of a rapid cellular analysis and cell type, morphologic correlation with smears, FNAC material, or histological sections is critical to determine the composition of the cell the suspension submitted for flow cytometry.

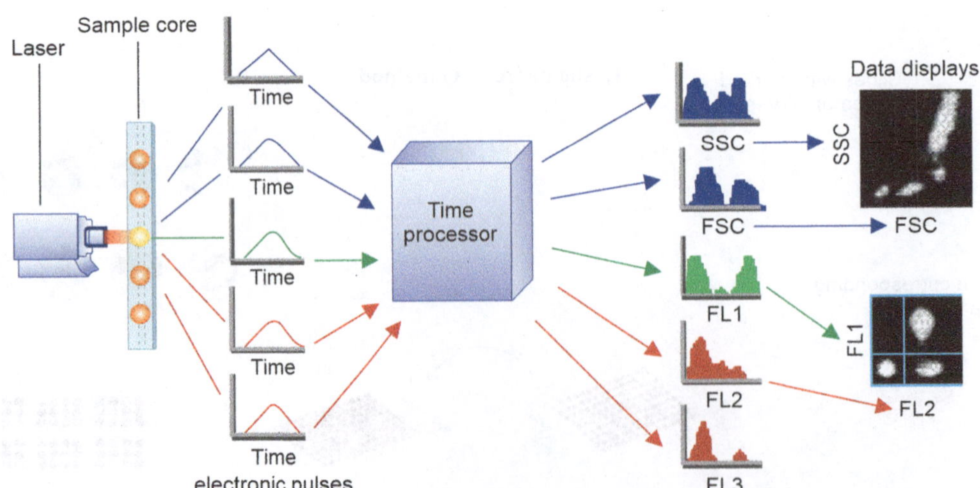

FIG. 5: Scattered and emitted light signals are converted to electronic pulses that can be processed by the computer.

Human Leukocyte Antigen Typing[22]

Human's major histocompatibility complex (MHC) proteins are encoded in the human leukocyte antigen (HLA) system. They are located in the cell membrane of cells. MHC is divided into two classes: (1) MHC class I and (2) MHC class II. The *HLA* gene complex is found on chromosome 6p21.

There are over 10,000 different HLA alleles identified to date and therefore an immune response to the HLA antigens varies significantly between individuals due to polymorphisms of genes. These antigens play a significant role in Transplant rejection and autoimmune diseases.

Human leukocyte antigen genotyping is the process of determining an individual's HLA class I and class II gene polymorphisms, which is required for transplant matching and other diseases.

Serologic Typing for HLA Antigens

The complement-mediated micro-lymphocytotoxicity technique has been used as the standard for serologic typing of HLA class I and class II antigens. HLA typing sera are mainly obtained from multiparous alloimmunized women, and their HLA-specific antigens are determined against a panel of lymphocytes with known HLA types. Some monoclonal antibody reagents derived from immunized mice are also used.

Peripheral blood lymphocytes (PBLs) express HLA class I antigens and are used for the serologic typing of HLA-A, HLA-B, and HLA-C. Magnetic beads are utilized to segregate B lymphocytes from blood or spleen for HLA class II typing. HLA class I typing can be done with the remaining leucocytes. HLA typing is performed in multiwell plastic trays (Terasaki plates) with each well containing a serum of known HLA specificity. Lymphocytes are plated in the well and incubated, and complement (rabbit serum as a source) is added to mediate the lysis of antibody-bound lymphocytes.

Flow Cytometry

This technique can also be used to detect HLA antibodies.

Freshly nucleated leucocytes are mixed with fluorescently labeled monoclonal antibodies in this procedure. Surface HLA antigens that bind to antibodies fluoresce, allowing flow cytometers to detect them as they pass through a laser beam.

CONCLUSION

Advances in medicine have known no bounds; the present era is of molecular pathology and maybe a day will come when the role of a cyto- and surgical pathologist will be reduced to a bare minimum of just signing out reports on molecular pathology inclusive of prognostication.

REFERENCES

1. Longtime JA, Fletcher JA, Sklar JL. Molecular genetic techniques in diagnosis and prognosis. In: Fletcher CDM (Ed). Diagnostic Histopathology of Tumors, 2nd edition. Amsterdam: Elsevier; 2000. pp. 1825-51.
2. Brooks JD. Translational genomics: the challenge of developing cancer biomarkers. Genome Res. 2012;22(2):183-7.
3. Mertens F, Tayebwa J. Evolving techniques for gene fusion detection in soft tissue tumours. Histopathology. 2014;64(1): 151-62.
4. Bonberg N, Taeger D, Gawrych K, Johnen G, Banek S, Schwentner C, et al. UroScreen Study Group. Chromosomal instability and bladder cancer: the UroVysion(TM) test in the UroScreen study. BJU Int. 2013;112(4):E372-82.
5. Lisa GS, Niels T; International Standing Committee on Human Cytogenetic Nomenclature. ISCN 2005: An International System for Human Cytogenetic Nomenclature. In: Shaffer LG, Tommerup N (Eds). Basel; Farmington, CT: Karger; 2005.
6. O'Connor C. Fluorescence in situ hybridization (FISH). Nat Educ. 2008;1(1):171.
7. National Human Genome Research Institute. Fluorescence In Situ Hybridization Fact Sheet. [online] Available from https://www.genome.gov/about-genomics/fact-sheets/Fluorescence-In-Situ-Hybridization [Last accessed March, 2024].
8. Lakowicz JR. Principles of Fluorescence Spectroscopy, 3rd edition. New York: Kluwer Academic; 1999.
9. Mullis KB, Faloona FA. Specific synthesis of DNA in vitro via a polymerase-catalyzed chain reaction. Methods Enzymol. 1987; 155:335-50.
10. In: Erlich HA (Ed). PCR Technology: Principles and applications for DNA amplification. New York: Stockton Press; 1989.
11. Rao PNS. Polymerase Chain Reaction (PCR). [online] Available from https://www.microrao.com/micronotes/pg/PCR.pdf [Last accessed March, 2024].
12. Yi X, Ma J, Guan Y, Chen R, Yang L, Xia X. The feasibility of using mutation detection in ctDNA to assess tumor dynamics. Int J Cancer. 2017;140(12):2642-7.
13. Fass L. Imaging and cancer: a review. Mol Oncol. 2008;2(2): 115-52.
14. Johnson KS, Conant EF, Soo MS. Molecular Subtypes of Breast Cancer: A Review for Breast Radiologists. J Breast Imaging. 2021;3(1):12-24.
15. van't Veer LJ, Dai H, van de Vijver MJ, He YD, Hart AA, Mao M, et al. Gene expression profiling predicts clinical outcome of breast cancer. Nature. 2002;415(6871):530-6.
16. Delahaye LJMJ, Drukker CA, Dreezen C, Witteveen A, Chan B, Snel M, et al. A breast cancer gene signature for indolent disease. Breast Cancer Res Treat. 2017;164(2):461-6.

17. Technologynetworks.com. (2020). Liquid biopsy: guide, applications and techniques. [online] Available from https://www.technologynetworks.com/diagnostics/articles/liquid-biopsy-guide-applications-and-techniques-328957 [Last accessed March, 2024].
18. Diaz LA, Bardelli A. Liquid biopsies: Genotyping circulating tumor DNA. J Clin Oncol. 2015;32(6):579-86.
19. Leon SA, Shapiro B, Sklaroff DM, Yaros MJ. Free DNA in the serum of cancer patients and the effect of therapy. Cancer Res. 1977;37(3):646-50.
20. Aktas S. Tissue microarray: Current perspectives in pathology. Aegean Pathol J. 2004;1:27-32.
21. Huh YO, Andreeff M. Flow cytometry. Clinical and research applications in hematologic malignancies. Hematol Oncol Clin North Am. 1994;8(1):703-23.
22. Bouças J. HLA typing: Introduction, methods, and applications. [online] Available from https://www.earlycountygin.com/markets/stocks.php?article=marketersmedia-2023-5-6-cd-genomics-to-host-online-webinar-on-bioinformatics-tool-flaski-with-guest-speaker-jorge-bouas [Last accessed March, 2024].

CHAPTER 27

Museum Techniques

INTRODUCTION

"The dead teach the living" is the English translation of the Latin "mortui vivos docent" used to justify dissections of human cadavers in order to understand the cause of death. The same can be applied aptly to all pathology and anatomy specimens displayed in museums.

An institutional museum is a place where a record of operated and resected specimens is kept. All teaching colleges and hospitals have museums attached to the department of pathology which serve many functions, including a permanent exhibition of surgical specimens for undergraduate and postgraduate teaching purposes, a display of the operating skills of the institutional surgeons, and an important repository for congenital and developmental anomalies. The saying "Here the dead teach the living" is apt for the museum wherein there are present organs and organ systems to enrich the knowledge of medical and science students. Organ demonstrations still hold value for teaching although e-learning is slowly replacing this.

In order to set up a worthwhile museum familiarity with techniques of preserving and mounting specimens is mandatory.

BASIC MUSEUM TECHNIQUES[1-4]

Any specimen for a museum should be handled by the following steps:

- Reception
- Choice of specimen for museum/mounting
- Preparation and fixation
- Restoration and preservation
- Mounting procedure
- Presentation and display

Reception of the Specimen

Any specimen received in the museum for purposes of mounting should be recorded in a reception book and given a specimen number—numbering should be, serial number, followed by year (e.g., 02/2017 is the second specimen received in the year 2017 for the museum). This number is the permanent specimen number for that particular specimen in the museum whether it is used as a wet specimen or mounted and displayed on the racks. This number is written on a tie-on type label in permanent ink and is stitched onto the specimen. The first column in the reception book will contain this number against which all necessary information about the specimen (surgical biopsy no., clinical, gross, and microscopic findings will be entered). The specimen may be used for display on the museum rack or as a collection as a wet specimen for the trainee or even mounted and given for display in other clinical departments.

Choice of Specimen and Categories for Museum/Mounting

Specimens in the museum may be channeled for various purposes. The ultimate use of the specimens will determine the best way to select or choose a specimen for the museum. The senior teaching staff of a department should be made responsible for the choice of the specimen for a specific purpose. For instance:

- Specimens intended for placement on museum racks (rarities and those for display) should be mounted in Perspex or glass jars which are sealed, and the specimen number and label be fixed on the jar.
- Specimens for demonstration/teaching of undergraduate medical students (where no handling of wet specimens by the students is needed); should be

completely enclosed in portable and nonbreakable containers, such as plastic bags **(Fig. 1)**, or they may be mounted in plastic jars which are sealed in order to avoid leakage and kept aside for this purpose. Specimens in plastic bags are easy to handle by students.

On the other hand, fixed and washed specimens are suitable for examination by pathologists-in-training **(Fig. 2)**, clinicians, and sometimes undergraduate medical students. These should be fixed and tagged with labels and kept aside in big bins with fixative for removal as and when needed. When put aside in bins, each specimen should have a long strong thread attached to it with the tie-on type of label in indelible ink attached both to the specimen and the loose end of the long thread **(Fig. 3)**.

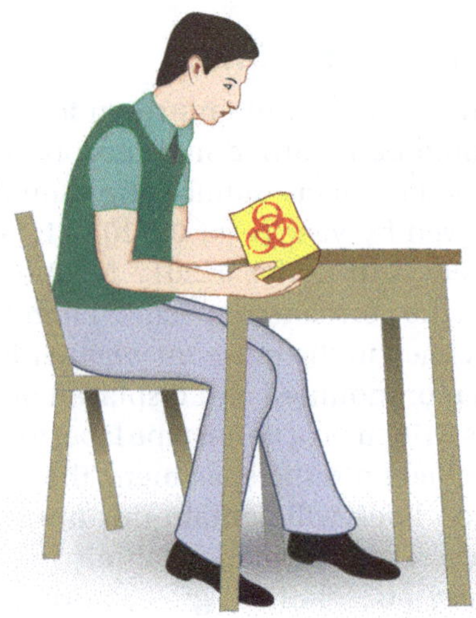

FIG. 1: Specimen mounted and sealed in a plastic bag for easy handling by the student.

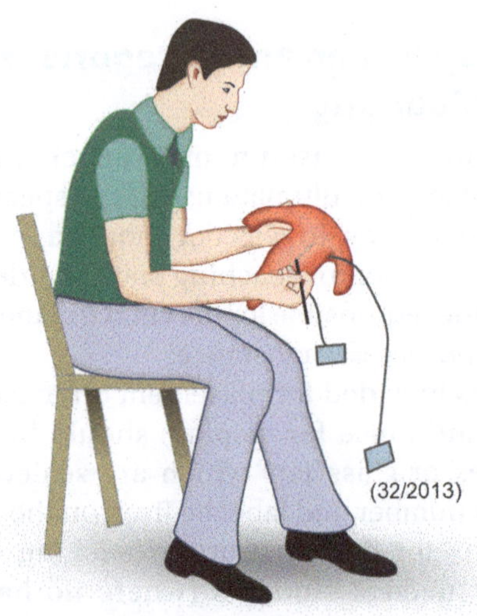

FIG. 2: Wet specimen handled by the trainee (postgraduate) in pathology.

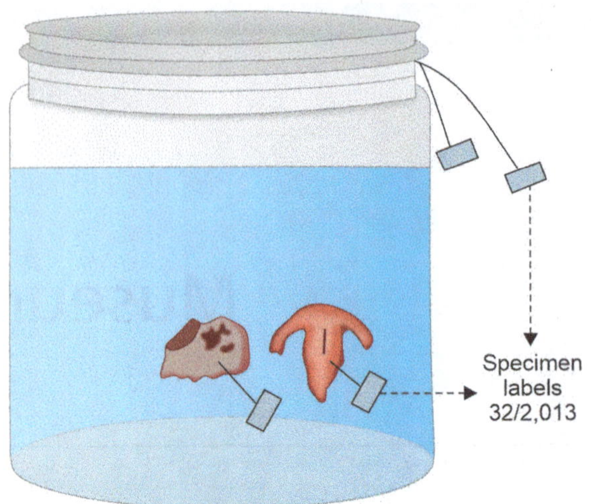

FIG. 3: Wet specimens stored in bins with labels attached to both the specimen and the end of a long thread.

The long end of the thread with the label should hang outside the closed bucket/large plastic container in order to read the number and identify a specimen easily. These specimens should be kept in running water for at least a few hours before handling and then reinserted after use in the same bucket with the thread tags hanging out. Bins or buckets should have adequate fixative, which should be checked and refilled from time to time.

Occasionally specimens are sent to the pathology department by surgical/gynecological departments with a request for mounting and transfer back to the clinical departments. Such specimens too should be entered in the reception register, mounted in sealed jars, and the detail mentioned against them with regard to its transfer to the said department, after mounting.

Preparation and Fixation

An ideal specimen for the museum is one that is obtained in a fresh unfixed state. However, most museums receive specimens from the pathology laboratory after being handled for grossing and so in formalin-fixed state. If an interesting specimen is seen at grossing to be used for a museum, the department policy should be that part of it (maybe one half) can be kept without disturbing it during grossing, e.g., in a kidney, it can be bisected, and one half kept aside for museum purposes; similarly, uterus and cervix. However, no compromise on the quality of the report should be made in order to preserve one-half. Any extra tissue/fat may be trimmed in order to optimize the specimen and its pathology. Fat-dissolving solutions such as chloroform and acetone may be used.

Fixation of the Specimen[1-4]

It is essential that all museum specimens be adequately fixed. Proper fixation preserves specimens in a life-like fashion for several years. The universal museum fixative is based on the principle of formalin fixation and derived from the "Kaiserling technique" and its modifications. Subsequently, many laboratories have had their own modifications (Meiller's, Lundquist's modifications, etc.).

As per *Kaiserling's technique*, the initial fixation is in a neutral formalin (K-I solution) and then the specimen passes through Kaiserling II and is then transferred to a final preserving glycerin solution (K-III) in which it is displayed. Color preservation is maintained with these solutions.

Kaiserling's Technique Fixation of Specimen

The specimen should be immersed in 10–20 times the volume of fixative in a spacious container that can accommodate the specimen and volume of fixative. The specimen is stored in the Kaiserling I solution for 1 month depending on the size of the specimen. Care should be taken such that the specimen does not rest on the bottom of the container, or else an artificial flat surface will result in hardening during fixation.

Kaiserling I solution:
- *Formalin*: 1 L
- *Potassium acetate*: 45 g
- *Potassium nitrate*: 25 g
- Distilled water makes up to 10 L

Restoration of Specimen[1-4]

After fixation, the specimen is transferred to Kaiserling II solution for restoration of color that it lost during fixation. Before immersing in solution II, the specimen is washed in running water and then transferred to 95% alcohol for 10 minutes to 1 hour depending on the size of the specimen. The specimen is then kept in solution II and observed for restoration of color for around 1–1.5 hours. Longer periods than this will fade the color and this change is irreversible. After this step, the specimen is ready for preservation.

Kaiserling II solution (rejuvenator solution)
- *Pyridine*: 100 mL
- *Sodium hydrosulfite*: 100 g
- *Distilled water*: 4 L

Preservation of Specimen

The recommended solution for preservation is Kaiserling III. This is the final solution in which the specimen will remain for display. It is a glycerin-based solution.

Kaiserling III solution
- *Potassium acetate*: 1,416 g
- *Glycerin*: 4 L
- Distilled water up to 10 L
- Thymol crystals were added as a preservative to prevent contamination with molds.

Leave solution to stand for 2–3 days before using to ensure proper mixing of chemicals. Add 1% pyridine as a stabilizer. This solution acts as a permanent fixative. This solution over time changes color to yellow and needs to be replaced to restore the color of the specimen.

A modification of K-III solution made by Pulvertaft3 replaces solution K-II and is as follows:
- *Pulvertaft–Kaiserling mounting fluid III*:
  - Glycerin: 300 mL
  - Sodium acetate 10% (pH 8): 100 g
  - 10% formalin: 5 mL
  - Tap water: 1,000 mL
  - Camphor/thymol can be added to prevent the growth of molds.

Immediately before sealing 0.4% sodium hydrosulfite is added. The amount of hydrosulfite should not normally exceed 0.4%. If color restoration must be rapid, 0.6% may be added, but this is to be avoided, as a white precipitate may form.

Mounting the Specimens

To support the specimen within its jar in the preservative, it is attached to a specimen plate (of Perspex or other plastic) by drilling holes into the Perspex sheet and tying the specimen with nylon threads through these holes. A rectangular bent glass rod can also support the specimen in the jar. This can be done by tying the specimen with nylon threads to the rod. Proper orientation should be supervised by the teaching staff.

Display/Presentation of the Specimen

Previously museum specimens were mounted in cylindrical jars and sealed with sheep bladder walls. Later they were replaced by rectangular glass jars; which afforded better viewing of the specimens. They were covered by rectangular glass plates and sealed. Nowadays, Perspex jars are available, which are lighter than glass jars and nonbreakable. Due to the convenience of usage, most laboratories use these for their mounting. However, they cannot be used to store specimens fixed in alcohol as this reacts with plastics over a prolonged period of time. It is advisable to bulk order these Perspex jars in various sizes and store them. They can be used from time-to-time depending on the size of the specimen. Departments with large museums often buy plastic Perspex sheets and train personnel to make jars in the department workshop itself; this is cost-effective. Specimen jars should not only have the specimen number clearly written on the jars but also provision be made in one corner for shelf no. (cupboard), rack no. (upper, middle, or lower horizontal rack), and placement serial no. starting from the right or left side of the horizontal rack. This helps in the easy replacement of the specimen even by personnel not familiar with placements after the specimen's usage. Separate shelves may be used to segregate specimens frequently taken out for undergraduate student demonstrations.

Other Methods of Specimen Display

Thin slices impregnated with gelatin or sealed between glass sheets, plasticated bronchial tree specimens, etc.

CATALOGS

These should be prepared so as to enable one to see the detail on a particular specimen. Each specimen should have in the catalog the specimen number with the following details: Shelf no., rack no., surgical biopsy no., gross specimen photograph, salient microscopic description with microphotograph, and finally the diagnosis. Most universities require such a complete picture to be maintained at least for the teaching specimens with a number of catalog copies to be made available for the students.

CONCLUSION

It is imperative that all laboratories strive to have a good display of all their surgical specimens not only for record purposes but also to enhance and motivate teaching to the younger generation. In order to have this documentation of the procedures used to enhance the quality of the specimens displayed should be undertaken in order to preserve these rare exhibits.

REFERENCES

1. Culling CFA, Dunn WL. Handbook of histopathological and histochemical techniques: (including museum techniques), 3rd edition. Oxford, United Kingdom: Butterworth-Heinemann; 2013.
2. NISO. Museum Techniques. [online] Available from http://www.nios.ac.in/media/documents/dmlt/HC/Lesson-20.pdf [Last accessed March, 2024].
3. Pulvertaft RJV. Museum techniques; a review. J Clin Pathol. 1950;3(1):1-23.
4. Waters BL. Museum techniques. [online] Available from https://link.springer.com/chapter/10.1007/978-1-59745-127-7_16#citeas [Last accessed February, 2020].

CHAPTER 28

Autopsy Techniques

INTRODUCTION

Clinical autopsies are carried out with the objective of finding out the disease process and cause of death in a patient who dies in the hospital during course of treatment. It is performed by the pathologist on request by the clinician with the consent given by the patient's close/blood relation.

OBJECTIVES OF A CLINICAL AUTOPSY

- To determine the cause of death
- To confirm or establish the clinical diagnosis
- To evaluate the effects of treatment given during life
- Study pathogenesis of disease
- Confirm or dismiss genetic implications for the family
- Prevent the spread of communicable disease
- Enhance research
- Educate medical personnel and students

DOCUMENTARY PREREQUISITES

- Clinical case chart of the patient maintained in the hospital ward
- Duly signed request from the concerned clinician
- Death certificate by the concerned clinician
- Consent from the next of kin or near relative for the autopsy and its procedures

Identification of the Body

The body should be correctly identified before a postmortem is begun. The name on the tag/label should match that in the case chart, death certificate and request for autopsy.

CLASSIC AUTOPSY TECHNIQUES[1,2]

Technique of Rudolf Virchow

The principle of the Virchow technique is to remove organs in sequential order in order to examine them. It begins with examination of the cranial cavity and brain, then spinal cord from the back. The body is then turned over and the organs of the thoracic cavity, cervical, and abdominal organs are examined. The anatomical-pathological relationship of the organs is not preserved.

Technique of Carl Rokitansky

This technique is characterized by in situ dissection, in part combined with the removal of organ blocks.

It is done in situations wherein to limit the spread of infection, e.g., human immunodeficiency virus (HIV) and hepatitis.

Disadvantage: Organs cannot be studied in detail.

Technique of A. Ghon

This is the "en bloc" removal of organs. The thoracic and cervical organs, abdominal organs, and the urogenital system in that order are removed as blocks so that relationship is maintained.

Technique of M. Letulle

This is the "en masse" removal. The trachea and esophagus are cut at the upper most limit, as much as the hand can be inserted in that direction, with the scalpel. Thoracic, cervical, abdominal, and pelvic organs are pulled out "en masse"; and subsequently dissected into organ blocks.

It is best for routine inspections and preservation of connection between organ and organ system. The organ blocks can then be studied in detail.

TYPES OF INCISIONS (FIG. 1)

- *"I"-shaped incision*: It starts from symphysis menti and extends straight to symphysis pubis right or left to umbilicus. It is routinely used as it is simple and convenient.
- *"Y"-shaped incision*: One limb of the "Y" starts near the acromion process, comes down obliquely, and medially passing below the breast up to the xiphoid process. It meets the other limb of the "Y" from the opposite side at the xiphoid and then the incision goes vertically down up to the symphysis pubis. This incision is used when detailed study of neck structures is required.
- *Modified "Y"-shaped incision*: It starts from acromion and goes up to the middle of the both sides, then it is carried over the clavicle and goes up to the suprasternal notch and then a straight down the middle up to the symphysis pubis.
- *Removal of brain*: Incision of the scalp is made from mastoid to mastoid process. Skin flaps are reflected to the front up to the eyebrows and behind up to the occiput. Bone saw is used and the skull cap removed. Meninges are opened longitudinally and reflected out. The brain is made to hang gently using hands by its own weight and the medulla oblongata severed at its junction to the spinal cord. The brain is then allowed to fix in a bucket of formalin by its weight using the basilar vessels as the anchoring loop.

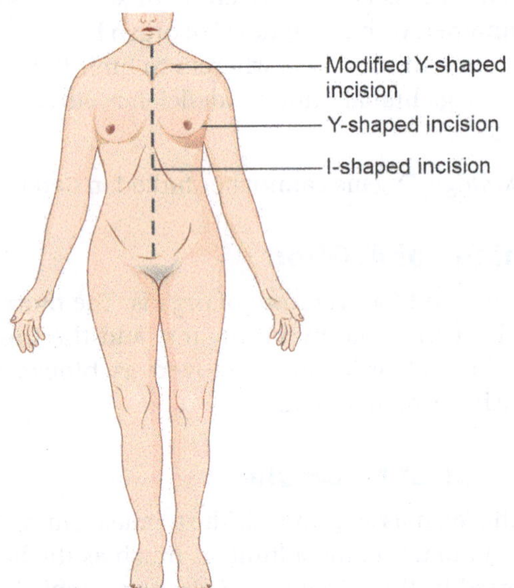

FIG. 1: Various types of incisions for performing an autopsy.

EXTERNAL EXAMINATION OF THE BODY

- The height and weight are recorded. Special weighing scales are available to record the height and weight with the body in the horizontal position.
- External appearance of the cadaver is examined carefully—for gender, build, skin color, and the presence of any scars, tattoos, or deformities and any other features which are recorded.
- Note of any cachexia, pallor, redness, jaundice, etc., is made.
- The under surface of the nails are inspected; color of skin is noted.
- Obvious intra-abdominal masses, or organomegaly or ascites is looked for and recorded. Girth of abdomen in ascites should be taken.
- Circumference of head and crown heel length should be measured in case of autopsy of infants/neonates.
- Injuries on the body
- Examination of body orifices/opening to look for injury or foreign body or exudates
- Physical changes that occur in the body after death like:
    - *Livor mortis (postmortem lividity)*: It is the staining of the dependent parts of the body due to gravitation of blood when circulation ceases. The external manifestation shows reddish erythema of the dependent skin surfaces, visible after 30–60 minutes in bright light.
    - *Rigor mortis (postmortem rigidity)*: The stiffness which occurs in a dead body is termed as "rigor mortis". The low-energy state of muscle fibers is manifested by stiffness. Rigor mortis is routinely detected in 2–4 hours after death. Onset reaches its peak in about 4–10 hours. The onset as well as passing off of rigor mortis are hastened by high temperature and delayed by cold ambient temperatures.
    - *Algor mortis (postmortem cooling)*: The rate of cooling of a dead body is dependent on the temperature difference between the body and the surrounding environment; also on the body mass in relation to surface area; the temperature of the air over the body surface; and the extent to which insulation is afforded to the body as a result of clothing, adipose tissue, etc.

Warm bodies mean death has occurred recently factors, such as sepsis, cocaine intoxication, and obesity play a role.

Cool bodies mean death has occurred sometime ago, and such bodies then exhibit either livor or rigor mortis.

ON TABLE TESTS[1-4]

Autopsy should always be done in bright daylight so as not to miss any findings.

Pneumothorax

Fill the space between ribs and thoracic skin flap with water and look for air bubbles.

Fat Embolism

Pulmonary artery is opened under water and look for escape of fat droplets.

Air Embolism

Pulmonary artery is opened under water and look for escape of air bubbles.

Myocardial Infarction

Myocardial infarction made visible by immersion of tissue in triphenyl tetrazolium chloride (TTC) and nitroblue tetrazolium test—stain imparts brick-red color to intact myocardium, infarcted area reveals unstained pale zone.

POSTMORTEM LESIONS IN TUBERCULOSIS

- Lesions of the size of millet seeds (1-2 mm) seen on cut sections of lungs, liver, and spleen in military tuberculosis; associated with caseating necrosis.
- Lymph nodes can be enlarged with tubercles and caseous necrosis.
- Cavities and fibrosis in the upper lobe (right) of lung in fibrocaseous tuberculosis
- Diffused distribution of subarachnoid to subcortical lesions with edematous enlargement of blood vessels is observed in tuberculosis of brain. Also seen is opacity of meninges at the base in meningitis; and also, subvertebral abscess are also observed.
- Spine—Pott's spine
- Transverse ulcers in small intestine
- Tuberculous pyelonephritis with caseous necrotic material in the pelvicalyceal system

POSTMORTEM CHANGES IN RHEUMATIC HEART DISEASE

- *Rheumatic endocarditis*: Thickening of valve leaflets and presence of small multiple warty vegetations along the lines of closure of the leaflets and cusps. In chronic stage due to fibrosis and calcification, mitral valve appears "fish-mouth or buttonhole stenosis".
- *Rheumatic mural endocarditis*: MacCallum's patch.
- *Rheumatic myocarditis*: Soft and flabby with dispersed Aschoff nodules/bodies.
- *Rheumatic pericarditis*: "Bread and butter" appearance due to thick fibrin.
- *Pan cardiac lesion at microscopy*: Aschoff bodies/nodules
- *Liver*: Cardiac cirrhosis due to mitral valve stenosis

POSTMORTEM CHANGES IN CIRRHOSIS

- *Skin*: Spider naevi
- *Liver*: Micronodular or macronodular cirrhosis depending on etiology; fatty change
- *Abdomen*: Ascites; caput medusae
- *Portal hypertension*: This is manifested by development of varices, i.e., large, swollen veins at the lower end of the esophagus, upper part of stomach, rectum, or umbilical area (caput medusa). Rupture of these could occur.
- *Gastrointestinal tract (GIT)*: Evidence of gastrointestinal bleeding

MINIMALLY INVASIVE AUTOPSY

The word "autopsy" derived from Greek, literally means "to see with one's own eyes!"

To the present day, the conventional autopsy (CA) has proven to be a valuable tool in clinical medicine. It is undoubtedly relevant and important for healthcare quality control and policy making; for the betterment of medical science and education; for ratifying cause of death, epidemiologic databases; and for obtaining human tissue specimens for museums and laboratory research.[5]

A CA also gave a feedback on clinical diagnostics and therapy for medical training and research. However, in spite of its immense benefits, autopsy rates have been declining in several countries the world over.[6] There could be various reasons for this—financial restraints on autopsy costs, consent from next of kin mandatory for autopsy, most times the next of kin fear disfigurement of the deceased's body and hold back on religious beliefs. Pathologists consider doing autopsies as additional duty! Reluctance among clinicians to be confronted with clinical "misdiagnoses" and the risk of lawsuits regarding alleged malpractice; lack of educational significance regarding autopsy in the general medical curriculum; dissatisfaction with the quality of autopsy reports, and the time period of reports being ready (3–4 weeks); surgical biopsies taking preference over these! There came a time, however, when a final diagnosis by autopsies had to be achieved against all odds of reasoning facing the dwindling autopsy rates. Aside from this, a growing misconception had crept in that the advanced diagnostic techniques used in today's clinical practice will hardly ever reveal new facts at autopsy!

A time came that the medical fraternity realized that the technology used on patients due to advancement could be translated for postmortem benefit resulting in nonperformance of autopsies. Imaging techniques have a long history in forensic pathology. Shortly after the discovery of X-rays by Roentgen, at the end of the 19th century, this technique was applied to localize bullets, detect fractures, and identify body age. In the clinical setting, the radiological techniques proved beneficial and were used primarily for perinatal autopsies. X-rays commonly complemented CA on fetuses or neonates, mainly for the detection of skeletal anomalies. But, the fact remained that just imaging by magnetic resonance imaging (MRI) and total body computed tomography (CT) after death did not suffice to establish true pathology; there had to be some means of a histological confirmation of these results at imaging.[7] This gave birth to the fancy term *"minimally invasive autopsy (MIA)"*, which satisfied the pathologists and clinicians to obtain tissue samples for diagnoses leading to less invasive, imaging-guided methods for obtaining these specimens. It also contributed to the need among the medical fraternity to develop methods that require less mutilation of the deceased's body thereby satisfying next of kin.

Studies proved that the diagnostic performance of a MIA (unenhanced whole-body CT and MRI scans, and image-guided biopsies) and CA performed equally well. In fact, according to studies in literature, a MIA technique using imaging and biopsies usually performs better than noninvasive methods.

Magnetic resonance imaging proved of immense benefit to identify pathologies of the internal organs and central nervous system. It was found that postmortem tissue biopsies were also of use for molecular translational research; and that MRI scans combined with targeted heart biopsies sufficed for establishing a cardiac cause of death. The benefits of MIAs in the face of steadily decreasing conventional autopsies can be summarized as:

- It is of immense use in an era of post acquired immunodeficiency syndrome (AIDS) and post-coronavirus disease (COVID) infections when pathologists dread doing autopsies on such disease afflicted bodies; considering the fact that majority of pathologists presently are ladies with family responsibilities.
- Guided needle biopsies serve equally well as tissue specimens particularly when image-guided; they can remove tissues from localized small lesions and deep-seated lesions. Both radiologists and pathologists will obtain better and adequate samples on dead versus living!
- Fluid samples can be obtained easily and provide immense information in confirming or ruling out disseminated cancer with effusions.
- Parenchymal organs—liver, kidney, and lung samples can be routinely collected with or without detecting lesions at imaging and processed; they give a good idea about disease/pathology in the body.
- Blood samples for microbiological culture can be removed under sterile conditions.
- Urine samples may be aspirated under sterile conditions.
- MRI can be used to examine congenital abnormalities or neurologic pathology in neonates, infants, and children, whereas CT will detect lung pathology in adults.
- Imaging data can easily be stored and subjected to second review, and used for clinical feedback and teaching purposes, whereas macroscopic autopsy findings have to be photographed or organs have to be preserved in order to do so.
- Just as in CA, one can collect extra tissue biopsies that can be frozen and stored in a tissue bank. Such frozen samples could be used for further diagnostic analyses on a molecular level, and for medical research.
- Postmortem angiographic studies[8] are feasible and not new; angiography of organs and tissues has been used as an adjunct to the autopsy procedure.
- Preliminary results are promising in establishing ischemic heart disease as the cause of death. Nonenhanced cardiac CT is also useful for detecting coronary artery calcifications.
- Postmortem MRI[9] without the use of contrast agents shows sufficient accuracy in detecting both acute and chronic myocardial infarction (MI). The age of an infarct can be diagnosed by evaluating the signal changes related to morphological alterations in the infarcted myocardium, such as the presence of myocardial edema, fibrosis, fat, etc.

- In the heart, standard biopsies (5–10 samples) are taken as a protocol from the lateral wall (mid and basal parts) and apex of the left ventricle. Additional biopsies can be taken from MRI signal abnormalities within the myocardium.
- Livor mortis is caused by blood settling in the dependent parts of the body due to gravity. This can be observed both internally, on imaging and autopsy, and externally upon visual inspection. External livores manifest as dark bluish (or livid) areas of the skin within several hours after death. Internal livores are noted as increased attenuation or signal changes of the dependent areas of organs.
- Putrefaction leads to gas formation, it is found intravascular in an early decomposition stage and in more advanced stages also in soft tissues and organ parenchyma at imaging.
- MIA outperforms CA in pathology where air/gas is involved, especially in cases of (massive) air embolism and pneumothorax.
- MIA provides a permanent auditable record that can be objectively consulted by pathologists, radiologists, and clinicians. All information including biopsy results can be digitally stored for teaching and other purposes.

CONCLUSION

In order to maintain autopsy rates, minimally invasive autopsies should replace full conventional ones.[10] The future of minimally invasive autopsies is bright, and these should be encouraged at all hospitals and institutions. However, for optimal contribution from these they are to be vigorously implemented in clinical practice; radiologists need an in-depth understanding of normal postmortem processes for correct acquisition and interpretation of the postmortem scans; pathologists should be well trained to read needle biopsies and aspirations, and finally the clinicians should accept the change in trend.

REFERENCES

1. Ludwig J. Handbook of Autopsy Practice. New Jersey: Humana Press; 2002.
2. Sheaff MT, Hopster DJ. Post Mortem Technique Handbook, 2nd edition. London: Springer-Verlag London Limited; 2005.
3. Kumar V, Abbas AK, Fausto N, Aster JC. Robbins and Cotran Pathologic Basis of Disease, 9th edition. Amsterdam, Netherlands: Elsevier Health Sciences; 2014.
4. Garg M, Aggarwal AD, Singh S, Kataria SP. Tuberculous lesions at autopsy. J Indian Acad Forensic Med. 2011;33:116-9.
5. Blokker BM, Wagensveld IM, Weustink AC, Oosterhuis JW, Hunink MG. Non-invasive or minimally invasive autopsy compared to conventional autopsy of suspected natural deaths in adults: a systematic review. Eur Radiol. 2016;26(4):1159-79.
6. King LS, Meehan MC. A history of the autopsy. A review. Am J Pathol. 1973;73(2):514-44.
7. Bernardi FD, Saldiva PH, Mauad T. Histological examination has a major impact on macroscopic necropsy diagnoses. J Clin Pathol 2005;58:1261-4.
8. Grabherr S, Gygax E, Sollberger B, Ross S, Oesterhelweg L, Bolliger S, et al. Two-step postmortem angiography with a modified heart-lung machine: preliminary results. AJR Am J Roentgenol. 2008;190(2):345-51.
9. Jackowski C, Hofmann K, Schwendener N, Schweitzer W, Keller-Sutter M. Coronary thrombus and peracute myocardial infarction visualized by unenhanced postmortem MRI prior to autopsy. Forensic Sci Int. 2012;214(1-3):e16-9.
10. Fryer EP, Traill ZC, Benamore RE, Roberts IS. High risk medicolegal autopsies: is a full postmortem examination necessary? J Clin Pathol. 2013;66(1):1-7.

CHAPTER 29

Laboratory Waste Management

INTRODUCTION

Hospital waste generated on a daily basis may be infectious and hazardous to the general population. Radioactive material may also be part of this waste. However, most of the waste generated in hospitals is nonhazardous or general waste; therefore, segregation of the waste will reduce the quantity of hazardous waste that needs special treatment for disposal to only about 15-20% of the total waste. This segregation will have to be done in different types of containers for easy and uniform identification of it. Rules for disposal of this should be in accordance with the Biomedical Waste (Management and Handling) Rules, of 1998 amended in 2016.[1,2]

BIOMEDICAL WASTE[1,2]

- *Definition*: Biomedical waste (BMW)/hospital waste refers to any waste generated while providing health care, performing research, and undertaking investigations or related procedures on human beings/animals in hospitals, clinics, laboratories, or similar establishments.
- The BMW is far more dangerous than domestic waste because it may be infectious, harming the patients and visitors. Sharps in BMW may cause injury. Chemicals and radioactive material in BMW may pollute soil, water, and air.
- In view of the hazardous effect of BMW, the Government of India has promulgated the BMW Rules 1998 which was later revised in 2016 and was amended in 2018 **(Table 1)**.
- *Waste generated in hospitals amounts to*: General waste—80%, hazardous infectious waste—15%, sharps—1%, and chemicals and other waste—3%. Hence, the segregation of BMW at source is very important.

TABLE 1: Regular biomedical waste will be disposed of as per Biomedical Waste Rules 2016 with 2018 and 2019 amendments.[3,4]

Category	Type of waste	Type of bag or container to be used	Treatment and disposal options
Yellow	*Human anatomical waste*: Human tissues, organs, body parts, and fetus below the viability period (as per the Medical Termination of Pregnancy Act 1971, amended from time to time)	Yellow-colored nonchlorinated plastic bags	Incineration or plasma pyrolysis or deep burial
	Animal anatomical waste: Experimental animal carcasses, body parts, organs, and tissues including the waste generated from animals used in experiments or testing in veterinary hospitals, colleges, or animal houses		

Continued

Continued

Category	Type of waste	Type of bag or container to be used	Treatment and disposal options
	Soiled waste: Items contaminated with blood, body fluids such as dressings, plaster casts, cotton swabs, and bags containing residual or discarded blood and blood components		• Incineration or plasma pyrolysis or deep burial • In the absence of the above facilities, autoclaving or microwaving/hydroclaving followed by shredding or mutilation or a combination of sterilization and shredding. Treated waste to be sent for energy recovery
	Expired or discarded medicines: Pharmaceutical waste such as antibiotics, and cytotoxic drugs including all items contaminated with cytotoxic drugs along with glass or plastic ampoules, vials, etc.	Yellow-colored nonchlorinated plastic bags or containers	Expired cytotoxic drugs and items contaminated with cytotoxic drugs are to be returned back to the manufacturer or supplier for incineration at a temperature > 1,200°C or to a common biomedical waste treatment facility or hazardous waste treatment, storage, and disposal facility for incineration at >1,200°C or encapsulation or plasma pyrolysis at >1,200°C. All other discarded medicines shall be either sent back to the manufacturer or disposed of by incineration
	Chemical waste: Chemicals used in the production of biological and used or discarded disinfectants	Yellow-colored containers or nonchlorinated plastic bags	Disposed of by incineration or plasma pyrolysis or encapsulation in hazardous waste treatment, storage, and disposal facility
	Chemical liquid waste: Liquid waste generated due to the use of chemicals in the production of biological and used or discarded disinfectants, silver X-ray film developing liquid, discarded formalin, infected secretions, aspirated body fluids, liquid from laboratories and floor washings, cleaning, house-keeping and disinfecting activities, etc.	Separate collection system leading to effluent treatment system	• After resource recovery, the chemical liquid waste shall be pretreated before mixing with other wastewater • The combined discharge shall conform to the discharge norms given in Schedule-III
	Discarded linen, mattresses, and beddings contaminated with blood or body fluid	Nonchlorinated yellow plastic bags or suitable packing material	• Nonchlorinated chemical disinfection followed by incineration or plasma pyrolysis or for energy recovery • In the absence of the above facilities, shredding or mutilation or a combination of sterilization and shredding. Treated waste to be sent for energy recovery or incineration or plasma pyrolysis
	Microbiology, biotechnology, and other clinical laboratory waste: Blood bags, laboratory cultures, stocks or specimens of microorganisms, live or attenuated vaccines, human and animal cell cultures used in research, industrial laboratories, production of biological, residual toxins, dishes, and devices used for cultures	Autoclave-safe plastic bags or containers	Pretreat to sterilize with nonchlorinated chemicals on site as per National AIDS Control Organization or World Health Organization (WHO) guidelines thereafter for incineration
Red	*Contaminated waste (recyclable)*: Wastes generated from disposable items such as tubing, bottles, intravenous tubes and sets, catheters, urine bags, syringes (without needles and fixed needle syringes), vacutainers with their needles cut, and gloves	Red-colored, nonchlorinated plastic bags or containers	• Autoclaving or microwaving/hydroclaving followed by shredding or mutilation or a combination of sterilization and shredding is preferred • Treated waste to be sent to registered or authorized recyclers or for energy recovery or plastics to diesel or fuel oil or for road making, whichever is possible. Plastic waste should not be sent to landfill sites

Continued

Continued

Category	Type of waste	Type of bag or container to be used	Treatment and disposal options
White (translucent)	*Waste sharps including metals*: Needles, syringes with fixed needles, needles from needle tip cutters or burners, scalpels, blades, or any other contaminated sharp object that may cause punctures and cuts. This includes used, discarded, and contaminated metal sharps	Puncture-proof, leakproof, and tamperproof containers	Autoclaving or dry heat sterilization followed by shredding or mutilation or encapsulation in a metal container or cement concrete; a combination of shredding cum autoclaving; and sent for final disposal to iron foundries (having consent to operate from the state pollution control boards or pollution control committees or sanitary landfill or designated concrete waste sharp pit)
Blue	• *Glassware*: Broken or discarded and contaminated glass including medicine vials and ampoules except those contaminated with cytotoxic wastes • Metallic body implants	Cardboard boxes with blue-colored marking	Disinfection (by soaking the washed glass waste after cleaning with detergent and sodium hypochlorite treatment) or through autoclaving or microwaving or hydroclaving and then sent for recycling

- The BMW generated in the hospital aims at three "*R's*," including (1) *r*educe, (2) *r*euse, and (3) *r*ecycle the BMW to minimize the quantity and is treated by various methods such as incineration and autoclave to make it noninfective and the waste, for example, sharps are also disposed in land field or damp yards.
- The BMW segregated at source has to be disposed of after the treatment. According to the nature of waste generated, it is segregated into different categories in different color-coded plastic bags and bins at the source and transported to the central storage area to be treated and disposed of. Treatment and disposal of the collected waste may be outsourced. The rules and regulations to treat and dispose of BMW which have been laid down by the Ministry of Environment and Forest of India is intern followed and controlled in all the states in India by the State Pollution Control Board.

CONCLUSION

The handling of BMW with appropriate technology is mandatory (by law). However, the type of technology that is suitable for any given institution, place, or country would largely depend on the finances available. Hence, in developing countries, those technologies that are cost-effective should be adopted rather than going for very high technology for which infrastructural facilities may not be available.

ACKNOWLEDGMENT

I wish to acknowledge the help of Dr Rama NK, Professor and Head, Department of Microbiology, MVJ Medical College and Research Hospital, Bengaluru, India, for her contribution to this chapter.

REFERENCES

1. Franklin WG. Cost Effective Waste Management for Large Hospitals: A Case Study of a Medical Teaching Hospital. India: Indian Society of Hospital Waste Management; 2002.
2. Ministry of Environment and Forests. (1998). Bio-Medical Waste (Management & Handling) Rules. [online] Available from http://www.igims.org/DataFiles/CMS/file/waste%20management/BIO-MEDICAL_WASTE__MANAGEMENT___HANDLING__RULE_-_1998.pdf. [Last accessed March, 2024].
3. Ministry of Environment, Forest and Climate Change. (2016). Amendment of the Bio-Medical Waste Management Rules, 2016. [online] Available from http://vikaspedia.in/energy/environment/waste-management/bio-medicalwaste-management/bio-medical-waste-management-rules#section-3 [Last accessed March, 2024].
4. World Health Organization. (2018). Treatment and Disposal Technologies for Health-care Waste. [online] Available from http://www.who.int/water_sanitation_health/medicalwaste/077to112.pdf. [Last accessed March, 2024].

CHAPTER 30

Microscope and Microscopy

INTRODUCTION

The first simple microscope was a glass globe filled with water and was described in the first century AD by Pliny. Lenses were used as spectacles since the 13th century.

Marcello Malpighi used a magnifying lens and described the structure of lung, capillaries, and breathing tubes of insects. Antonie van Leeuwenhoek (1632–1723), a Dutchman, was the first to describe microorganisms in the tartar of his own teeth as "animalcules". All these pioneers used single lenses of short focal length which had their limitations. The discovery of using multiple lenses together was accidental when the children of two Dutch spectacle makers Johan and Zacharias Janssen while playing viewed the church spires through putting together a convex and a concave lens. The church spires appeared very near and their shouts of joy attracted their elders; subsequent to this, the Janssen made the first telescope and presented it to prince Maurice of Nassau. Galileo copied the discovery and discovered the four moons of Jupiter! The enormous potential of the microscope was realized with the invention of the compound microscope. These consist of a lens toward the eye called the eyepiece and a lens toward the object called the objective, an important aspect of the microscope. Several technical giant steps had to be taken before the compound microscope became a reality.

COMPOUND MICROSCOPE[1-3]

Lenses and Principle of Image Formation

The lens is the basic component of a microscope and its aberrations or faults place most of the limitations on a microscope.

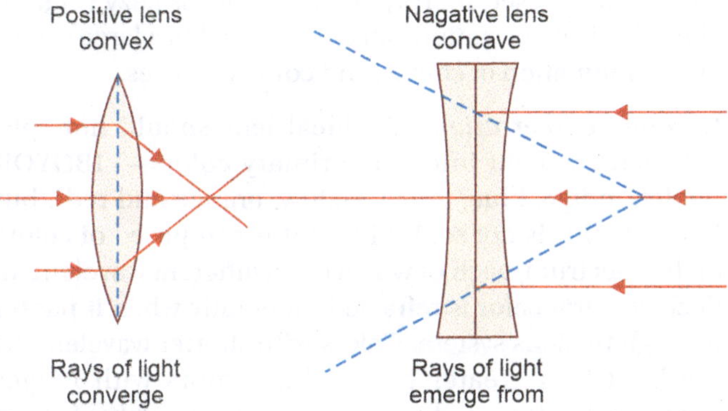

FIG. 1: Convex lens with rays converging and concave lens with divergent rays.

Lens refers to a piece of glass or other transparent material, usually circular, which has its faces ground and polished in such a manner that rays of light passing through it is either converge or diverge. Lenses which converge light rays and form images are called positive lenses; those that cause rays to diverge and which do not form real images are called negative lenses **(Fig. 1)**.

The principle focus in a lens is that point at which a lens forms a sharp image. In addition to the principle focus, positive lenses also have conjugate foci, i.e., they form sharp images on a screen at a distance which is dependent upon the distance of the object from the lens, i.e., distance from the top of the eye piece slot to the nose piece where the objective screws in. Moving the object really close to the lens causes the image to disappear (to form at infinity) and finally reappear as a virtual image on the same side as the object. *It is the virtual image on that we see when looking through the microscope.*

Bringing the object closer to a lens causes the image to be more distant and therefore more magnified. Therefore,

$$\text{Magnification} = \frac{\text{Screen distance from the lens}}{\text{Object distance from the lens}}$$

Example: In the case of a high dry objective lens of a 4 mm, the magnification is 160 mm (distance from the top of the eyepiece to the nose piece) divided by 4 mm, i.e., 40 mm.

Aberrations

Spherical aberrations: This occurs in a convex lens. The cause of this defect is the curvature of the lens. Rays passing through periphery of the lens are bent more than rays passing through the central parts of the lens. The rays bent more will therefore come to focus nearer the lens than those that are bent less. Hence, a point source of light will not be focused sharply and the image is hazy **(Fig. 2)**. The spherical aberration can be corrected to a large extent by a combination of convex and concave lenses.

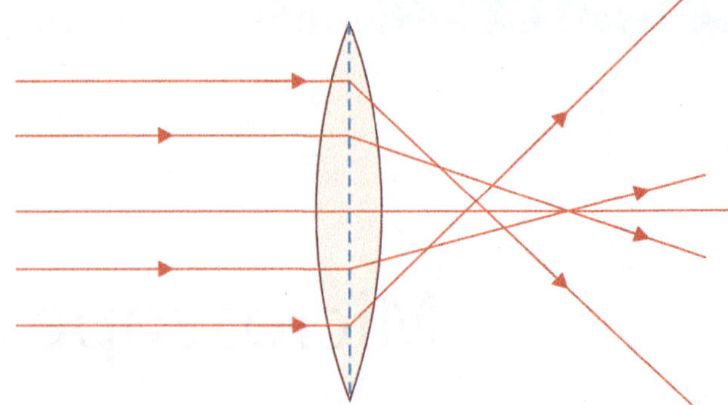

FIG. 2: Spherical aberration in a convex lens.

Chromatic aberrations: An ideal lens should not split the incident light into true primary colors—VIBGYOR (violet, indigo, blue, green, yellow, orange and red), but in reality this is not so. White light is composed of colors of the spectrum, each of which has a different wavelength. Each spectral color is refracted differently when it passes through the lens system. Colors with shorter wavelengths are bent to a greater extent than colors with longer wavelengths. Thus, red is bent the least while blue is bent the most **(Fig. 3)**.

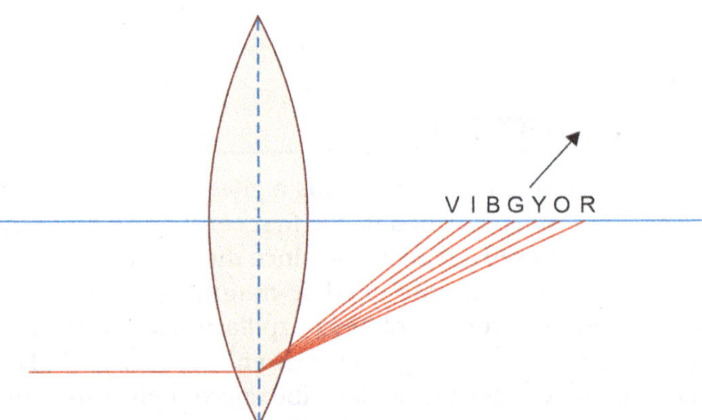

FIG. 3: Split of white light into colors as it passes through the convex lens.

Thus, blue comes to focus nearer the lens while red color comes to focus further away. The image formed has a red fringe surrounding a blue fringe or vice versa.

A lens which is corrected for two wavelengths of light in the green-blue region is called an "achromatic lens". The incorporation of fluorite allows correction of three wavelengths of light and such lenses are known as "fluorite lenses". If they are corrected for all wave lengths, they are called "apochromatic lenses".

Compound Microscope

In the compound microscope, a combination of lenses—the objective lens system (lens closer to the object) and the ocular lens system (lens closer to the eye) are used in combination to form the image to retina which is a virtual image disappearing below the plane of the object **(Fig. 4)**.

Objective

Objective lenses in wide use today are the achromatic which fulfil all requirements for ordinary work. The objective screws into the bottom of the body tube by means of a standard thread. This makes all objectives interchangeable.

Objectives usually are marked with their magnifying power (×2.5, ×10, ×40, ×100), but this only applies when they are used at a fixed tube length which is normally 160 mm. Dividing the tube length by the focal length will give the magnifying power of the lens, e.g., the high dry lens has a focal length of 4 mm which divides 160 mm to give 40×, which is its magnification.

Information which may be marked on an objective are its magnification, numerical aperture (NA), mechanical tube length, (at which it should be fixed) and the cover glass thickness (as shown in **Table 1**).

Numerical Aperture (Fig. 5)

The quality of an image is dependent upon the amount of light admitted by a lens and this is directly dependent upon the aperture of the lens. The NA of a lens is defined as $n(\sin \theta)$, where n is the refractive index (RI) of the medium between the specimen and the coverslip [such as air (RI = 1) or immersion oil (RI = 1.51)] and θ is the half angle of light acceptance (Keller, 2006).

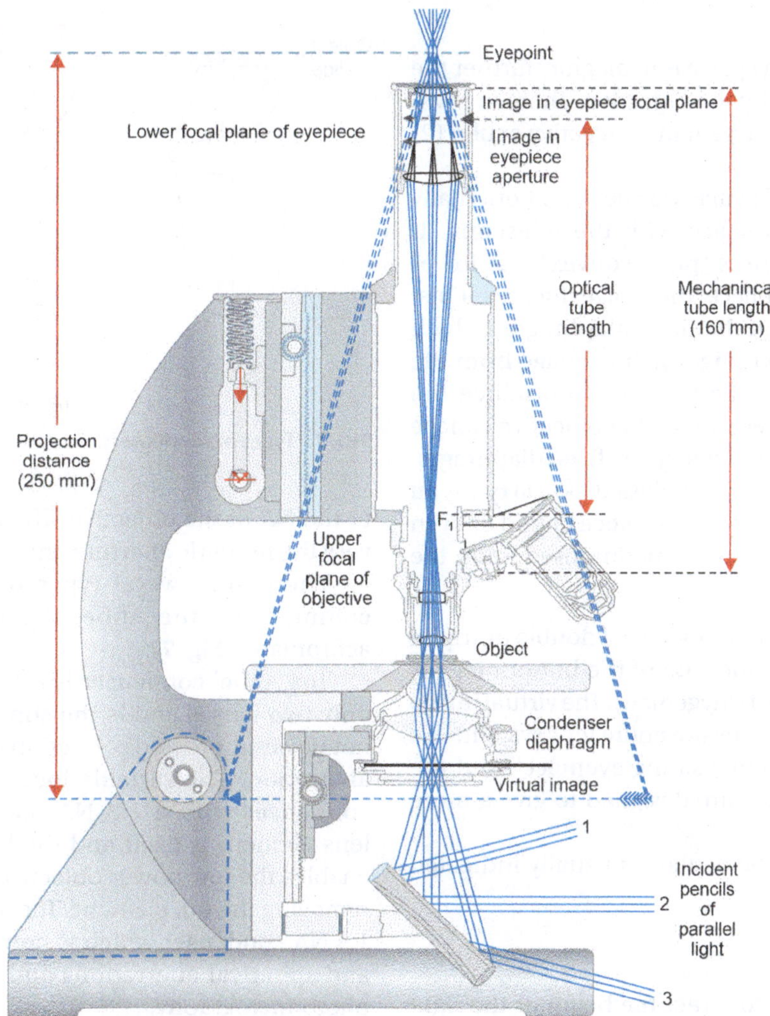

FIG. 4: Path of light through the microscope with formation of the "virtual image".

TABLE 1: Magnification, numerical aperture, and mechanical tube length.

40/0.65	40	Magnification
	0.65	Numerical aperture
160/0.17	160	Mechanical tube length
	0.17	Cover glass thickness

The NA of high dry objective should theoretically be "one" and of oil immersion with an RI of 1.51 should be 1.51. However, in practice, these values are usually 0.65 and 0.95, respectively.

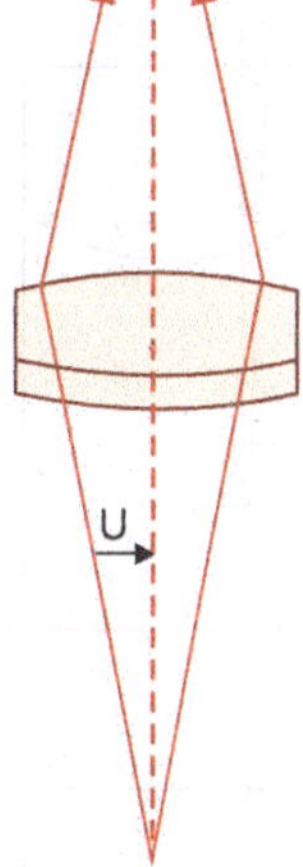

FIG. 5: Numerical aperture of the lens.

Resolution

Resolution is the ability to differentiate two points as separate and this resolving power is related to (1) NA of the objective and (2) wavelength of the light used. The shorter the wavelength and greater the NA, the more will be the resolution. In bright-field microscopy, blue filter is used as blue light has a shorter wavelength than others in the visible spectrum.

Oculars

The main function of the eyepiece is to magnify further the primary image produced by the objective. There are two basic types of oculars (1) Huygenian or negative ocular (2) Ramsden or positive ocular.

The *Huygenian type* of ocular was designed originally by Christiaan Huygens for use with the telescope. It consists of two simple lenses (planoconvex), the lower of which (the field lens) collects the image, focuses it just slightly above the plane of the fixed diaphragm (which is between the two lenses) **(Fig. 6)**. This image from the field lens is magnified by the top lens to produce the virtual image seen by the eye. Since the objective (image from field lens) is focused just above the fixed diaphragm, it follows that an optically plane glass disk, carrying an engraved scale, e.g., a micrometer eyepiece or grid or even a pointer will be seen (in focus) superimposed upon the object image.

Ramsden oculars: These are composed of double or triplet component lenses. The plane side of the bottom lens is toward the object (reverse of Huygenian). The virtual image from the objective is formed by the entire lens system. The other oculars are the "compensating eyepiece" and the "wide field eyepiece", which are designed to give a more flat field.

The magnification of the oculars is usually indicated on them, e.g., 5×, 10×, etc.

Condensers

The condenser functions to direct the beam of the light of the designed numeric aperture and field sizes onto the specimen. The NA of the condenser must be always equal to the NA of the objective. The iris diaphragm is used to vary the numeric aperture and not to cut down light.

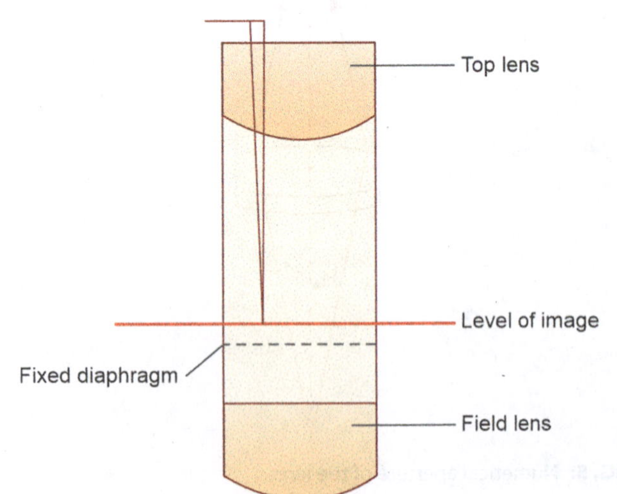

FIG. 6: Huygenian type of ocular.

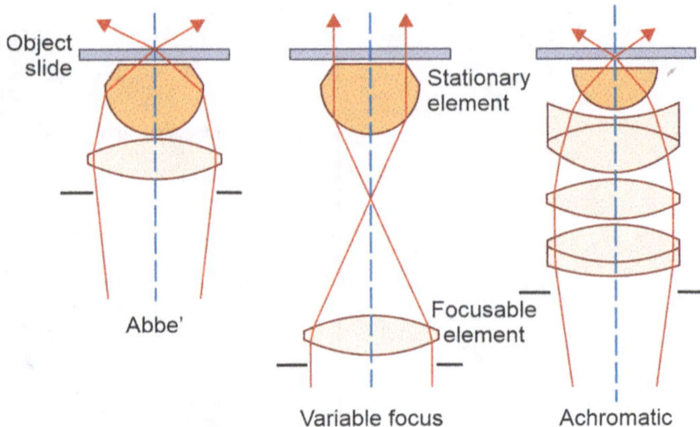

FIG. 7: Types of condensers.

There are several types of condensers. The most common are the Abbe', the variable focus, and the achromatic **(Fig. 7)**.

The Abbe' condenser is a 1.3 NA condenser utilizing only two lenses and is the simplest of the three. It does not however provide correction for spherical or chromatic aberration. The variable focus condenser is a two lens condenser with a 1.3 NA maximum, in which upper lens element is fixed and the lower one focusable. This enables the low power objective field to be filled without removing the top element. The achromatic condenser is a 1.4 NA condenser which is corrected for both chromatic and spherical aberrations and is used usually for color photomicrography.

To obtain numeric apertures over 0.95 in the condenser system for critical work, it is necessary to bring the condenser and the specimen slide into contact with an oil drop. It is very important that the condenser be centered accurately in the optical axis of the instrument and most instruments have centering screws or adjustment knobs for this.

Use of Mirrors to Direct Light

- Plane mirrors are used to (1) reflect light from infinity (daylight) and (2) when substage is being used.
- Concave mirrors are used (1) to direct light from an artificial source and (2) when substage lens is not available.

Filters

Usually blue filters are supplied with microscopes. These cut off yellow light which is abundant in light sources made of tungsten filaments.

Magnification in a Microscope

The greatest magnification that can be obtained is about 1,000 times the NA, and the higher the NA the more complex (and expensive) the lens system becomes. With a high dry having a numeric aperture of 0.65, it should therefore, be $0.65 \times 1{,}000 = 650$ times. This is never achieved in practice because beyond a limit, the magnification becomes empty since no more details are seen.

The magnification of a microscope may be calculated as follows:

$$\text{Magnification} = \frac{\text{Tube length} \times \text{NA of eye piece}}{\text{Focal length of objective}}$$

$$= \frac{160 \times 10}{4} = 400$$

Magnification is usually increased by using a higher power objective because the resolving power is also increased. Changing the ocular lenses has limited use because the resolving power is not increased leading to empty magnification.

Illumination

Two types of illumination are used in microscopy:

1. *Nelson or critical system* **(Fig. 8A)** where the light source is imaged directly on the specimen.
2. *Kohler illumination (Fig. 8B)*: The latter system is more commonly used and requires a field diaphragm control where the source is imaged in the aperture of the system. It is also the system of choice for photomicrography.

Use of Microscope

Guidelines

- Both eyes should be kept open.
- Focus upward
- Fine adjustments only for exact focusing; not to be turned more than one revolution.
- Work with the low power objective as far as possible
- Objects should be centered for clarity.
- External illumination should be subdued.
- Use vernier scale to mark objects or use object markers on slide
- A slight disturbance also causes harm to the microscope. Even a slight resistance should never be forced.
- Should be kept scrupulously clean and dust free. Use xylol sparingly. Lens to be cleaned by lens paper. Do not allow oil to dry on objectives.

Maintenance of Microscope

Daily Maintenance

- Dust it daily. Polish the outer surface of lens with lens paper.
- Polish the top lens of ocular with lens paper to remove finger marks
- Set the microscope for correct illumination
- Rotate the eyepiece. If any dust is seen to rotate with the eye piece, then clean the lens of ocular.
- Clean the substage condenser lens and mirror. If dust is allowed to remain on the lens, some of the particles being chemically corrosive may damage the lens.

Weekly Maintenance

- The sides of coarse adjustment, mechanical stage, and substage condenser should be wiped with a cloth dampened with xylene to remove the dust. Oil supplied by the manufacturer should be applied and the sides replaced. The latest models do not require this.
- The lens system should be checked and cleaned.
- Clean the oculars
- Clean the interocular adjustment once a month. Take care not to disturb the prism arrangement.

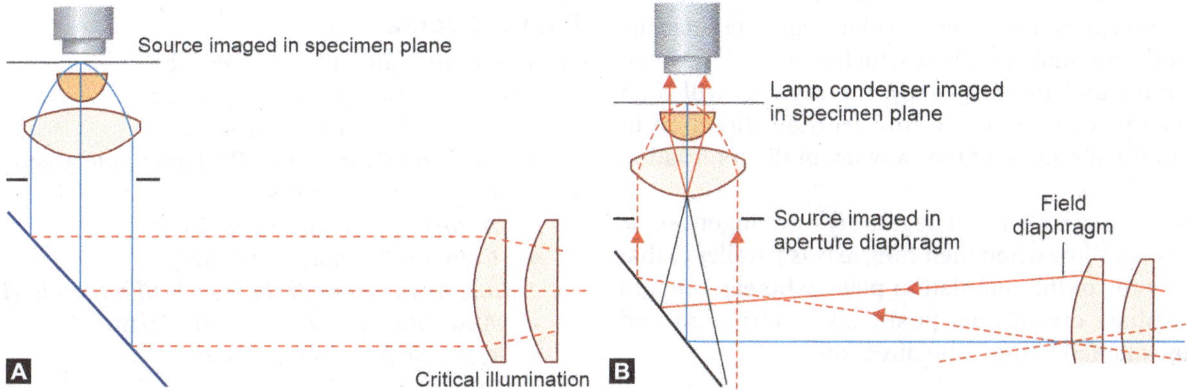

FIGS. 8A AND B: (A) Nelson illumination; and (B) Kohler illumination.

VARIOUS TYPES OF MICROSCOPY[1,3]

Dark-field Microscopy

It is achieved by blocking out the central rays of light and directing the peripheral rays against the microscope against the objective from the side. Only those rays that strike the object and are reflected upward pass into the objective lens; the object thus appears on a black ground. This type of illumination is most frequently used in the detection of *Treponema pallidum*. Dark-field condensers depend upon the use of high numeric aperture with a hollow cone of light.

Bright-field Microscopy

It is the examination under subdued light using a bright-field objective and condenser to delineate more translucent elements in a given specimen.

Phase-contrast Microscopy (Fig. 9)

The *phase-contrast microscopy* is based on the *principle* that small *phase* changes in the light rays, induced by differences in the thickness and RI of the different parts of an object, can be transformed into differences in brightness or light intensity.

Phase-contrast microscopy was developed for the microscopy of particularly transparent objects. Transparent objects are, for the most part, optically denser than the surrounding medium and therefore create more resistance to the light. The light is therefore slowed down, which results in a phase shift when it exits the object again. This phase shift is used to create a brightness contrast. This also requires a ring aperture in the condenser and a phase ring in the objective which must be calibrated to each other.

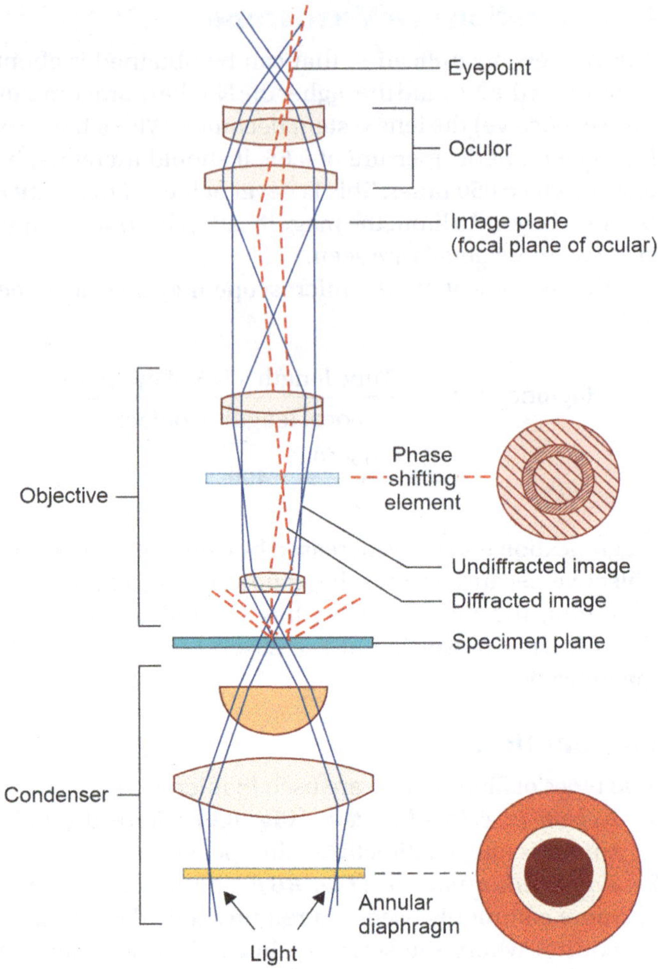

FIG. 9: Phase-contrast: Illumination is controlled by the annular diaphragm and the phase shifting results in the retardation of the image.

Polarizing Microscope

It is used mainly for viewing crystals in a fluid. It has a retardation plate which is placed between the polarizer (filter which is placed between the object and the substage condenser) and analyzer (filter which is placed between the objective and the eyepiece); the crystals will then appear yellow or blue depending on their direction in relation to the direction of the slow ray of the retardation plate.

Urate crystals are termed negatively birefringent since their color is yellow when their long axis is parallel to that of the slow ray of the retardation plate, whereas calcium pyrophosphate crystals are positively birefringent and blue when aligned in the same direction.

Fluorescence Microscope

The essential components for fluorescent microscopy[4] include the fluorochrome dye, the ultraviolet light source, the fluorescence microscope, the exciter filter system, and the suppressor filter system.

Fluorochrome Dye

The common fluorochrome dyes are:

- *Fluorescein isothiocyanate (FITC)*:
  - *Absorption maximum*: 495 nm
  - *Color on fluorescence*: Brilliant apple green
- *Lissamine rhodamine B*:
  - *Absorption maximum*: 575 nm
  - *Color on fluorescence*: Orange
- *1-dimethylaminonaphthalene-5 sulfonic acid (DANS)*:
  - *Absorption maximum*: 310–370 nm
  - *Color on fluorescence*: Green

- *Tetramethylrhodamine (TRITC)*:
  - *Absorption maximum range*: 510–545 nm
  - *Color on fluorescence*: Orange

It is important to know that the absorption maximum for these common fluorochromes, so that the correct exciter filters may be used.

Ultraviolet Light Source

- *High-pressure mercury vapor lamp 50–1000 watts (common usage 200 watts)*: It utilizes electrodes housed in a quartz (containing mercury and argon). The lamp has a limited time and blackens with time and has a potential for explosion.
- Iodine—quartz lamp (tungsten-halogen) 100 watts (Toshiba, Japan)
- *Others*: Xenon-mercury arc lamp; cadmium lamp. Emission spectrum 365, 405, 445, and 546.

Advantage

A wide range of ultraviolet light for various fluorochromes of different absorption spectrum is made use of with a single mercury bulb.

Disadvantages

- Excessive heat; likelihood of spontaneous bursting
- Maximum emission is usually reached after 30 minutes of putting on.
- Bulb life span is usually about 200 hours, after which if light is emitted, the ultraviolet range may not be satisfactory.
- Bulb life span is also governed by the number of putting-off and putting-on. The more the putting off, the shorter the life.

Fluorescence Microscopy

It is a technique of microscopy that uses a fluorescing material to produce better contrast resulting in an image of very high resolution, i.e., very good quality. The fluorescence microscope generates the strongest possible fluorescent radiation emitted by the specimen.

The basic task of the fluorescence microscope is to let excitation light radiate the specimen and then sort out the much weaker emitted light from the image.

Uses and applications of fluorescence microscopy: This technique can be used to detect viral, parasitic, tumor antigens from patient specimens, or monolayer of cells **(Fig. 10)**.

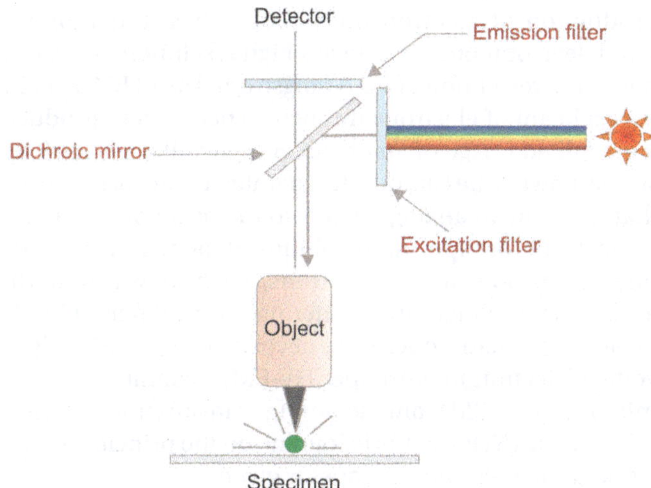

FIG. 10: Fluorescence microscopy.

Direct Immunofluorescence

- Cutaneous/mucosal biopsies for direct immunofluorescence are stained with fluorescence-labeled antibodies immunoglobulins (IgG, IgA, and IgM), complement (C3), and collagen IV, e.g., bullous pemphigoid, pemphigus vulgaris, dermatitis herpetiformis, vasculitis, and lupus.
- *Kidney*: Evaluation with antibodies against IgG, IgM, IgA, C3, C1q, fibrinogen, albumin, kappa, and lambda are performed by direct immunofluorescence. Transplant kidney biopsies are stained for C4d to assess the presence of humoral injection.

Indirect Immunofluorescence

Blood without anticoagulant is required. The serum is separated and serial dilutions (1:20 to 1:280) of serum are inoculated onto the tissue substrate along with fluorescence-labeled IgG, e.g., bullous pemphigoid, paraneoplastic pemphigus, pemphigus vulgaris, and dermatitis herpetiformis.

Disadvantages of Fluorescence Microscopy

- Incapability of detecting minute quantities of an antigen, antibody, or antigen-antibody complex.
- Lack of stability over prolonged ultraviolet exposure resulting in fading of fluorescence called quenching.
- Difficulty in recording results, as ultraviolet emissions from fluorochromes are low with consequent long film exposure times.
- Most fluorochrome preparations are unstable and must be used fresh.

Electron Microscope

Electron microscope is a high-resolution microscopy.[5] The resolving power which is the limit where two closely spaced points can be distinguished as two distinct entities, is much higher in an electron microscope as compared with that achieved by light microscope. Since the time, the first transmission electron microscope (TEM) was produced (Ruska, 1934) with the advanced technology;

production of electron microscopes has undergone a rapid development to achieve a high resolution. Now, it is possible a resolution of 2.5 Å (angstroms) in a TEM. A TEM uses a beam of electrons through a specimen to produce a magnified image of an object. A high-voltage electricity supply powers the cathode. It generates a beam of electrons that works in an analogous way to the beam of light in an optical microscope. As resolution depends on various physical properties of electrons, such as wavelength, accelerating voltage, and scattering power, different kinds of electron microscopes have developed, e.g., TEM, high-voltage electron microscope (HV-EM), scanning electron microscope (SEM), and scanning transmission electron microscope (STEM). A brief outline on the principle of the workings of these microscopes is given.

Basic Principles of Electron Microscope

Electron microscopes were developed due to the limitations of light microscopes, which depend on the physics of light. Ernst Ruska understood that electron wavelengths are far shorter than light wavelengths and used this principle to assemble the electron microscope.

Electron microscopes use signals arising from the interaction of an electron beam with the sample to obtain information about structure, morphology, and composition. Electrons are such small particles that, like photons in light, they act as waves. A beam of electrons passes through the specimen, then through a series of lenses that magnify the image. The image results from a scattering of electrons by atoms in the specimen. A heavy atom is more effective in scattering than one of low atomic number, and the presence of heavy atoms will increase the image contrast.

- *Scanning electron microscope*:
  - *Principle*: A SEM is chiefly a surface reading microscope and the backscatter of electrons on the surface of the object creates an image which is read. The electrons that are reflected off the specimen (known as secondary electrons) are directed at a screen, similar to a cathode-ray TV screen, where they create a TV-like picture. Its resolution (100–200 Å) is about 10 times more than that of a light microscope and 50 times less than that of a TEM. The magnification is between 100 and 1,000 folds and rarely reaches 10,000 or more.
  - *Uses:* The signals give information about the sample including the external morphology (texture), chemical composition, and crystalline structure. In most applications, data are collected over a selected area of the surface of the sample and a two-dimensional image is generated. Distances ranging from 5 μm to 1 cm can be imaged in a scanning mode. The SEM is also capable of performing analyses of selected areas on the sample; this approach is particularly useful in qualitatively and semiqualitatively determining not only morphology but also chemical composition, crystalline structure, and crystal orientation.
  - *The SEM helps select areas to be studied by the TEM.*
- *Transmission electron microscope*: The forward scattering of the electrons is used to construct the image.
  - *Uses*:
    - TEMs are the most powerful electron microscopes which are used to see things just 1 nm in size, so they effectively magnify by a million times or more.
    - TEMs have a wide-range of applications and can be utilized in a variety of different scientific, educational, and industrial fields.
    - TEMs provide information on element and compound structure with images of high-quality and detailed structure.
    - TEMs are able to yield information of surface features, shape, size, and structure.
    - They are easy to operate with proper training.
    - Their most significant application in medicine is in the study of renal biopsies, tumors of neural and central nervous system besides several other areas.

Confocal Microscopy

A confocal microscopy[6] creates sharp images of a specimen that would otherwise appear blurred when viewed with a conventional microscope. This is achieved by excluding most of the light from the specimen that is not from the microscope's focal plane. The image has less haze and better contrast that of conventional microscope and represents a thin cross section of the specimen. Thus, apart from allowing better observation of fine details, it is possible to build three-dimensional (3D) reconstructions of a volume of the specimen by assembling a series of thin slices taken along the vertical axis.

Modern Confocal Microscopy

Modern confocal microscopy has kept the elements of Minsky's design: The pinhole apertures and point by point illumination of the specimen. Advances in optics and electronics have been incorporated into current designs and provide improvements in speed, image quality, and storage of the generated images.

The majority of confocal microscopes image either by reflecting light off the specimen or by stimulating fluorescence from dyes (fluorochromes) applied to the specimen. The focus of this entry will be on fluorescent confocal microscopy as it is the mode which is most commonly used in biological applications.

These microscopes are often used for:
- Imaging structural components of small specimens such as cells
- Conducting viability studies on cell populations (are they alive or dead?)
- Imaging the genetic material within a cell [deoxyribonucleic acid (DNA) and ribonucleic acid (RNA)]
- Viewing specific cells within a larger population with techniques such as fluorescence in situ hybridization (FISH)

Basic step of confocal microscope: Light from the laser is scanned through the specimen by the scanning mirrors. Optical sectioning occurs as the light passes through the pinhole as it passes through the detector **(Fig. 11)**.

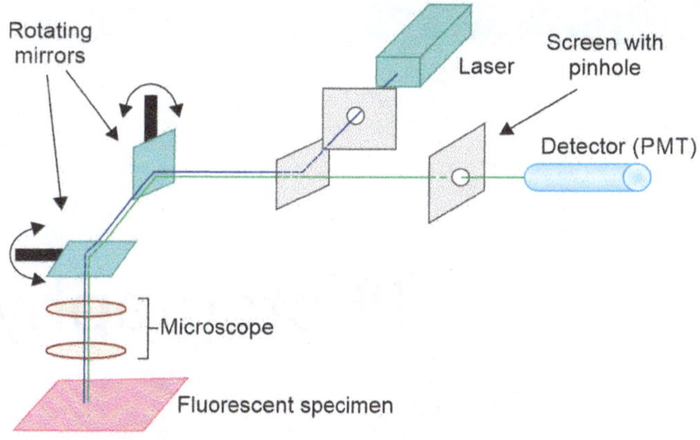

FIG. 11: Basic steps in confocal microscopy.
(PMT: photomultiplier tube)

CONCLUSION

The journey of the microscope as an aid in diagnosis has come a long way; and in all practical purposes, this will continue making this instrument indispensable as a pathologist's friend.

REFERENCES

1. Bancroft JD, Gamble M. Theory and Practice of Histological Techniques, 5th edition. London: Churchill Livingstone; 2002.
2. Shariff S. Laboratory Techniques in Surgical Pathology. Bengaluru: Prism Books Pvt Ltd.; 1999.
3. ScienceDirect. (2014). Numerical Aperture: an overview. [online] Available from https://www.sciencedirect.com/topics/neuroscience/neuroscience [Last accessed March, 2024].
4. Wikipedia. (2006). Fluorescence Microscopy. [online] Available from https://en.wikipedia.org/?title=Fluorescence_microscopy&redirect=no [Last accessed March, 2024].
5. Watt IM. The Principles and Practice of Electron Microscopy. Cambridge University Press; 1997. pp. 136-188. https://doi.org/10.1017/CBO9781139170529.006
6. Semwogerere D, Weeks ER. (2005). Confocal Microscopy. [online] Available from https://physics.emory.edu/faculty/weeks/lab/papers/ebbe05.pdf [Last accessed March, 2024].

CHAPTER 31

Photography in Pathology

INTRODUCTION

Photography has an essential role in pathology. Photographs of surgical pathology and autopsy specimens as well as photomicrographs is of invaluable benefit to patient care, clinicians, colleagues, and residents in pathology.

Photographic documentation of clinical specimens during cut up/grossing and microscopic pictures attached to histopathology reports are essential for the effective practice of surgical pathology; the reasons for such documentation being:

- Complete record of the case with gross and microscopic features
- Documentation and comparison with diagrammatic representative figures drawn during "cut up" to demonstrate the location of bits taken.
- Documentation for educational, teaching, and study purposes.
- Transfer of images in consultation and telepathology across the globe.

CONVENTATIONAL PHOTOGRAPHY

Specimen photography[1] may be either conventional using cameras with manual adjustments; a feature used in the past and still practiced by photography lovers. For these regular cameras with adjustable distances from short to distant levels are sufficient. A great reduction in aperture achieves more depth of field particularly for objects placed in the center, i.e., the targeted specimen; alternatively, lenses made especially for this purpose get good quality close-up photographs. They are designed in such a way as to provide sharp definition from a short distance of say 25 cm to great lengths; the optical computations of such lenses make them mainly suitable for close-up photography. The thrill of taking these photographs by skillful adjustments, and subsequent development of the pictures in a darkroom set up on the premises itself has a satisfaction of its own. Good quality black and white or even color prints to supplement the description of the pathology reports can be obtained. However, we rarely see this in present-day pathology departments and the practice is now considered a thing of the past.

Kodachrome, a color reversal film was extremely popular for color photography about three decades ago and was used in routine cameras to obtain gross and microscopic illustrations, projection, and teaching purposes. Slides could be projected on a white screen using easily available projectors. Due to the growth and popularity of alternative cheaper photography material, its complex processing requirements, and the widespread use of digital photography, Kodachrome has now lost its market value.

DIGITAL PHOTOGRAPHY

Digital photography[2,3] has changed the world of histopathologists. Presently most labs incorporate prints of the gross specimen as well as relevant colored microscopic features using this facility while issuing reports; greatly enhancing the nature and accuracy of the findings in histopathology. It is put to use as a popular commercial advantage to reporting.

As the investment factor is minimal in digital photography, there is no limit to the number of images taken and in the selection of the best possible images for the record. Images can be erased and reinstated within no time. The development of digital photography and the affordable prices of digital cameras have made a major breakthrough in the traditional way of documenting pathology findings at both the gross and microscopic levels.

Dedicated digital microscopy cameras generally do not have a lens within themselves but an attachment to the microscope via a common tube with easy fixability and removal from time to time. The images can be transferred directly onto computers within seconds or stored on cards incorporated in the camera.

High-quality photographic images can be rapidly and conveniently acquired with high-resolution cameras, for photomicrography and video capture at the same time, while viewing slides. Digital cameras do not use photography films, images are created by captured light which focuses via the lens onto a sensor made of silicon. This has several pixels that capture the image. These images are immediately available for incorporation into digital publications, transfer to other individuals by email, or as a result of internet other applications such as use and transfer in anatomical telepathy. The images are essentially indistinguishable from conventional film images; and can also be printed with reasonable accuracy.

Digital pathology is now considered a subfield of pathology that focuses on data management through the use of computer-based technology and virtual microscopy. Glass slides are converted into digital slides that can be viewed, managed, shared, and analyzed. The field of digital pathology has grown and has prongs in diagnostic medicine and the prediction of diseases in the field of artificial intelligence.

When photographs are taken the best possible effort should be made to achieve optimal results, both for gross and microscopic photography. Efforts should be made to streamline the procedures.

GROSS SPECIMEN PHOTOGRAPHY

A dedicated corner of the laboratory should be identified where natural light is maximum, or provision made for artificial light.

Specimen preparation for photographs is as follows:

- Proper lighting and background. The background for placing the specimen is usually green or royal ink blue devoid of wrinkles. A plastic sheet should not cover the background to avoid any light reflection.
- As far as possible take the specimen photograph before mutilating the specimen during cut-up.
- Wiping the surface of the specimen from excess fluid, and blood, and removing material such as plaster, fragments of tissue, tubes, or bandages. The specimen may be kept in running water for some time in order to remove these. The background surface where the photograph is being taken should be wiped of blood or other material.
- Orienting the specimen in the proper anatomical fashion, framing the specimen to fill the screen, positioning probes, and using a visible right-sized scale either vertically or horizontally as the case may be.
- The height of the specimen and scale should be at the same level.
- Use the zoom lens to adjust the magnification.
- Take the external as well as relevant cut surfaces of the specimen.

PHOTOMICROGRAPHY

The broad outlines of this practice are as follows:

- A thin section well stained with hematoxylin and eosin (H&E) should be chosen. The area of interest or lesion should be studied.
- Take the low power view (2.5× or 4×) to show the number of fragments or orientation.
- Zoom down using the 10×, then 40×, and oil immersion if necessary to show a closer view.
- Special stains should also be photographed for additional confirmation but after the H&E stain.
- Slides may be marked after the pictures with either arrows or circles as the case may be to highlight features.
- Appropriate legends for figures should accompany all pictures with the magnification and stain used.

Mobile Phone Photomicrography

Mobile phone photomicrography has presently become an easy way of documenting photomicrographs at the reporting table. It needs practice and a steady hand in performing it. Pathardhan, 2021[4] has outlined step by step a detailed procedure for the capturing of images by a mobile phone. The ease of documenting images using the mobile phone is now the fashion of the day for all younger generation pathologists.

CONCLUSION

Specimen and slide photography has invaluable weightage in surgical pathology. Digital imaging has made inroads into the routine practice of anatomical pathology and has replaced to a large extent conventional prints and Kodachromes for consultation and conference purposes. More advanced systems and computers have provided greater versatility in incorporating macroscopic and microscopic pictures into pathology reports and publications. Digital images allow telepathology transmission to remote sites via the Internet for expert consultation and educational purposes. Total slide digitization is now a reality and will replace glass slides to a large extent in the future. Three-dimensional images of gross specimens can be posted on websites for educational programs. A permanent record of rare specimens is thereby maintained. Gross and photomicrography can be used for research purposes.

REFERENCES

1. Rampy BA, Glassy EF. Pathology Gross Photography: The Beginning of Digital Pathology. Surg Pathol Clin. 2015;8(2):195-211.
2. Leong FJW-M, Leong ASY. Digital photography in anatomical pathology.z J Postgrad Med. 2004;50(1):62-9.
3. Riley RS, Ben-Ezra JM, Massey D, Slyter RL, Romagnoli G. Digital photography: A primer for pathologists. J Clin Lab Anal. 2004;18(2):91-128.
4. Patwardhan SY. Microphotography of mobile simplified. Pathology News. [online] Available from http://Pathoindia.com PathoIndia, the e-pathologists of India. [Last accessed March, 2024].

APPENDICES

APPENDIX 1: COMPOSITION OF FIXATIVES

- *10% formalin*: The most commonly used form in laboratories is *10% formalin*, which is prepared as follows:
  - *Formalin (40% of formaldehyde dissolved in water)*: 10 mL
  - *Water*: 90 mL

  (This in essence is 4% formaldehyde).
- *10% formol saline*:
  - *Distilled water*: 90 mL
  - *Formalin*: 10 mL
  - *Sodium chloride*: 0.9 g
- *10% neutral buffered formalin*:
  - Formalin: 100 mL
  - *Distilled water/tap water*: 900 mL
  - Sodium phosphate monobasic monohydrate: 4 g
  - *Sodium phosphate dibasic anhydrous*: 6.5 g

  (pH should be 7.2–7.4).
- *10% formol calcium acetate*:
  - *Tap water*: 900 mL
  - *Formalin*: 100 mL
  - *Calcium acetate*: 20 g

  (Calcium acetate is used in Lillie's formula and calcium chloride in Baker's formula. Both serve the same purpose other than the fact that calcium acetate gives a more alkaline solution).
- *Flemming's fluid*:
  - *1% aqueous chromic acid*: 15 mL
  - *2% osmium tetroxide*: 4 mL
  - *Glacial acetic acid*: 1 mL

  Specimens fixed should be washed and stored in 80% alcohol.
- *Zenker's fluid*:
  - *Composition*:
    - *Distilled water*: 100 mL
    - *Mercury chloride*: 5 g
    - *Potassium dichromate*: 2.5 g
    - *Sodium sulfate*: 1 g
    - Add 5 mL of glacial acetic acid immediately before use.
- *Helly's fluid (Syn–Spuler's or Maximow's fluid)*: This fixative has the same composition as Zenker's fluid but differs from it in that 5 mL of formalin is added immediately before use instead of acetic acid.
- *B-5 fixative*:
  - *Stock reagent A*:
    - *Mercury chloride*: 12 g
    - *Sodium acetate*: 2.5 g
    - *Distilled water*: 200 mL
  - *Stock reagent B*:
    - 10% buffered neutral formalin.

  To prepare the working solution, mix 90 mL stock reagent A with 10 mL stock reagent B.
- *Bouin's fluid*:
  - *Picric acid, saturated aqueous solution*: 75 mL
  - *Formalin*: 25 mL
  - *Glacial acetic acid*: 5 mL
- *Gendre's fluid*:
  - *Picric acid saturated solution in 95% alcohol*: 80 mL
  - *Formalin*: 15 mL
  - *Glacial acetic acid*: 5 mL

- *Rossman's fluid*:
  - *Formalin (neutralized)*: 10 mL
  - Absolute ethyl alcohol saturated with picric acid (approximately 8.5–9%): 90 mL
  - It is similar to Gendre's but without acetic acid.
- *Regaud's fluid or Moller's solution*:
  - *Potassium dichromate*: 3 g
  - *Distilled water*: 80 mL
  - *At the time of use add 10% formalin*: 20 mL

  (Solutions to be mixed immediately before use).
- *Champy's fluid*:
  - *3% potassium dichromate*: 7 mL
  - *1% chromic acid*: 7 mL
  - *2% osmium tetroxide*: 4 mL

  (And fluids should be freshly prepared each time).
- *Orth's fluid*:
  - *Potassium dichromate*: 2.5 g
  - *Sodium sulfate*: 1 g
  - *Distilled water*: 90 mL

  (At the time of use add 10 mL of formaldehyde).
- *Carnoy's fixative*:
  - *Absolute alcohol*: 60 mL
  - *Chloroform*: 30 mL
  - *Glacial acetic acid*: 10 mL
- *Clarke's fluid*:
  - *Absolute alcohol*: 75 mL
  - *Glacial acetic acid*: 25 mL
- *Newcomer's fluid*:
  - *Isopropanol/isopropyl alcohol*: 60 mL
  - *Propionic acid*: 30 mL
  - *Petroleum ether*: 10 mL
  - *Acetone*: 10 mL
  - *Dioxane*: 10 mL
- *Acetic alcohol formalin (AAF) fixative*:
  - *Formalin*: 5 mL
  - *Glacial acetic acid*: 5 mL
  - *70% alcohol*: 90 mL
- *Alcohol-formalin*:
  - *Ethanol 95%*: 90 mL
  - *Formalin*: 10 mL
  - If desired 0.5 g of calcium acetate may be added for neutrality
- *Davidson's fixative (Hartmann's fixative)*:
  - *Strong formalin (37%)*: Two parts or 500 mL
  - *Alcohol*: Three parts or 750 mL
  - *Glacial acetic acid*: One part or 250 mL
  - *Tap water*: Three parts or 750 mL
  - *Eosin*: Enough to color

[Second formula (John L): Davidson's solution: Davidson's fixative (DF): 2% of a 37–40% solution of formaldehyde, 35% ethanol, 10% glacial acetic acid, and 53% distilled H_2O].

- *Modified Davidson's fixative (mDF)*: 30% of a 37–40% solution of formaldehyde, 15% ethanol, 5% glacial acetic acid, and 50% distilled H_2O.

APPENDIX 2: DIFFICULTIES IN PARAFFIN SECTIONING, RELEVANT CAUSES OF THE SAME, AND RECTIFICATION[1,2]

Section problem	Cause	Rectification
Thick/thin section	• Insufficient tilt of knife causing too more or too little of the clearance angle • Clamping screws on the block and knife holder may not be tightened adequately • Large blocks • Block too hard	• Correct tilt and clearance angle • Clamp screw tightly • Trim block • Use softer paraffin for embedding

Continued

Continued

Section problem	Cause	Rectification
• Scored grooved, smeared, and deformed sections • Regular length-wise scratches and tears in the ribbon 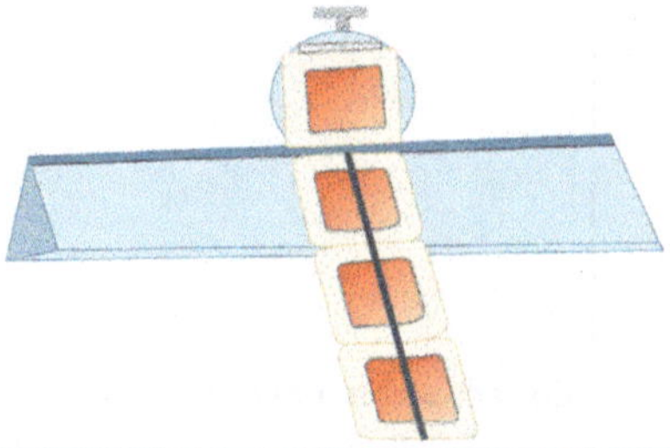	• Dull knife • Defective knife edge with knicks, dirt, or hard material on it • Hard material in the tissue itself, e.g., calcium or mercury salts and crystals • Hard material in paraffin	• Sharpen • Clean knife, check edge, and sharpen • Decalcify tissue wherever necessary • Check block for dirt
Sections fall out after being mounted on a slide	Embedding medium is of inadequate support/consistency compared to the processed tissue	Reblock tissue or if tissue is hard, cool the block
• Torn sections • Mushy sections and crumbly sections 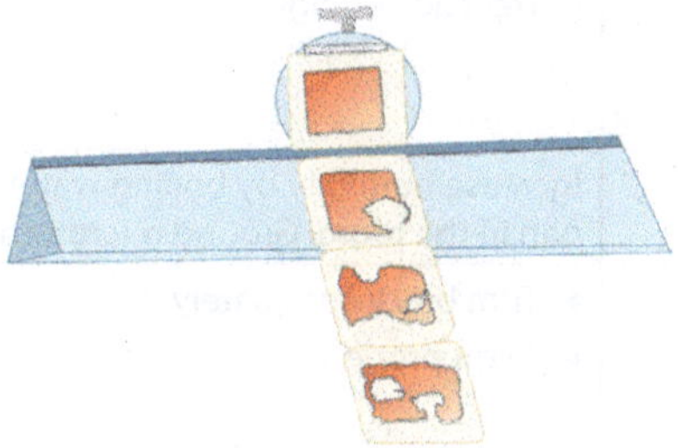	• Improper fixation • Insufficient dehydration • Insufficient clearing • Paraffin too hot at infiltration	Reprocess tissue
• Tissue jumps out of the block • Fragmented sections	• Hard brittle tissue in blocks due to prolonged fixation (Zenker's, Helly's, and Bouin's fluid) • Prolonged treatment in xylene	Take fresh bits or soak the block surface with an alkaline solution, such as 10% ammonium hydroxide. This will soften the tissue, prevent cracking, and facilitate sectioning
Crooked or uneven ribbons 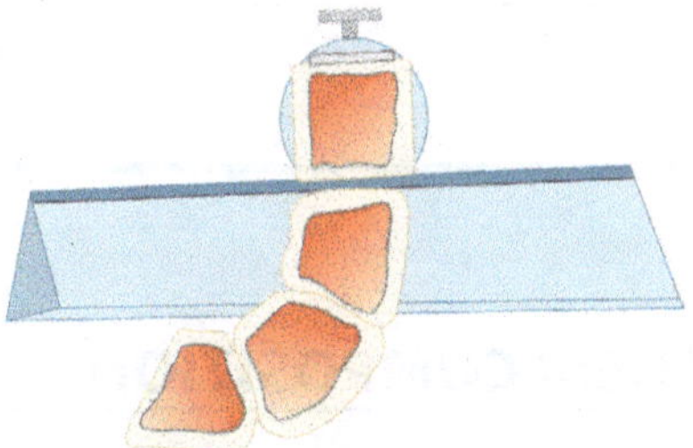	• Edges of block not parallel to the knife • Block not trimmed parallel • Irregular but sharp knife edge • Paraffin of different constituencies in different portions of the block as occurs in re-embedding • One side of the block warmer than the other (e.g., spirit lamp near microtome)	Correct accordingly
Ribbons fail to form 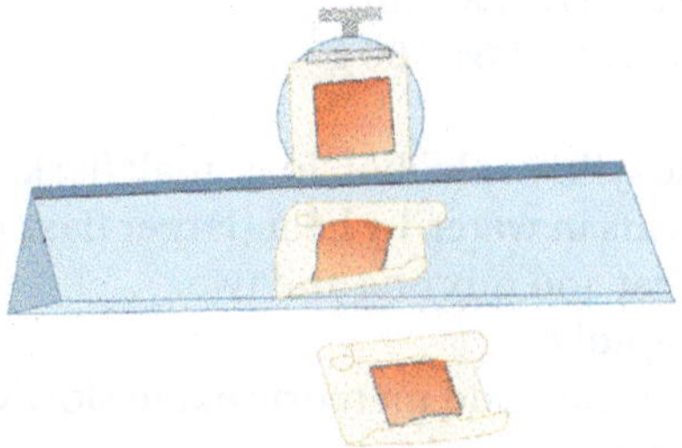	• Room too cold, paraffin too hard • *Incorrect knife angle*: Tilt may be too much • Section thick • Knife too dull	• Use softer paraffin with a lower melting point; warm knife • Lesson tilt of knife • Thinner sections • Sharpen the knife, and unroll the section with a brush, do not detach from the knife as a ribbon may form

Continued

Continued

Section problem	Cause	Rectification
Wrinkled, compressed, crushed, and jammed sections	• Blunt or dull knife (knife tilt slightly; knife edge coated with paraffin) • Cutting too rapidly • Room warm • Clearance angle too much • Micrometer screw set too thin for wax hardness	Rectify accordingly
Knife rings and sections scratched	• Increased knife tilt • Material too hard • Knife too thin	Correct accordingly
Sections lifted from knife	• Increased knife tilt • Room too warm • Knife may be dull	Correct accordingly
Sections stick to the knife	• Knife edge dirty • Knife tilt too little • Dull knife	Correct accordingly
Sections fly and stick to microtomes or nearby objects	Static electricity due to dry air	Increase humidity by boiling water in a pan in the room. Ground microtome
Unequal sized sections	• Block not trimmed uniformly • Knife and block not aligned	• Trim block adequately • Align properly

APPENDIX 3: VARIOUS TYPES OF HEMATOXYLINS AND THEIR COMPOSITION

The hematoxylins are grouped according to the mordant used: whether alum (ammonium or potash alum) or iron:

- Alum hematoxylin, e.g., Delafield's, Ehrlich's, Mayer's, Harris's, and Coles.
- Iron hematoxylins (uses ferric ammonium sulfate and ferric chloride), e.g., Weigert's iron hematoxylin.

The formula of commonly used hematoxylins:

- *Alum hematoxylins*:
    - *Harris hematoxylin*:
        - *Hematoxylin crystals*: 5.0 g
        - *Absolute ethyl alcohol*: 50 mL
        - *Ammonium or potash alum*: 100 g
        - *Distilled water*: 1,000 mL
        - *Red mercuric oxide*: 2.50 g

Preparation:

- Dissolve hematoxylin in alcohol. In a small flask.
- Dissolve alum salts in water, by heat (larger flask).
- Remove from heat and mix one and two.
- Bring to a boil rapidly.
- Remove from heat and add mercuric oxide slowly.
- Reheat until dark purple color.

- Remove and plunge the vessel into cold water until cool.
- The stain is ready for use.

Note: 2–4 mL of glacial acetic acid added to every 100 mL stain increases the nuclear stain precision. To be filtered before use.

Results: Nuclei—blue and background—as counterstain or unstained.

- *Mayers hematoxylin*:
  - *Hematoxylin*: 1 g
  - *Distilled water*: 1,000 mL
  - *Potash or ammonium alum*: 50 g
  - *Sodium iodate*: 0.2 g
  - *Citric acid*: 1 g
  - *Chloral hydrate SLR*: 50 g
  - This is used as both a progressive and regressive stain.

Preparation: Dissolve the alum in distilled water using a magnetic stirrer. When this has dissolved completely, hematoxylin crystals are added, after this dissolve, sodium iodate is added. It is stirred for about 10 minutes before adding citric acid; again, stirred for 10 minutes before adding chloral hydrate. After all these dissolves, the resulting color will be a deep wine color and for testing one mL is dropped into tepid water when it will immediately turn blue.

The main differences between Harris's and Mayer's hematoxylins are:

Mayer's	Harris
Hematoxylin is dissolved in water	Hematoxylin is dissolved in absolute alcohol
The quantity of the dye is less	The quantity of the dye is more
Sodium iodate is used as an oxidizer	Mercuric oxide is used as an oxidizer
Citric acid used to sharpen the staining	Acetic acid used to sharpen the staining

- *Ehrlich's alum hematoxylin*:
  - *Hematoxylin*: 5 g
  - *Absolute ethyl alcohol*: 250 mL
  - *Glycerol*: 250 mL
  - *Distilled water*: 250 mL
  - *Glacial acetic acid*: 25 mL
  - *Potash alum*: 50 g
  - It is an excellent nuclear stain.
  - Dissolve the crystals of hematoxylin in absolute ethyl alcohol, then add the glacial acetic and the glycerin. In a 2,000 mL flask, dissolve the potash alum in distilled water. When dissolved completely add hematoxylin, alcohol, glycerin, and acetic acid mixture. Loosely cover the mouth with filter paper. Allow it to ripen for about 3 months, avoid sunlight. This is a stock solution. For the working solution, stock 20–30 drops and 300 mL of distilled water.
- *Gill's hematoxylin*:
  - *Distilled water*: 730 mL
  - *Ethylene glycol*: 250 mL
  - *Hematoxylin*: 2 g
  - *Sodium iodate*: 20 g
  - *Aluminum sulfate*: 17.6 g
  - *Glacial acetic acid*: 20 mL

(Combine reagents in the order given, mix, and keep for 1 hour at room temperature. The stain can be used immediately).

Examples of other alum hematoxylins are: *Delafield's hematoxylin*—naturally ripened alum hematoxylin, *Cole's hematoxylin*—artificially ripened hematoxylin, used in frozen section, and *Carazzi's hematoxylin*—progressive nuclear stain with a short staining time.

- *Iron hematoxylins*: Iron salts are used in these hematoxylins.
  - *Weigert's iron hematoxylins*: The most commonly used Weigert's hematoxylin is as a nuclear stain in techniques where acidic staining solutions are to be applied to the sections, e.g., Van Gieson stain. But a more convenient celestine blue alum hematoxylin has largely replaced Weigert's hematoxylin in this stain. It is a useful stain with eosin in central nervous system (CNS) tissues. It is used as a progressive stain.
    - *Solution A*:
      - *Hematoxylins 1% in ethyl alcohol*: 95%
    - *Solution B*:
      - *Ferric chloride aqueous—29%*: 4 mL
      - *Distilled water*: 95 mL
      - *Hydrochloric acid concentrated*: 1.0 mL
    - *Working solution*:
      - Mix equal parts of A and B
      - The mixture should be a violet-black color and must be discarded if it is brown.
  - *Heidenhain's iron hematoxylin*: This is a regressive stain.
    - *Hematoxylin solution*:
      - *Hematoxylin*: 0.5 g
      - *Absolute alcohol*: 10 mL
      - *Distilled water*: 90 mL

        (The solution must be allowed to ripen for 4–5 weeks).
    - *Iron solution*:
      - *Ferric ammonium sulfate (violet crystals)*: 5 g
      - *Distilled water*: 100 mL

Verhoeff's hematoxylin: It was used primarily as a stain for elastic fibers. It also gives a high contrast for photomicrography, to demonstrate nuclei and myelin and can be adapted for electron microscopy.

Preparation of stain: Dissolve 1 g of hematoxylin in 22 mL of absolute alcohol in an open dish on a hot plate. Cool, filter, and add 8 mL of a 10% aqueous solution of ferric chloride and 8 mL of iodine solution (2 g of iodine plus 4 g of potassium iodide dissolved in 100 mL of distilled water).

For better results make up fresh solutions just before use.

Ferric chloride solution:

- *Ferric chloride*: 2 g
- *Distilled water*: 1,000 mL

Sodium thiosulfate (hypo) solution: Removes excess of iron

- *Sodium thiosulfate*: 5 g
- *Distilled water*: 1,000 mL

The counterstain used is Van Gieson's stain.

Results:

- Elastic fibers and nuclei—black to blue-black
- Cytoplasm and muscle—yellow
- Collagen—red

Tungsten hematoxylins: They have the most satisfactory method of preparation and can be ripened naturally or artificially. This process is time-consuming, takes months to ripen but remains stable for some months.

Its use applies to both CNS material and general tissue structure. Staining is more precise after the sections have been treated with an acid dichromate solution. Good results are obtained with buffered formalin fixative.

Mallory's phosphotungstic acid hematoxylin (PTAH):

- *Hematoxylin*: 1.0 g
- *Phosphotungstic acid*: 20.0 g
- *Distilled water*: 1,000 mL

Dissolve the hematoxylin in about 300 mL of water with the aid of gentle heat. Dissolve the phosphotungstic acid in the remainder of the water and when cool combine the two solutions. The stain will ripen in 5–7 weeks if placed in warm sunshine. Alternatively, it may be ripened instantly by the addition of 0.177 g of potassium permanganate or 2 mL of (3%) hydrogen peroxide. But with artificial ripening agents (i.e., chemical oxidation) the stain may not reach peak efficiency.

Results:

- Nuclei, centrioles, neuroglia, fibrin, and cross-striations of muscle fibers—blue
- Collagen, reticulin and bone, cartilage, and ground substance—yellow to red.

APPENDIX 4: IHC MARKERS

Histogenesis and typing of neoplasia: In the typing of neoplasia, immunohistochemistry has gained widespread popularity. A variety of markers are available for use in the market which include epithelial and nonepithelial markers, hormones- and related proteins, intermediate filament proteins, leukocyte markers, and hormone receptors.

In the identification of surface and Intracytoplasmic B-cell immunoglobulins and T-cell markers in lymphoid hyperplasia.

Monoclonal antibodies:

B-lineage	CD19, CD79a, CD20, and CD22
T-lineage	CD2, CD3, CD5, and CD7
Myeloid	CD13, CD33, CD15, CD117, and MPO
Hematopoietic precursors	CD41 and CD61
Monocytic	CD14 and CD11
Erythroid	CD36, CD7, and glycophorin A

Continued

Continued

For subclassification of *acute leukemias*: Monoclonal antibodies for acute leukemia:

Pan-B cell	CD10, CD19, CD20, CD21, CD22, Cd23, CD79a, CD37, and CD32
Pan-T	CD1, CD2, CD3, CD4, CD5, CD7, CD8, CD43, CD57, and CD45RO
Monocyte-macrophage system	CD11c, CD13, CD14, CD15, CD33, and D64
N-K cell	CD16 and CD56

To differentiate *lymphomas* from other small cell neoplasms, such as carcinomas and rhabdomyosarcomas:

Histogenetic classification	Markers
Epithelial origin	CK, EMA, CEA, and NSE
Mesenchymal origin	Vimentin, desmin, and S-100
Neuroendocrine origin	NSE and chromogranin
Lymphomas	LCA, Pan-B, and Pan-T
Melanomas	S-100, vimentin, NSE, and HMB-45
(CEA: carcinoembryonic antigen; CK: cytokeratin; EMA: epithelial membrane antigen; NSE: neuron-specific enolase)	

In the subclassification of *soft tissue neoplasia*:

Myogenic	SMA, desmin, MyoD, and myogenin
Nerve sheath	S-100, CD56, and CD57
Vascular	CD34, CD31, vWF, and factor VIII
GIST	CD117, CD34, DOG-1, PDGFRA, SDH-subunit B
Melanocytic	S-100, HMB-45, and Melan A
Adipocytic	CD34, MDM2, and CDK4
(CDK4: cyclin-dependent kinase 4; HMB: human melanoma black; PDGFRA: platelet-derived growth factor receptor alpha; SDH: succinate dehydrogenase; SMA: smooth muscle actin; vWF: von Willebrand factor)	

In the specific diagnosis of *small round cell tumors*:

	CK	CD45	S-100	CD99	Desmin	MyoD1/myogenin	CD56	WT1
EWS/PNET	+/–	–	–	+	–	–	–	–
RMS	–	–	–	–	+	+	+	–
DSRCT	+	–	–	+/–	+	–	+/–	+
WT	+/–	–	–	–	+	+/–	+	+
NB	–	–	+	–	–	–	+	–
SmCC	+	–	–	–	–	–	+	–
Melanoma	–	–	+	+/–	–	–	–	–
(CK: cytokeratin; DSRCT: desmoplastic small round cell tumors; EWS: Ewing's sarcoma; NB: neuroblastoma; PNET: peripheral neuroectodermal tumor; RMS: rhabdomyosarcoma; SmCC: small cell carcinoma; WT: Wilms' tumor)								

Tumor-specific markers and their staining patterns:

Marker	Tumor	Staining pattern
TTF-1	Lung and thyroid	Nuclear
Thyroglobulin	Thyroid	Cytoplasmic
Villin	Gastrointestinal (epithelia)	Membranous
CDX2	Colorectal	Nuclear
HepPar-1	Hepatocellular	Cytoplasmic
GCDFP-15	Breast	Cytoplasmic
ER/PR	Breast, ovary, and endometrium	Nuclear
Mammaglobin	Breast	Cytoplasmic
PSA	Prostate	Cytoplasmic
PAP	Prostate	Cytoplasmic
Uroplakin III	Urothelium	Membranous
RCC marker	Renal	Membranous
Inhibin	Sex-cord-stromal and adrenocortical	Cytoplasmic
Melan A	Adrenocortical and melanoma	Cytoplasmic

Continued

Continued

Marker	Tumor	Staining pattern
Calretinin	Mesothelioma, sex-cord-stromal, and adrenocortical	Nuclear/cytoplasmic
WT-1	Wilms, ovarian serous, mesothelioma, desmoplastic small round cell	Nuclear/cytoplasmic/membranous
Mesothelin	Mesothelioma	Cytoplasmic/membranous
D2-40	Mesothelioma and lymphatic endothelial cell marker	Membranous

Modified McCarthy's H-scoring system/histoscore: The whole stained section is scanned under low power and an estimation is made on the percentage of tumor cells that are negative, weakly, moderately, or strongly positive. Positive staining is indicated by the presence of brown nuclear stain. Each percentage is multiplied by a number: 0, 1, 2, and 3 respectively, reflecting the intensity of their staining. This gives a total score varying from 0 to 300 which is expressed as negative (negative: H-score 50 or less), weakly positive (positive: H-score 50-100); moderately positive (++ve: H-score 101–200), or strongly positive (+++ve: H-score 201–300). There is a good correlation between this and other similar semiquantitative scoring systems and quantitative biochemical assays.

Interpretation by McCarthy's histoscore:
100 cells have to be counted:

- % of cells with strong positivity × 3 = 20% × 3 = 60
- % of cells with mod positivity × 2 = 60 × 2 = 120
- % of cells with weak positivity × 1 = 10 × 1 = 10
- % of cells with neg staining = 10 × 0 = 0
  Score = 190/300 (maximum score)

Scores < 50 are considered negative and such tumors will not show a response to tamoxifen. The score for PR receptors is calculated similarly.

Alfred's quick score: This takes into account two criteria while scoring the percentage of cells stained and the intensity of staining.

Percentage of positive cells	Score	Intensity of stain	Score
NIL	0	Nil	0
1–25	1	Mild	1
26–50	2	Moderate	2
51–75	3	Intense	3
76–100	4		

The total score is calculated by adding the 2 scores. Maximum is 7 scores above 3 are considered positive.

Her2neu stain: The interpretation of the IHC staining is done as follows:

- >10% of cells show weak staining of the cell membrane 1+
- >10% of cells show moderate staining of the cell membrane 2+
- >10% of cells show a continuous strong staining of the cell membrane 3+
- It is recommended that all 2+ results need to be confirmed by the fluorescence in situ hybridization (FISH) technique

APPENDIX 5: SNOP CODING ON SALIENT ANATOMICAL AREAS (TOPOGRAPHY) AND MORPHOLOGICAL CODES COMBINED WITH CYTOLOGICAL DIAGNOSIS

NOS is "not otherwise specified"

- T-Y4: Abdomen including retroperitoneal
  - M0001: No pathological diagnosis
  - M4000: Inflammation
  - M8013: Carcinoma
- T-Y5: Abdominal visceral—general
  - MNOS
- T-Y4: Ascitis
  - M0001: No pathological diagnosis
  - M3880: NOS
  - M4100: Acute inflammation
  - M4014: Lymphocytic inflammation
  - M8013: Carcinoma NOS
  - M8016: Carcinoma, metastatic

- M9051: Mesotheliomas, NOS
- 6971: Cytological alteration, suspicious
- 6972: Cytological alteration, positive
- 6973: Cytological alteration, deferred classification

- T-1100: Bone
  - M0001: No pathological diagnosis
  - F9492: Tuberculosis
  - M4000: Osteomyelitis
  - M9251: Giant cell tumor
  - M9223: Chondrosarcoma
  - M9260: Aneurysmal bone cyst
  - M9733: Myeloma and plasma cell
  - M9593: Malignant lymphoma
  - M9183: Osteogenic sarcoma
  - M8016: Metastatic carcinoma
  - 6971: Cytological alteration, suspicious
  - 6972: Cytological alteration, positive
  - 6973: Cytological alteration, deferred classification
- T-0400: Breast
  - M0001: No pathological diagnosis
  - M7816: Lactation alteration
  - M4000: Mastitis
  - F9492: Tuberculosis
  - M7631: Mammary dysplasia
  - M7631: Cystic disease and chronic cystic mastitis
  - M9010: Fibroadenoma
  - M9020: Giant fibroadenoma
  - M8513: Medullary carcinoma
  - M8023: Anaplastic carcinoma
  - M8016: Metastatic carcinoma
  - 6971: Cytological alteration, suspicious
  - 6972: Cytological alteration, positive
  - 6973: Cytological alteration, deferred classification
- T-X1: Cerebrospinal fluid
  - M0001: No pathological diagnosis
  - M4000: Inflammation, NOS
  - M9383: Glioma, NOS
  - M8013: Carcinoma, NOS
  - 6971: Cytological alteration, suspicious
  - 6972: Cytological alteration, positive
  - 6973: Cytological alteration, deferred classification
- T-83: Cervix uteri
  - M0001: No pathological diagnosis
  - M4000: Cervicitis
  - M7500: Metaplasia
  - M7600: Dysplasia
  - M8012: Carcinoma in situ
  - M8072: Squamous cell carcinoma
  - M7100: Atrophy
  - E3141: Herpes simplex virus
  - 6971: Cytological alteration, suspicious
  - 6972: Cytological alteration, positive
  - 6973: Cytological alteration, deferred classification
- T-5600: Liver
  - M0001: No pathological diagnosis
  - M4174: Abscess
  - E4420: Amoeba
  - E4725: Echinococcus
  - M4850: Cirrhosis
  - M8173: Liver cell carcinoma
  - M8023: Anaplastic cell carcinoma
  - M8016: Metastatic carcinoma
  - 6971: Cytological alteration, suspicious
  - 6972: Cytological alteration, positive
  - 6973: Cytological alteration, deferred classification
- T-28: Lung
  - M0001: No pathological diagnosis
  - M8013: Carcinoma, NOS
  - M8016: Carcinoma, metastatic
  - 6971: Cytological alteration, suspicious
  - 6972: Cytological alteration, positive
  - 6973: Cytological alteration, deferred classification
- T-08: Lymph nodes
  - M0001: No pathological diagnosis
  - M4000: Lymphadenitis including reactive changes
  - F9492: Tuberculosis
  - M9633: Hodgkin's lymphoma
  - M9823: Lymphocytic leukemia
  - M8016: Metastatic carcinoma
  - 6971: Cytological alteration, suspicious
  - 6972: Cytological alteration, positive
  - 6973: Cytological alteration, deferred classification
- T-87: Ovary
  - M8013: Carcinoma, NOS
  - 6971: Cytological alteration, suspicious
  - 6972: Cytological alteration, positive
  - 6973: Cytological alteration, deferred classification
- T-3X: Pericardial fluid
  - M4000: Inflammation
  - M0001: No pathological diagnosis
  - M9051: Mesothelioma, NOS
  - 6971: Cytological alteration, suspicious
  - 6972: Cytological alteration, positive
  - 6973: Cytological alteration, deferred classification
- T-29: Pleura
  - M0001: No pathological diagnosis
  - M4150: Pleuritis
  - M9051: Mesothelioma, NOS
  - 6971: Cytological alteration, suspicious
  - 6972: Cytological alteration, positive
  - 6973: Cytological alteration, deferred classification
- T-2Y: Pleural fluid
  - M0001: No pathological diagnosis
  - M4000: Inflammation
  - M8013: Carcinoma NOS
  - M9051: Mesothelioma, NOS

    - 6971: Cytological alteration, suspicious
    - 6972: Cytological alteration, positive
    - 6973: Cytological alteration, deferred classification
- T-7700: Prostate
    - M0001: No pathological diagnosis
    - M8013: Carcinoma NOS
    - M7300: Benign hyperplasia
    - 6971: Cytological alteration, suspicious
    - 6972: Cytological alteration, positive
    - 6973: Cytological alteration, deferred classification
- T-55: Salivary gland
    - M4000: Sialadenitis
    - M8940: Pleomorphic adenoma
    - M8433: Mucoepidermoid carcinoma
    - M8013: Carcinoma, NOS
    - M8560: Papillary cyst adenoma lymphomatosum
    - 6971: Cytological alteration, suspicious
    - 6972: Cytological alteration, positive
    - 6973: Cytological alteration, deferred classification
- T-01-02: Skin
    - M8013: Carcinoma
    - M8073: Squamous cell carcinoma
    - F9391: Leprosy
    - 6971: Cytological alteration, suspicious
    - 6972: Cytological alteration, positive
    - 6973: Cytological alteration, deferred classification
- T-1900: Soft tissue
    - M0001: No pathological diagnosis
    - M4000: Inflammation
    - F9492: Tuberculosis
    - M9300 to 9500: Miscellaneous specific infectious diseases
    - M8850: Lipoma/fibrolipoma
    - M8810: Fibroma
    - M8853: Fibroliposarcoma
    - M8873: Leiomyosarcoma
    - 6971: Cytological alteration, suspicious
    - 6972: Cytological alteration, positive
    - 6973: Cytological alteration, deferred classification
- T-1Y: Synovial fluid
    - M4000: NOS
    - M9043: Synovial sarcoma
    - M9040: Synovial benign
    - 6971: Cytological alteration, suspicious
    - 6972: Cytological alteration, positive
    - 6973: Cytological alteration, deferred classification
- T-78:Testis
    - M-NOS
    - M4000: Inflammation, NOS
    - M8013: Carcinoma NOS
    - 6971: Cytological alteration, suspicious
    - 6972: Cytological alteration, positive
    - 6973: Cytological alteration, deferred classification
- T-9600: Thyroid
    - M0001: No pathological diagnosis
    - M4000: Thyroiditis
    - M7661: Thyroiditis—Hashimoto's
    - F4621: Thyrotoxicosis
    - M7233: Goiter—colloid
    - M7234: Goiter—adenomatous
    - M8001: Neoplasm
    - M8330: Follicular adenoma
    - M8140: Adenoma
    - M8333: Follicular carcinoma
    - M8053: Papillary carcinoma
    - M8513: Medullary carcinoma
    - M8023: Undifferentiated carcinoma
    - 6971: Cytological alteration, suspicious
    - 6972: Cytological alteration, positive
    - 6973: Cytological alteration, deferred classification
- T-8100: Vagina
    - M0001: No pathological diagnosis
    - M4000: Vaginitis
    - M4464: *Trichomonas vaginalis*
    - M7821: Proliferative
    - M7822: Secretory
    - F0101: Pregnancy NOS
    - M7100: NOS
    - 6971: Cytological alteration, suspicious
    - 6972: Cytological alteration, positive
    - 6973: Cytological alteration, deferred classification

REFERENCES

1. Culling CF. Histopathological and Histochemical Techniques, 3rd edition. Oxford, United Kingdom: Butterworth-Heinemann; 1976.
2. Prophet EB, Mills B, Arrington JB, Sobin LH (Eds). Armed Forces Institute of Pathology: Laboratory Methods in Histotechnology. Washington DC: Armed Forces Institute of Pathology, American Registry of Pathology; 1994.

INDEX

Page numbers followed by *b* refer to box, *f* refer to figure and *t* refer to table.

A

C

D

E

F

G

H

I

J

K

L

M

N

P

Q

R

S

T

U

V

W

X

Y

Z